P9-DUA-053

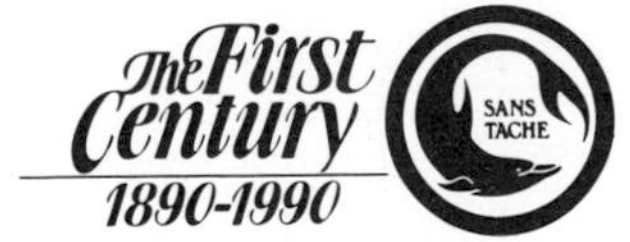
The First Century
1890-1990
SANS TACHE

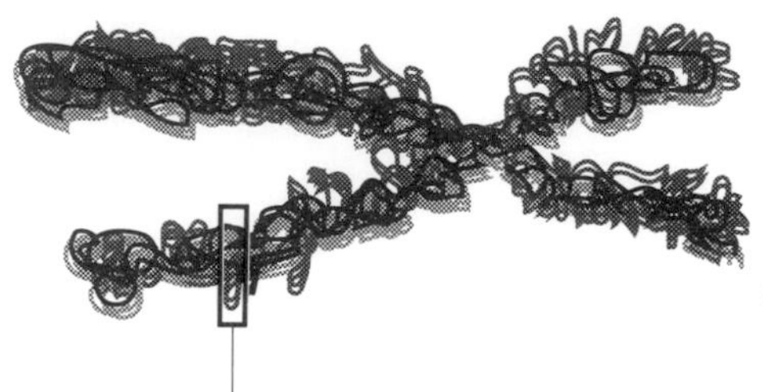

Principles of MEDICAL

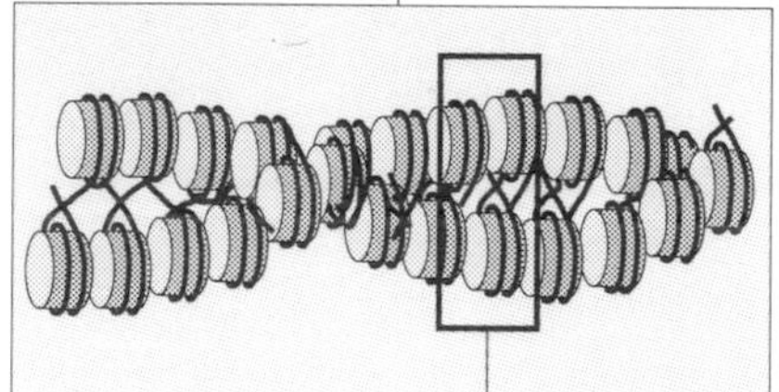

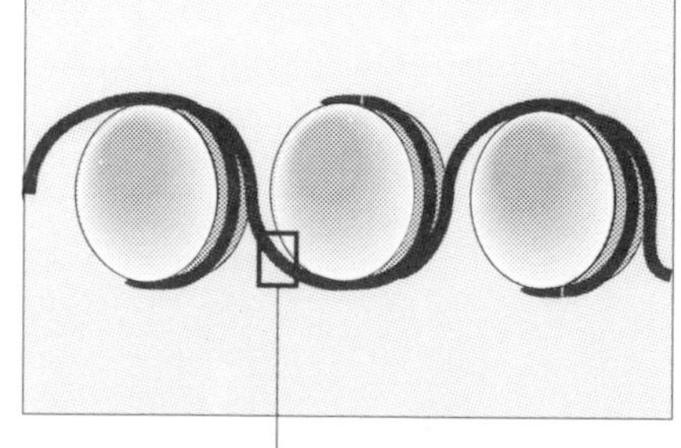

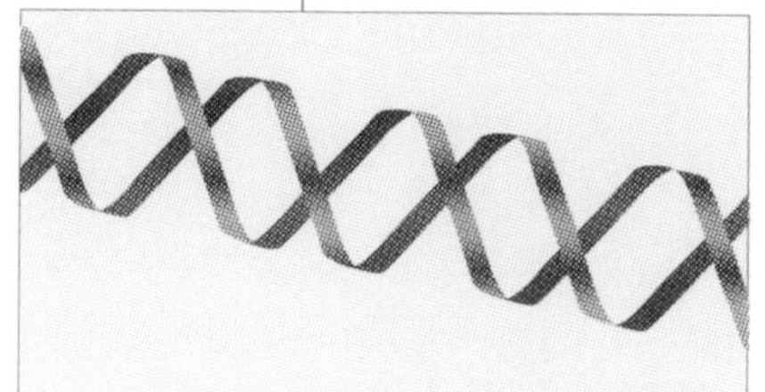

GENETICS

Thomas D. Gelehrter, M.D.

Professor and Chairman
Department of Human Genetics
Professor of Internal Medicine
University of Michigan Medical School
Ann Arbor, Michigan

Francis S. Collins, M.D., Ph.D.

Associate Professor of Internal Medicine and of Human Genetics
Director, Division of Medical Genetics
Associate Investigator, Howard Hughes Medical Institute
University of Michigan Medical School
Ann Arbor, Michigan

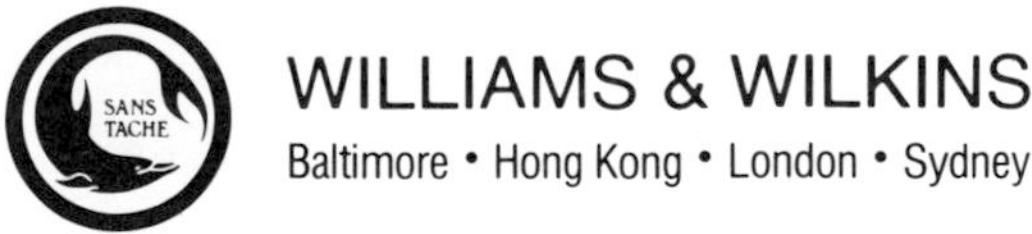

WILLIAMS & WILKINS
Baltimore • Hong Kong • London • Sydney

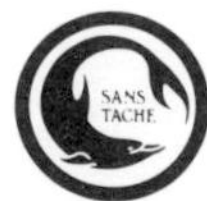

Editor: John N. Gardner
Managing Editor: Linda Napora
Copy Editor: Klementyna L. Bryte
Designer: Wilma Rosenberger
Production Coordinator: Charles E. Zeller
Illustrators: Mollie Dunker and Jacqueline A. Schaffer

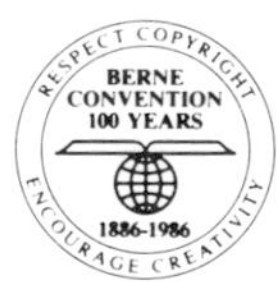

Accurate indications, adverse reactions, and dosage schedules for drugs are provided in this book, but it is possible that they may change. The reader is urged to review the package information data of the manufacturers of the medications mentioned.

Printed in the United States of America

Library of Congress Cataloging-in-Publication Data

Gelehrter, Thomas D.
Principles of medical genetics / Thomas D. Gelehrter, Francis S. Collins.
p. cm.
ISBN 0-683-03447-2
1. Medical genetics. I. Collins, Francis S. II. Title.
[DNLM: 1. Genetics, Medical. QZ 50 G316p]
RB155.G358 1990
616'.042—dc20
DNLM/DLC
for Library of Congress 89-21487
CIP

90 91 92 93
1 2 3 4 5 6 7 8 9 10

Foreword

What is medical genetics? Starting with the usual definition of genetics as the science of biological variation, one can say that human genetics is the science of biological variation in humans, and medical genetics is the science of human biologic variation as it relates to health and disease. Clinical genetics is that part of medical genetics concerned with the health of individual humans and their families. It can be argued that medical genetics is a more extensive discipline than human genetics because it is impossible to think of any aspect of human genetics that is not relevant to medical genetics, but the converse is not true. Indeed, medical genetics might be defined as "all of medicine that is genetic and all of genetics that is medical."

Another definition of clinical genetics is, "The science and practice ('art') of the diagnosis, prevention, and treatment of genetic disease." Some years ago I heard British biostatistician Bradford Hill suggest that the practice of medicine consists of seeking the answers to three questions: What is wrong? (The answer is diagnosis.) What is going to happen? (The answer is prognosis.) What can be done about it? (The answer is treatment.) I would add a fourth question, Why did it happen? On the answer to this question depend prevention and the advancement of science.

Diagnoses are of great importance in dealing with genetic disorders because of the large number of different disorders and because appropriate genetic counseling and other aspects of management may be quite different depending on the mode of inheritance and the natural history of the specific disorder. Prognosis in medical genetics is the basis of genetic counseling. Treatment in genetic disorders is not as hopeless as sometimes thought, particularly as understanding of genetic disease at an increasingly basic level progresses. The study of genetic disease has contributed heavily to our understanding of many aspects of human biology.

It has been customary to think of disease as falling into three main categories as far as the role of genetic factors is concerned: single gene disorders, multifactorial disorders, and chromosomal disorders. Today we are inclined to include two additional categories. A fourth category is that of somatic cell genetic disorders, of which all cancers appear to be examples, as well as some congenital malformations. A fifth category of genetic disease is comprised of disorders due to mutation in the mitochondrial chromosome—mitochondrial genetic disease.

The human has become a leading object for genetic study. It is true that human genetic analysis is hampered by long generation time and small families; however, it is an advantage that anatomical, chemical, physiological, and pathological descriptions of phenotype in the human are both extensive and intensive. Many physicians and workers in paramedical professions collect information of genetic significance that can be exploited by competent students of the science. Furthermore, in recent decades, surrogate methods of genetic study, such as the study of the genetics of cultured cells and genetic analysis at the level of the gene itself, have obviated some of the handicaps to genetic analysis based on family studies alone. Although studies in other organisms have been powerfully contributory in our understanding of human genetics, the science of human heredity cannot depend only on extrapolation from findings in other species. Some aspects can be studied conclusively only in humans, forcing one to agree, although for different reasons, with Pope: "The proper study of mankind is man."

Genetics is to biology what the atomic theory is to the physical sciences. Human genetics has implications not only for all aspects of human biology, but also for the cultural, political, and social aspects of human activity.

Great areas of ignorance about the detailed genetics of many of the important human disorders, such as major mental diseases, remain. An optimistic attitude toward long range accomplishments is justified, however, on the basis of the progress made to date. Drs. Gelehrter and Collins convey to their readers the excitement of discovery in the rapidly advancing field of medical genetics. I hope that the readers will also be aware of what is not yet known and will be challenged by these gaps in our knowledge.

Victor A. McKusick, M.D.
University Professor of Medical Genetics
The Johns Hopkins University School of Medicine
Baltimore, Maryland

Preface

Increasing awareness of the role of genetic factors in the causation of human disease has made clinical genetics one of the fastest growing fields in medicine during the past two decades. Our objective here is to present the basic principles of medical genetics and their application to clinical medicine; our emphasis is on molecular genetics because we believe that advances in this area have provided the major impetus to the rapid development of medical genetics, especially in the areas of diagnosis and prevention of disease. The intent of *Principles of Medical Genetics* is to allow students and physicians to understand ongoing developments in genetics and to apply them to patient care. This book is aimed primarily at first or second year medical students taking a course in medical genetics. We anticipate that the book will also prove useful to house officers who wish to review basic principles of medical genetics, to physicians whose training preceded current advances in medical genetics, to genetic counselors, and to nurses and other allied health professionals.

Although this is not a book about clinical medicine, human diseases are used to illustrate basic genetic principles. Furthermore, we have used certain diseases repeatedly because they illustrate several aspects of medical genetics and serve as useful paradigms. Our choice of examples reflects more than 25 years' combined experience as clinical geneticists.

Principles of Medical Genetics covers basic principles of chromosome structure and function, Mendelian patterns of inheritance, mitochondrial diseases, and multifactorial inheritance and its role in human variation and human disease. We have included a detailed discussion of the molecular structure of the gene, regulation of its expression, and techniques for manipulation of genetic material. A detailed discussion of the hemoglobinopathies serves as a model for the molecular genetics of human disease. Other single gene disorders, however, are also discussed from the clinical to the molecular level as paradigms of molecular diseases. Human biochemical genetics, including pharmacogenetics, and cytogenetic disorders are also covered. Gene mapping is considered from the perspective of a background in molecular genetics, cytogenetics, and population genetics to provide a modern approach to this important area. There is a chapter devoted to the genetics of cancer due to the significant advances in cytogenetic and molecular genetic understanding of this group of disorders. Important aspects of the practice of clinical genetics, such as obtaining and interpreting a family history, genetic counseling, and genetic screening, are discussed as are current and future approaches to prenatal diagnosis and treatment. The final chapter points to further areas in which major advances can be expected and to which the basic principles learned can be applied.

In a field that changes and progresses so rapidly, the role of a textbook might be questioned. The intent of this book is not simply to present a body of facts, but rather to present the principles that allow one to keep up with rapid progress in the laboratory and its applications at the bedside.

Each chapter is followed by a group of study questions. These are of two types: First, there are questions that can be answered, either directly by studying the material contained in that chapter, or indirectly by applying the principles learned to areas not specifically covered in the text. A second class of questions, indicated by an asterisk, may not necessarily have any simple, straightforward, or correct answers. Rather, these questions are designed to stimulate thought and discussion, to encourage the reader to extend his/her analysis beyond that presented in the text, and hopefully, to apply the principles included herein to new situations with uncertain outcomes.

We wish to acknowledge the help of many colleagues who have made major contributions to the preparation of this book. First, we thank Drs. Richard King (University of Minnesota), Margretta Seashore (Yale University), and Claire Leonard (University of Utah) for reviewing the text and providing constructive criticisms. We thank Professor Peter Smouse (Rutgers University), formerly of the University of Michigan, for his help with the chapter on population genetics and multifactorial inheritance, and Dr. Thomas Glover of the University of Michigan for his review of the cytogenetics chapter. We thank Drs. Glover and Constance Stein and Beth Cox of the University of Michigan Clinical Cytogenetics Service for the excellent chromosome photomicrographs. We owe special thanks to Dr. Robert Nussbaum (University of Pennsylvania) for preparing the study questions, to Mollie Dunker and Jacqueline A. Schaffer for preparing the illustrations, to Dr. Pamela Talalay for help in preparing the glossary, and Lee Marks, Danielle Paille, June McGee, and Bernice Sandri for secretarial help. We especially thank our editor, John Gardner, and managing editor, Linda Napora, for their support, encouragement, threats, and other interactions that kept this project going during the years of its creation. A textbook is a teaching device, and teaching has no meaning without students. The first-year medical students at the University of Michigan were our laboratory, our critics, and, ultimately, our reason for writing this book. Finally, we thank our families: our parents for providing the support and nurture to bring us to our professional calling, and, most of all, our spouses and children whose forbearance, patience, and support throughout this project were essential for its completion.

Contents

1

The Role of Genetics in Medicine

"Nature is nowhere accustomed more openly to display her secret mysteries than in cases where she shows traces of her workings apart from the beaten path; nor is there any better way to advance the proper practice of medicine than to give our minds to the discovery of the usual law of Nature by careful investigation of cases of rare forms of diseases. For it has been found in almost all things, that what they contain of useful or applicable nature is hardly perceived unless we are deprived of them, or they become deranged in some way."

—William Harvey, 1657

The recognition of the role of genetic factors in the causation of human disease has made clinical genetics one of the most rapidly developing fields in medicine. With the marked reduction in nutritional and infectious diseases in the developed countries, there has been an increasing awareness of the role of genetic determinants of human disease. Important genetic contributions to the etiology of major diseases such as coronary artery disease, diabetes mellitus, hypertension, and the major psychoses have been identified. At the same time, there has been a veritable explosion of knowledge in basic genetics. Much of this progress has been propelled by recent advances in the area of molecular genetics, which in turn have been applied directly to a better understanding of the pathogenesis of disease and to improved diagnosis and management of patients. Appropriately, a major contribution of these new developments in genetics has been in the area of *prevention and/or avoidance of disease,* the aspect of medicine that must become the focus of modern medicine. Genetic screening programs to detect individuals at risk, genetic counseling, and prenatal diagnosis are some of these current applications of new genetic knowledge to medical practice.

IMPACT OF GENETIC DISEASES

Contrary to common belief, many genetic diseases are far from rare and, in fact, are a significant cause of illness and death. Even those individually rare conditions are, in aggregate, a major cause of morbidity and mortality. Approximately 3% of all pregnancies result in the birth of a child with a significant genetic disease or birth defect that can cause crippling, mental retardation, or early death. A recent survey of more than 1 million consecutive births in British Columbia indicated that at least 1 in 20 individuals younger than 25 years of age developed a serious disease with an important genetic component (1). The chronic nature of many genetic diseases imposes a heavy medical, financial, and emotional burden on affected patients and their families, as well as on society at large.

Two studies of the causes of death of more than 1200 children admitted to hospitals in the United Kingdom (2, 3) identified genetically determined diseases as contributing 38 and 42% of the total mortality (Table 1.1). In two North American studies of nearly 17,000 pediatric hospital admissions (4, 5), clearly genetic disorders accounted for 5–10% of the admissions. When diseases in which genetic factors are thought to play a role were included, a third to more than half of the admissions were the result of genetic disorders (Table 1.2). Furthermore, patients with genetic diseases were hospitalized more frequently and for longer periods. Although the frequency of genetically caused diseases in the adult population is less clear, it is estimated that about 10% of adult hospital admissions are due to genetic diseases. Thus, the financial and medical burdens of genetic diseases are indeed significant.

Aside from trauma, the term "nongenetic" may be a misnomer, for it is hard to conceive of any disease as being wholly nongenetic. The development of any individual depends on the interplay of genetic and environmental influences. Genetic factors are present from conception although their expression varies throughout development; whereas environmental influences are constantly changing. Since all human variation in both health and disease is to some extent genetic, all diseases are therefore genetic (6). Infectious diseases were once thought to represent clear examples of nongenetic diseases because specific exogenous agents of disease could be identified. However, it is now appreciated that host defense factors, many of them genetically determined, play an important role in susceptibility to infection and in the nature of the immune response to infectious agents. Thus, even in diseases with well-defined exogenous causes, genetic factors may play a critical role. More subtle examples of this same principle may be involved in the causation of such common problems as alcoholism.

Table 1.1. Genetic Components of Childhood Mortality in the United Kingdom[a]

Cause of Death	Newcastle	London
Chromosomal	2.5%	12.0% (Chromosomal and Single gene combined)
Single gene	8.5%	
Polygenic	31.0%	25.5%
Nongenetic/unknown	58.0%	62.5%
Total deaths	1041	200

[a]Adapted from Roberts DF, Chavez J, Court SDM: The genetic component in child mortality. Arch Dis Child 45:33–38, 1970 and Carter CO: Changing patterns in the causes of death at the Hospital for Sick Children. Great Ormond St J 11:65–68, 1956.

Table 1.2. Frequency of Genetic Disorders among Pediatric Hospital Admissions in North America[a]

Cause	Seattle	Montreal
Chromosomal	0.6%	0.4%
Single gene	3.9%	6.9%
Polygenic	48.9%	29.0%
Nongenetic	46.6%	63.7%
No. of admissions	4,115	12,801

[a]Adapted from Hall JG, Powers EK, McIlvaine RT, Ean VH: The frequency and financial burden of genetic disease in a pediatric hospital. Am J Med Genet 1:417–436, 1978 and Scriver CR, Neal JL, Saginur R, Clow A: The frequency of genetic disease and congenital malformation among patients in a pediatric hospital. Can Med Assoc J 108:1111–1115, 1973.

The nature and extent of the genetic contribution to human variation and disease is the substance of the fields of human and medical genetics. Identification of genetic factors predisposing to disease and identification of genetically predisposed individuals are powerful keys for discovering the critical environmental agents of disease. Paradoxically, one of the most important benefits of identifying the genetic factors in disease susceptibility may not be the potential for gene therapy, but rather the opportunity for treatment and prevention of clinical disease by manipulating the environment of individuals genetically at risk.

MAJOR TYPES OF GENETIC DISEASE

Genetically determined diseases are often classified into three major categories: chromosomal, single gene defects, and polygenic diseases. Each of these will be discussed briefly below and more extensively in subsequent chapters. Recent studies on the genetics of human cancer require a fourth category, somatic cell genetic defects.

Chromosomal Disorders

These diseases are the result of the addition or deletion of entire chromosomes or parts of chromosomes and will be discussed in detail in Chapter 8. Because each chromosome contains tens of thousands of genes, physical manifestations of chromosome disorders are often quite striking. Most major chromosome disorders are characterized by growth retardation, mental retardation, and a variety of somatic abnormalities. The loss or gain of whole chromosomes other than the sex chromosomes is often incompatible with survival, and such abnormalities are a major cause of spontaneous abortions or miscarriages. Clinically significant chromosome abnormalities occur in nearly 1% of liveborn babies and account for about 1% of pediatric hospital admissions and 2.5% of childhood deaths. Major chromosomal anomalies are found in almost half of spontaneous abortuses. Since approximately 15% of recognized pregnancies end in a miscarriage and it is estimated that 50% of conceptions do so, it appears that a quarter of conceptions may suffer from major chromosome problems.

A typical example of a major chromosomal disease is Down syndrome, which is secondary to trisomy 21, or three copies of chromosome 21 instead of the usual two copies. This abnormality occurs in approximately 1 in 800 liveborn infants and increases in frequency with advancing maternal age. It is characterized by growth retardation, variable but often severe mental retardation, and characteristic physical abnormalities including the upward-slanting eyes that have in the past given the condition the unfortunate name "mongolism." Most significant among the congenital abnormalities associated with this condition are congenital heart defects, which are the major cause of death in children with Down syndrome. Trisomy 21 also significantly decreases intrauterine viability and the majority of affected fetuses are spontaneously aborted. Down syndrome was the first chromosomal disease defined in humans and demonstrated for the first time that alterations in chromosomal material could cause mental retardation and severe congenital anomalies. Down syndrome was also one of the first diseases amenable to prenatal diagnosis by amniocentesis.

Single Gene Disorders

These disorders are due to single mutant genes with a large effect on the patient's health. As might be expected, single gene disorders are inherited in a simple Mendelian fashion (discussed in Chapter 3) and are also referred to as Mendelian diseases. Some 3000 distinct disorders are now known or suspected to be single gene diseases inherited in autosomal dominant, autosomal recessive, or X-linked fashion. Some of these disorders will be discussed in greater detail in subsequent chapters. Single gene disorders account for approximately 5–10% of pediatric hospital admissions and childhood mortality. Although many single gene disorders are rare, others are common and pose major health problems. Familial hypercholesterolemia with its attendant high risk of premature coronary artery disease occurs in 1 in 500 individuals. Sickle cell anemia affects 1 in 400 blacks in the United States, and cystic fibrosis affects 1 in 2000 whites. Sickle cell anemia was the first genetic disease to be defined at the molecular level, and its study serves as a model for the application of modern molecular genetic analysis to clinical disease. Single gene disorders have thus far proven to be the area in which advances in molecular genetics have made the major contribution to understanding and managing disease.

Polygenic Diseases

These diseases result from the interaction of multiple genes, each of which may have a relatively minor effect. This group of diseases is both the most common and the least understood of human genetic disease. Examples of such polygenic diseases are diabetes mellitus, hypertension, schizophrenia, and a variety of common congenital defects such as cleft lip, cleft palate, and most congenital heart diseases. These diseases account for 25–50% of pediatric hospital admissions, approximately 25–35% of childhood mortality, and because of the chronicity of many of these conditions, perhaps an even greater component of disease burden in the adult population. Conceptually, this group of diseases poses the challenge of sorting out the ways in which the additive or interactive effects of multiple genes create the predisposition to disease, which in turn is manifest only in the presence of appropriate environmental triggers. It is hoped that molecular genetic approaches will allow a clearer definition of these genetic determinants and of the genetic heterogeneity underlying disease susceptibility. Models for how such interactions can cause disease, and methods for identifying the nature and contribution of genetic factors in such diseases will be discussed in Chapter 4.

Somatic Cell Genetic Disorders

In contrast to the above three categories in which the genetic abnormality is found in the DNA of all cells in the body including germ cells (sperm and egg) and can be transmitted to subsequent generations, somatic cell genetic disorders arise only in specific somatic cells. The paradigm for somatic cell genetic diseases is cancer, in which development of malignancy is the consequence of mutations in genes that control cellular growth. The various genetic mechanisms that can result in cancer are discussed in Chapter 10.

GENETICS AND MEDICINE: THE DYNAMIC INTERFACE

The interaction between the basic science of genetics and the clinical science of medicine has been bidirectional and highly productive over the past several decades. In its early stages, genetics was more the province of the botanist and the entomologist than the physician. Mendel, working in the 1860s, was able to formulate the concept of the gene from his experiments with pea plants, and his ability to perform planned matings and observe multiple generations provided crucial elements not so easily achieved when studying humans. Similarly, the work of Thomas Hunt Morgan and others on the fruit fly, *Drosophila melanogaster,* was much benefitted by the short generation time and relatively simple genome (compared with the same factors in mammals) of the fruit fly. However, as interest in human genetics began to blossom in the 20th century, important concepts began to be recognized and explored in greater depth for humans than they had been for other species. Prominent examples include population genetics, the study of polymorphism (see Chapter 9), and biochemical genetics (see Chapter 7). In more recent times, the trend has continued and the spin-offs from one discipline to another have multiplied. As will be described in Chapter 10, for example, the newly emerging field of the genetics of human cancer has demonstrated that human cells carry a variety of genes called "oncogenes," which normally participate in growth control. Certain mutations of these oncogenes can contribute to the uncontrolled growth pattern we recognize as cancer. The discovery of oncogenes has demonstrated an unexpected link between cancer, virology, and genetics and has brought together several diverse fields of biology. Furthermore, by using the strong evolutionary conservation of these genes, this discovery has led directly to the cloning of important growth-regulating genes in yeast!

Thus, efforts in medicine have yielded continuing insights in genetics and basic biology. In the other direction, the contribution of research in genetics to medicine is even easier to appreciate. It is easy to forget in today's technological medical care system that medicine for most of its history has been a descriptive discipline. Although the descriptive approach is a valuable one for determining the natural history of disease and describing the effects of various therapeutic maneuvers, fundamental advances in medicine generally have come instead from an elucidation of more basic scientific principles and their subsequent application to a clinical situation. Medical genetics deals with human disease at the most fundamental level—that of the gene itself. It is thus natural that developments in genetics have had profound implications for clinical medicine, and the magnitude of those implications will continue to grow.

A prime example is the concept of molecular disease, which was first clearly enunciated by Pauling with regard to sickle cell anemia.

Known for centuries in West Africa as a lifelong disease causing anemia and pain in the bones, joints, and abdomen, the actual pathogenesis remained unknown until 1910 when James Herrick, a cardiologist in Chicago, first noted the abnormally shaped red blood cells in an affected individual. Four decades later Pauling demonstrated that hemoglobin from patients with sickle cell anemia was electrophoretically different from normal hemoglobin and that parents of affected children showed both normal and abnormal hemoglobins. In 1956, Ingram, using a peptide fingerprinting technique, showed that the difference was due to the substitution of valine for glutamic acid as the sixth amino acid of the β chain of hemoglobin. Subsequently the mutation has been identified at the nucleic acid level as a single base substitution of A to T, and prenatal diagnosis is now available based on DNA analysis (see Chapter 6 for more details). The fact that such a severe and clinically complex disorder could be caused by alteration of only one nucleotide in 3 billion would not have been predicted by the descriptive approach that characterized medicine in previous centuries. This demonstration was powerful evidence that the genetic approach to medicine could be extremely revealing. It also illustrates an important paradigm: a single gene alteration can have complex clinical effects on multiple organ systems. Medical genetics is thus a broad specialty with wide areas of overlap with all other clinical disciplines.

The example of hemoglobin also demonstrates a second paradigm: the study of mutation can yield important insights about structure-function relationships. Subsequent to the description of sickle hemoglobin, which we now know creates its havoc by favoring the intracellular polymerization of hemoglobin, more than 300 other mutant hemoglobins have been described. Some of these, presumably located in noncritical parts of the hemoglobin polypeptide chain, have no functional consequences. Others, located near the site for heme binding, can lead to oxidation of the iron carried by the molecule (methemoglobinemia). Mutations that affect the equilibrium between the high and low oxygen affinity forms can lead to high affinity hemoglobins, which release oxygen poorly. By determining the position of the mutations in these various conditions, the functional role of the various parts of the globin molecule begins to emerge (7).

The contribution of the study of hemoglobin to our understanding of human biology is difficult to overstate and is the reason for the dedication of an entire chapter of this text (Chapter 6) to this topic. Another important principle is thus revealed: what one learns from an intensive study of a particular gene-protein system often provides critical insights for other systems.

The concept of molecular medicine has continued to broaden. For example, coronary artery disease is one of the leading causes of death in the Western world. The association of high serum cholesterol with an increased risk of coronary artery thrombosis has been noted for decades, but the inheritance pattern was not clear and the metabolic pathways leading to elevated cholesterol were obscure. Families with very high cholesterol levels, deposits of cholesterol in the skin and tendons, and an extremely high risk of heart attacks were discovered (see Chapter 7). Focusing their studies on such families, Goldstein and Brown (8) were able to demonstrate the existence of a cell surface receptor for a cholesterol-rich lipoprotein called low-density lipoprotein (LDL) and found that the LDL receptor was defective in these patients. The elucidation of this important pathway by a genetic approach has contributed greatly to our understanding of cholesterol metabolism and of the cause of atherosclerosis in general. Even more than that, it has led to a rapid expansion in understanding of the whole phenomenon of cell surface receptor biology, including how such receptors are synthesized, how they are localized in the cell membrane, and how they carry their ligands into the cell interior (a process known as receptor-mediated endocytosis). This example illustrates another important paradigm, one recognized clearly by William Harvey in the quotation which began this chapter (9): the study of rare genetic mutations provides a powerful way to understand normal function. Many examples of the success of this approach can be found in modern medicine.

Only a few years ago courses in medical genetics were given in only a small number of medical schools. Today most medical students are given some direct instruction in medical genetics, and the trend is to increase this emphasis. The direct relevance to clinical medicine, and the scientific undergirding of much of medical science that genetics provides, has made an understanding of this area essential to the modern physician. Fortunately, the grasp of a basic set of principles, which this text endeavors to present, allows the derivation of conclusions in complex situations. For the medical student burdened with a massive body of information to be memorized, genetics can be a welcome respite—a truly rational, logical, satisfying discipline.

REFERENCES

Impact of Genetic Diseases

1. Baird PA, Anderson TW, Newcombe HB, Lowry RB: Genetic disorders in children and young adults: A population study. *Am J Hum Genet* 42:677–693, 1988.
2. Roberts DF, Chavez J, Court SDM: The genetic component in child mortality. *Arch Dis Child* 45:33–38, 1970.
3. Carter CO: Changing patterns in the causes of death at the Hospital for Sick Children. *Great Ormond St J* 11:65–68, 1956.
4. Hall JG, Powers EK, McIlvaine RT, Ean VH: The frequency and financial burden of genetic disease in a pediatric hospital. *Am J Med Genet* 1:417–436, 1978.
5. Scriver CR, Neal JL, Saginur R, Clow A: The frequency of genetic disease and congenital malformation among patients in a pediatric hospital. *Can Med Assoc J* 108:1111–1115, 1973.
6. Edwards JH: The importance of genetic disease and the need for prevention. *Phil Trans R Soc Lond B* 319:211–227, 1988.

Genetics and Medicine: The Dynamic Interface

7. Bunn HF, Forget BG: *Hemoglobin: Molecular, Genetic and Clinical Aspects.* Philadelphia, WB Saunders, 1986.
8. Motulsky AG: Michael Brown and Joseph Goldstein. The 1985 Nobel Prize in Physiology or Medicine. Science 231:126–129, 1986.
9. Harvey W, quoted by Garrod A: The lesson of rare maladies. Lancet 1:1055–1066, 1928.

1/ Study Questions

1/ Discuss the relative contributions of heredity and environment in the following clinical cases:

a. Mental retardation in a boy with phenylketonuria
b. Squamous cell carcinoma of the cheek in an English farmer on a penal colony in Australia
c. Intellectual regression in a child with Tay-Sachs disease
d. Death in an automobile accident of a Navajo teenager with a blood alcohol of 225 mg/dl
e. Myocardial infarction in a 52-year-old male cigarette smoker
f. Faintness and syncope in a middle-aged hypertensive patient 1 day after starting therapeutic doses of a new blood pressure medication

2/ How can mutations in the same gene result in a number of different clinical disorders or in no disease at all?

2

Structure and Behavior of Genes and Chromosomes

"In the next day or so Crick and I shall send a note to* Nature *proposing our structure (of DNA) as a possible model, at the same time emphasizing its provisional nature and the lack of proof in its favor. Even if wrong, I believe it to be interesting since it provides a concrete example of a structure composed of complementary chains. If, by chance, it is right, then I suspect we may be making a slight dent into the manner in which DNA can reproduce itself."

—James Watson,
from a letter
to Max Delbrück,
March 12, 1953

To begin a description of the basic principles of human genetics, we must start with DNA. DNA, or deoxyribonucleic acid, is the ultimate molecule of life. The instructions that direct human cells to grow, to differentiate into specialized structures, to divide, and to respond to environmental changes are all encoded within the elegant simplicity of the human DNA genome. Furthermore, the basis of all genetic disease ultimately is founded on changes in this DNA sequence. An understanding of the structure and behavior of DNA and of the chromosomes into which it is packaged is thus fundamental to medical genetics and to medicine in general, especially as these fields have moved from descriptive into molecular sciences.

Some readers of this text are already very familiar with the contents of this chapter and the next. We include this basic information, however, recognizing that those with an interest in medical genetics have diverse backgrounds.

DNA IS THE HEREDITARY MATERIAL

That chromosomes contain DNA and are responsible for hereditary traits has been known since the 1860s. However, in the earlier part of the 20th century most biologists who were more familiar with the informational possibilities of proteins and their 20 amino acid building blocks tended to assume that a protein constituent of the chromosomes would be the true hereditary material. Resolution of this problem awaited the development of a biologic assay for genetic molecules, which was eventually provided by the Pneumococcus, a bacterial agent that causes pneumonia. Pneumococci that cause human disease grow as smooth, glistening, mucoid colonies, whereas those that do not are rough in appearance (now known to be due to the presence or absence of the thick polysaccharide cell wall). Heat-killed smooth bacteria, when mixed with living rough cells, are able to transform a small percentage to a smooth appearance. By investigating the nature of this "transforming factor," Avery, MacLeod, and McCarty showed definitively in 1944 that it was not protein but DNA. This seminal observation provided a new fundamental paradigm and set the stage for the modern revolution in genetics.

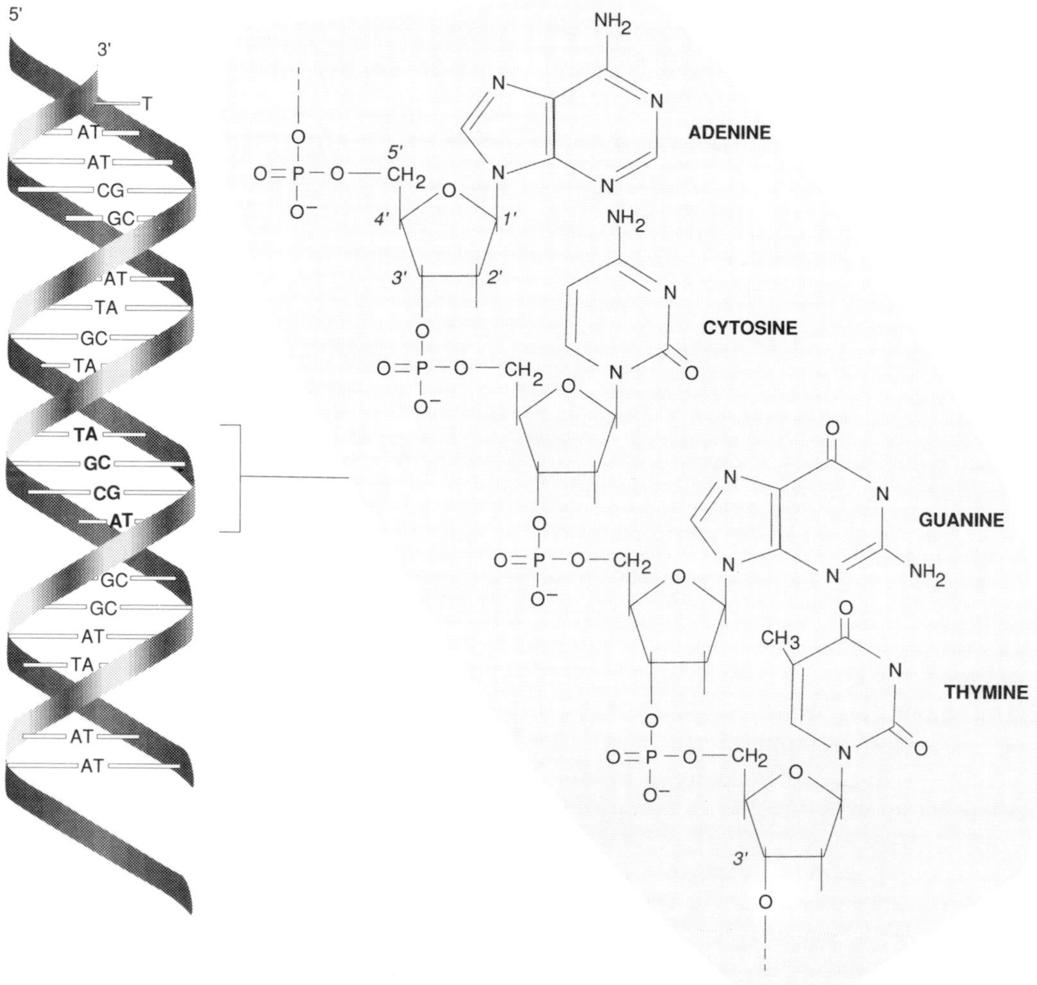

Figure 2.1. **The structure of DNA.** At the *left* is a schematic drawing of the DNA double helix, showing the sugar-phosphate backbone as a ribbon, with the bases arranged toward the middle. Note that A always pairs with T, and C always pairs with G. At the *right* is an expanded view of four nucleotides along one strand, showing the complete chemical structure of the sequence 5′-ACGT-3′. (A nucleotide consists of a sugar, a phosphate group, and an attached base.) Note that the 5′ and 3′ designations, used to indicate the polarity of a DNA strand, refer to the numbering of carbons on the deoxyribose ring.

STRUCTURE OF DNA

With the demonstration that DNA itself carries genetic information, a number of laboratories at the end of World War II turned their attention to its physical structure. Using the careful x-ray crystallographic data of Wilkins and Franklin, Watson and Crick deduced the correct structure in 1953 (Fig. 2.1). That DNA was a long polymer was in itself not surprising. What no one had predicted was that DNA consists of *two* intertwined chains, running in opposite directions.

The molecular structure of DNA, depicted schematically in Figure 2.1 and in a space-filling model in Figure 2.2, consists of a double helix. The "backbone" of each strand of the helix consists of an invariant sugar-phosphate-sugar-phosphate polymer, with the sugar being deoxyribose and the phosphates being attached through ester bonds to its 3′- and 5′-hydroxyl groups. Attached to the 1′ position of the sugar ring is one of four nitrogen-containing "bases." Two of these, adenine (A) and guanine (G), are purines, whereas the other two, cytosine (C) and thymine (T), are the less bulky pyrimidines. Watson and Crick correctly deduced that the bases lie almost flat within the interior of the double helix, like a stack of coins spaced 3.4 Å apart. The double helix is held together by hydrogen bonds, which can form between A and T bases and between G and C bases (Fig. 2.3), each of which is called a "base pair." Thus, the two strands of DNA are "complementary"; if one is 5′-ATGCCAG-3′, the other must be 5′-CTGGCAT-3′, with the full double-stranded structure of 7 base pairs (bp) being written as follows:

5′-ATGCCAG-3′
3′-TACGGTC-5′

This pairing of A with T and G with C explains the basis of Chargaff's rule, which was deduced before the structure of DNA was elucidated and states that the percentage of A and T bases in a given species' DNA is the same, and the percentage of G and C is the same.

There are a number of features of this structure that should be carefully noted:

1. It provides a means of storing and coding vast amounts of information, based on the sequence of the bases present in the DNA strand; for a molecule N bases long, there are 4^N possible sequences. The complete DNA sequence of an organism, containing its complete genetic information, is called its genome. The smallest viruses have genomes of only a few thousand base pairs and contain only a small number of genes. The size and complexity of the genome increase in a nonlinear fashion, however, as one moves along the evolutionary tree, from 4×10^6 bp in a bacterium to 3×10^9 bp in humans. A representative sample of genome sizes is shown in Table 2.1.

2. As noted by Watson and Crick, the double helical complementary structure immediately suggests a mechanism of DNA replication. Each strand contains the full informational content of the DNA molecule and can serve as a template for synthesis of a new complementary strand as the helix unwinds and replicates (Fig. 2.4). This mode of replication is denoted "semiconservative" because each daughter DNA strand contains one parental strand and one newly synthesized strand.

3. The complementary structure also provides a defense against information loss by DNA damage. A base on one strand that is damaged or lost can be replaced using the complementary strand to direct its

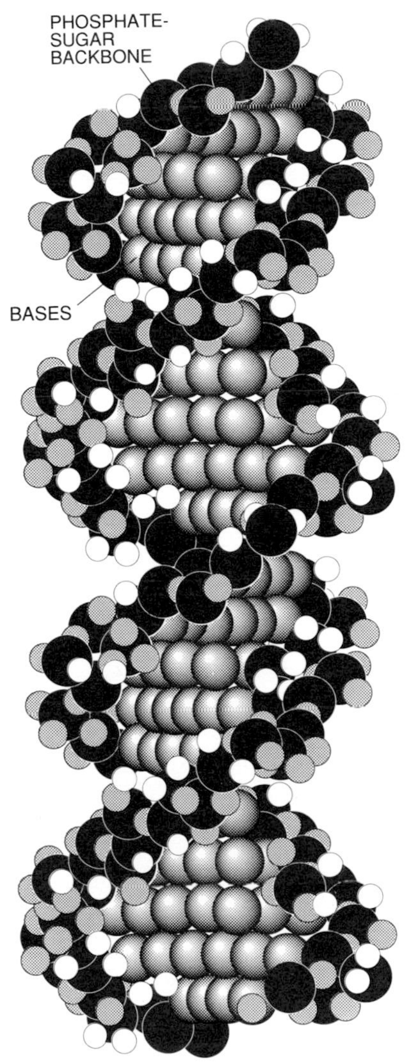

Figure 2.2. Space-filling model of DNA.

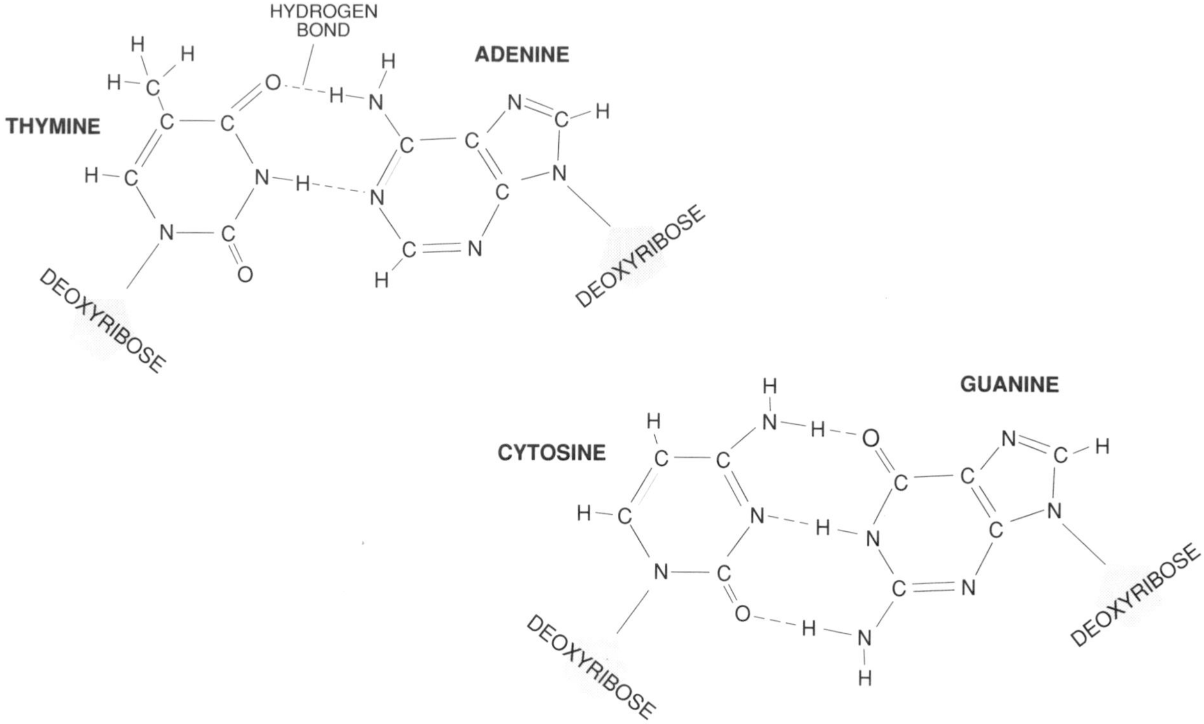

Figure 2.3. Hydrogen bonding between the adenine-thymine and guanine-cytosine base pairs. Note that two hydrogen bonds can form in A-T pairs, and three in C-G pairs.

repair. Similarly, a break in the sugar-phosphate backbone, which would be nearly impossible to correctly reconnect in a single-stranded molecule, can be repaired in a double-stranded molecule without any loss of contiguity.

4. The complementarity of DNA strands also allows them to find each other in a complex mixture of molecules. This "reannealing" or "hybridization" process is used in some situations by the nuclear machinery to regulate gene expression. Furthermore, this phenomenon has been heavily exploited in molecular biology, as we shall see in Chapter 5, and is at the heart of its current success.

TRANSCRIPTION INTO RNA

Even as early as the 19th century, another nucleic acid was known to exist within cells. This nucleic acid is present in the cytoplasm, particularly in association with polyribosomes, the protein synthesis factories of the cells. Chemical and structural analysis revealed this nucleic

Table 2.1. Representative Genome Sizes in Base Pairs

SV40, a mammalian DNA virus	4×10^3
λ, a bacterial virus	5×10^4
Escherichia coli, a bacterium	4×10^6
Saccharomyces cerevisiae, a yeast	2×10^7
Caennorhabitis elegans, a nematode	5×10^7
Drosophilia melanogaster, the fruit fly	1×10^8
Human chromosome 21	5×10^7
Human chromosome 1	3×10^8
Entire human genome[a]	3×10^9

[a]This is actually the *haploid* genome, or *half* the size of the number of base pairs of DNA in a human somatic cell. As will become clear in Chapter 3, the human is a *diploid* organism, with two copies of each chromosome, except for the sex chromosomes in males. Thus, there are actually 6×10^9 bp of DNA in each human somatic cell.

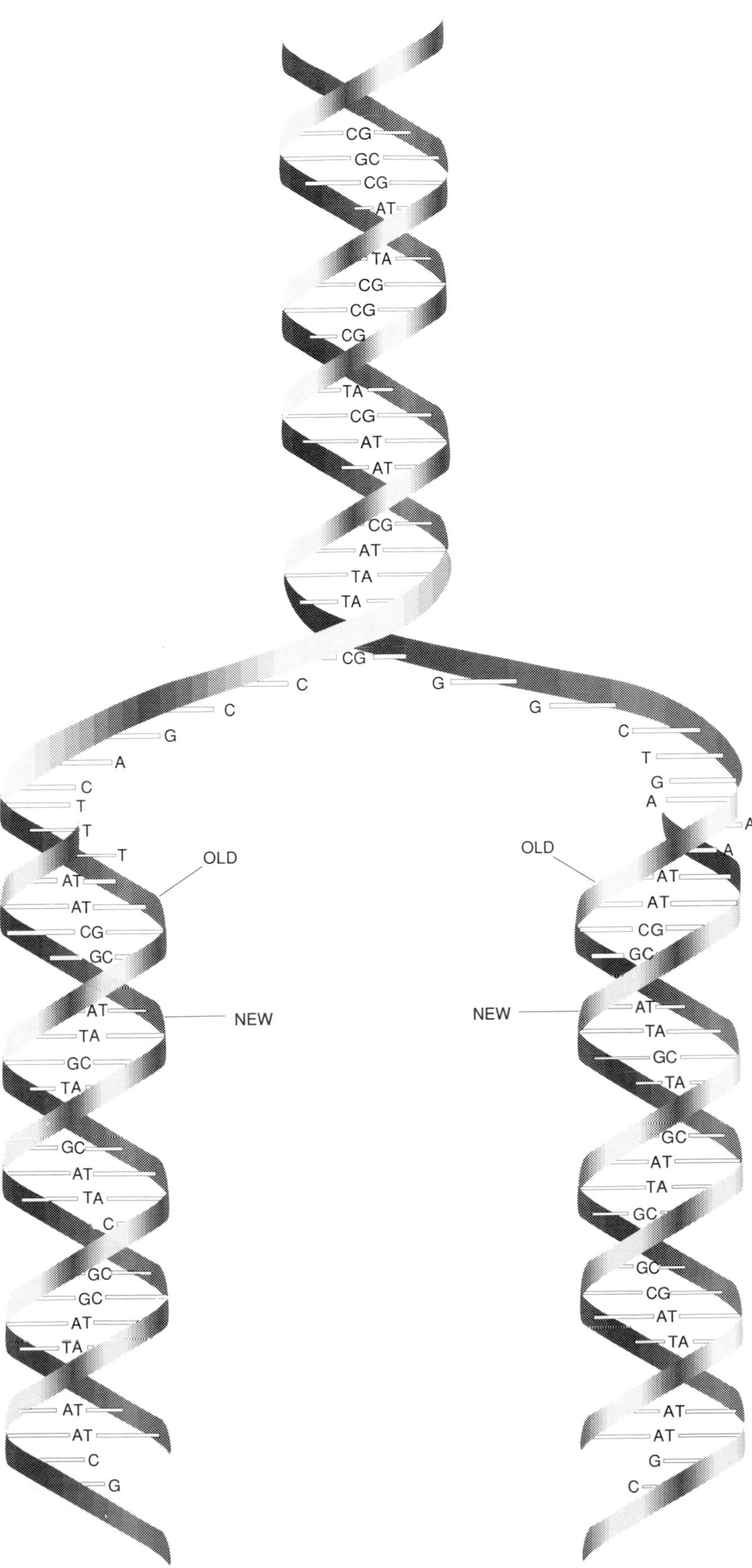

Figure 2.4. Replication of DNA. Identical daughter DNA molecules are generated by unwinding of the parental molecule, with each strand acting as a template for synthesis of a new strand using base pairing rules.

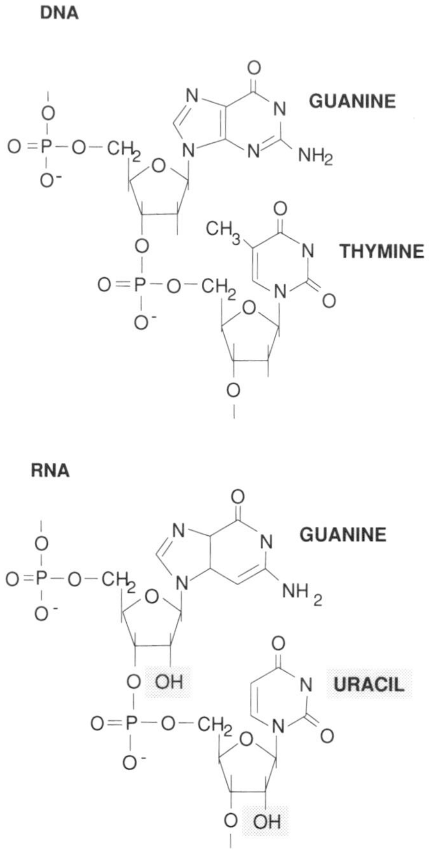

acid to be similar to DNA, but with three crucial differences (Fig. 2.5): (*a*) it is single-stranded; (*b*) the sugar is ribose, not deoxyribose; and (*c*) the pyrimidine base uracil replaces thymine.

This ribonucleic acid (RNA) has many roles in the cell. Certain RNAs, called ribosomal RNAs, make up a part of the polyribosomes and are synthesized in the nucleolus. Small molecules called transfer RNAs (tRNAs) are crucial elements in the translation of genetic information into protein molecules (see below). Other RNAs are involved in transcript processing functions. But the major RNA species of concern to biologists and geneticists is messenger RNA (mRNA), which occupies the essential connecting link between information contained in a gene and its end result as the specific amino acid sequence of a protein.

We will save a complete presentation of the transcriptional process for Chapter 5, where a description of the tools of the molecular biologist will allow more details to be included. For the time being, however, it is useful to consider transcription as the generation of a single-stranded RNA molecule from a double-stranded DNA template in the cell nucleus. This process, carried out by the enzyme RNA polymerase II, always occurs in the 5′ to 3′ direction; that is, new ribonucleotides are added to the 3′ end of the growing strand according to the DNA instructions (Fig. 2.6). In order for this process to be successful, some signal must be present in the DNA (the promoter) to indicate to the transcriptional machinery where to start. Similarly, transcription must not con-

Figure 2.5. Comparison of the chemical structures of DNA and RNA. The DNA sequence would be written 5′-GT-3′; the RNA sequence would be written 5′-GU-3′. The additional 2′ hydroxyl on the ribose ring of RNA is highlighted. The DNA base thymine is replaced in RNA by uracil, which lacks the methyl group on the pyrimidine ring. Not shown is the additional difference that DNA is ordinarily double-stranded whereas RNA is ordinarily single-stranded.

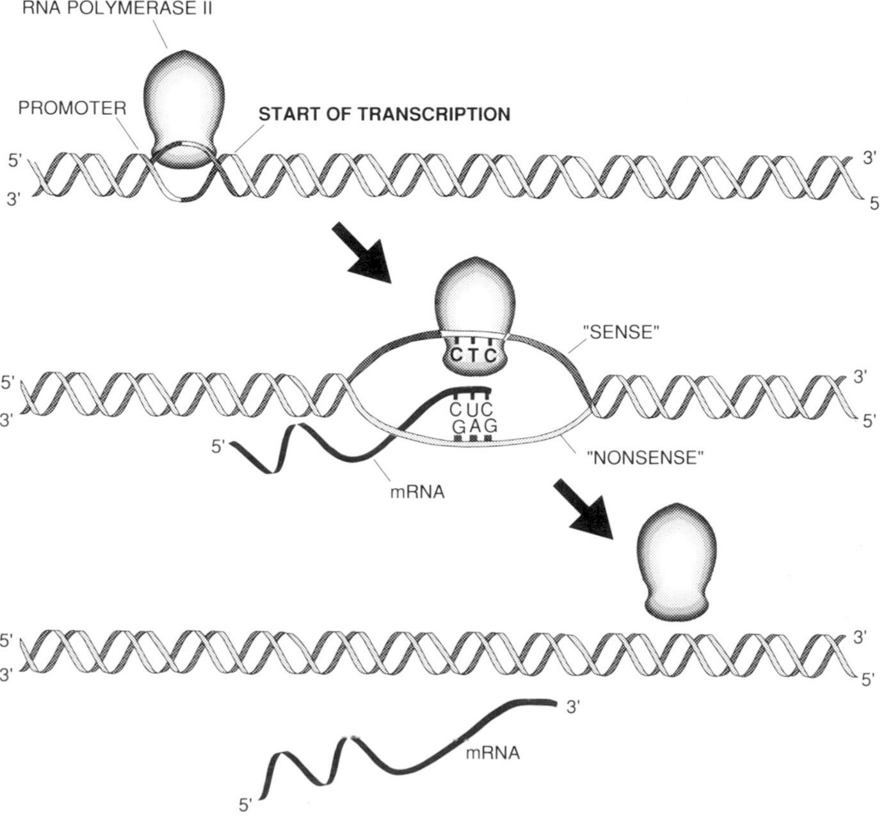

Figure 2.6. Schematic drawing of the transcription process. RNA polymerase II recognizes a specific sequence at the 5′ end of a gene (the promoter) and begins to transcribe it into messenger RNA (mRNA). The mRNA is synthesized in the 5′ to 3′ direction and has the same sequence as the 5′ to 3′ DNA strand, also known as the "sense" strand. The mechanism of RNA formation presumably depends on base pairing of the newly formed RNA with the "nonsense" strand of the DNA, which acts as a template for copying.

tinue indefinitely, but must end after the necessary sequence has been transcribed.

TRANSLATION INTO PROTEINS

The messenger RNA produced by transcription must make its way out of the nucleus to ribosomes where it can be translated into a protein sequence. One of the great achievements of the past 30 years has been the deduction of the mechanism of translation and the "language" used in the process, commonly referred to as the genetic code. Because there are only 4 bases in DNA and RNA, but 20 amino acids in proteins, at least 3 bases ($4^2 = 16$, $4^3 = 64$) would be needed to unambiguously specify an amino acid. A series of careful experiments performed between 1961 and 1966 deduced that the 3-base word, or "codon," is correct and led to determination of the genetic code, as shown in Table 2.2. Note that there is "degeneracy" in this code, so that several codons may result in the same amino acid. Codons UUA, UUG, UCU, UCC, UCA, and UCG, for example, all code for leucine. Three codons, UAA, UAG, and UGA, do not encode amino acids but result in a termination of translation and are called stop codons.

The machinery that carries out the translation process on the ribosome is complex. An array of amino acid-specific adaptor molecules, called transfer RNAs, covalently bind a particular amino acid. The 3-base "anticodon" is complementary to the codon specifying that amino acid and allows it to be accurately added to the growing polypeptide chain, as depicted in Fig. 2.7. This process continues until the stop codon is reached, which leads to release of the polypeptide chain from the ribosome. The order of addition of amino acids is such that the 5′ end of the mRNA corresponds to the amino (NH_2) terminus of the protein, and the 3′ end of the mRNA corresponds to the carboxy (COOH) terminus of the protein.

Table 2.2. The Genetic Code[a]

	Second Position				
First Position (5′ end)	U	C	A	G	Third Position (3′ end)
U	Phe	Ser	Tyr	Cys	U
	Phe	Ser	Tyr	Cys	C
	Leu	Ser	STOP	STOP	A
	Leu	Ser	STOP	Trp	G
C	Leu	Pro	His	Arg	U
	Leu	Pro	His	Arg	C
	Leu	Pro	Gln	Arg	A
	Leu	Pro	Gln	Arg	G
A	Ile	Thr	Asn	Ser	U
	Ile	Thr	Asn	Ser	C
	Ile	Thr	Lys	Arg	A
	Met	Thr	Lys	Arg	G
G	Val	Ala	Asp	Gly	U
	Val	Ala	Asp	Gly	C
	Val	Ala	Glu	Gly	A
	Val	Ala	Glu	Gly	G

[a]Amino acid abbreviations are: Ala, alanine; Arg, arginine; Asn, asparagine; Asp, aspartic acid; Cys, cysteine; Gln, glutamine; Glu, glutamic acid; Gly, glycine; His, histidine; Ile, isoleucine; Leu, leucine; Lys, lysine; Met, methionine; Phe, phenylalanine; Pro, proline; Ser, serine; Thr, threonine; Trp, tryptophan; Tyr, tyrosine; Val, valine.

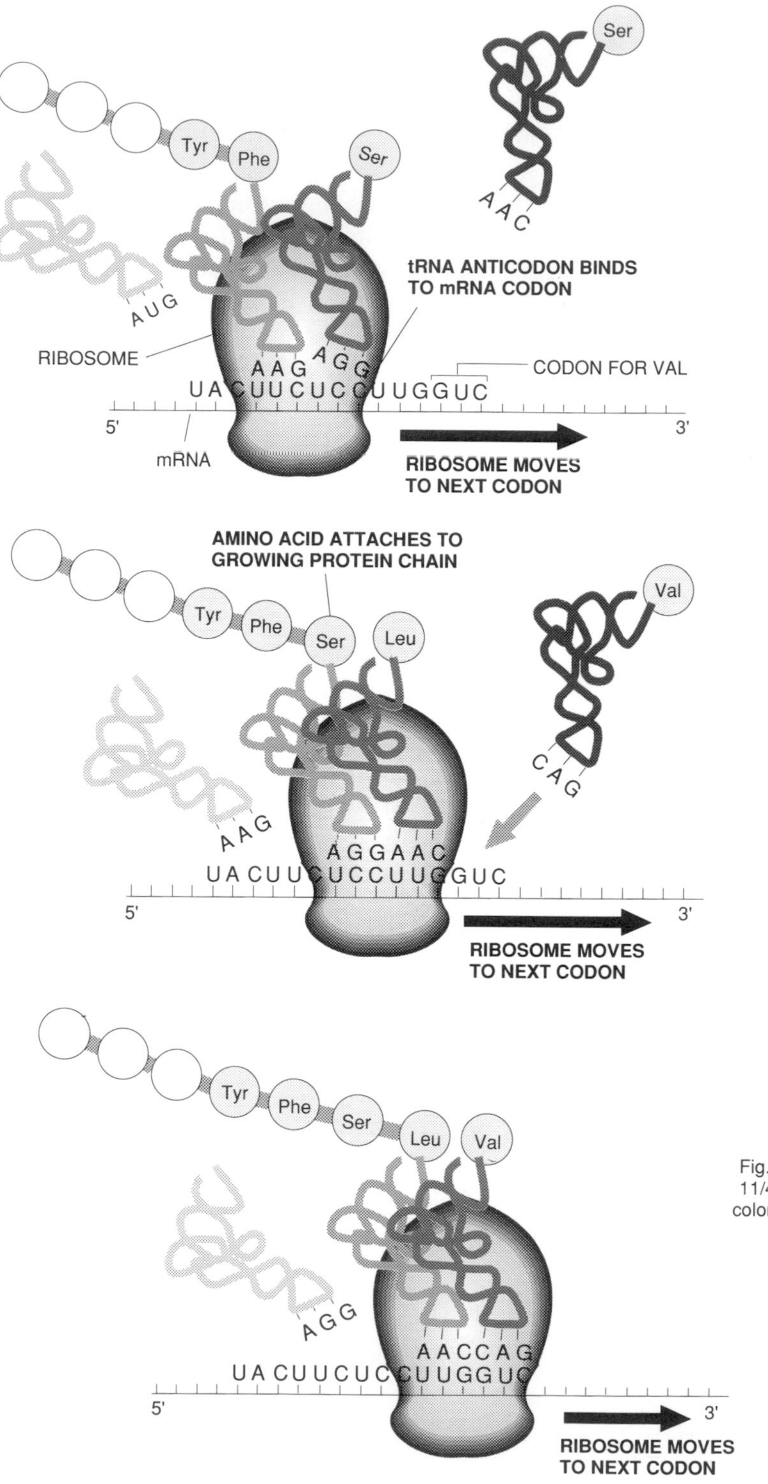

Figure 2.7. Translation of mRNA into protein by a ribosome. The mRNA sequence 5′-UAC-UUCUCCUUGGUC-3′ is translated to the amino acid sequence Tyr-Phe-Ser-Leu-Val, using the tRNA molecules and their anticodons as adaptors.

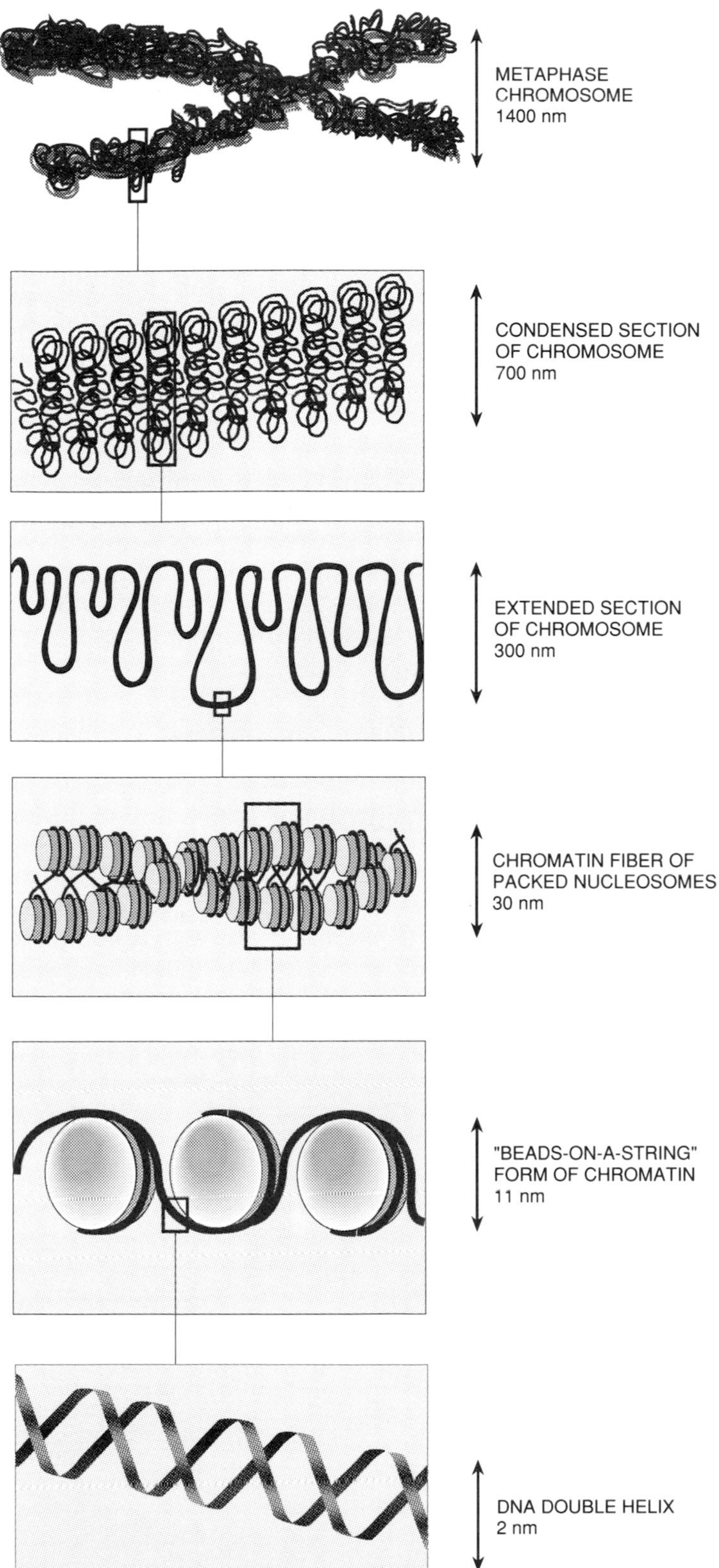

Figure 2.8. Coiling of DNA, arranged in increasing order of organization from *bottom* to *top*. In *each panel* a size marker in nanometers (nm) indicates the scale.

HIGHER ORDER COILING OF DNA

It is likely that each of the 46 chromosomes of humans is made up of a single molecule of double-stranded DNA. If stretched out, the DNA from a single cell would extend approximately 2 meters in length. Obviously an efficient method of packaging must be used by cells in order to deal with a molecule of such complexity. An elaborate system of coiling, which also seems to be involved in the control of gene expression in as yet poorly understood ways, is present in mammalian cells. Basic proteins called histones provide a core around which DNA is wound in a double loop composing approximately 146 bp of DNA (Fig. 2.8). This unit is referred to as a nucleosome; the tight evolutionary conservation of the histone structure implies an important functional role. The resulting "beads-on-a-string" DNA structure results in a compaction of length of about a factor of 7; further organization occurs by arrangement of the nucleosomes in a solenoid fashion and by higher order structural complexities (Fig. 2.8).

The mechanism by which factors responsible for regulation of gene expression interact with this monotonous histone-DNA complex represents an important area of current investigation. There is evidence that regions of the DNA molecule that are involved in regulation may be locally free of histones. For example, certain areas (especially the 5′ ends) of actively expressed genes are unusually sensitive to cleavage by enzymes that cut DNA (nucleases), which do not efficiently cut histone-bound DNA.

HUMAN CHROMOSOMES

The highest order of DNA coiling is the chromosome. Each species has a characteristic number and size of chromosomes, known as the karyotype. The human karyotype, to be discussed in more detail in Chapter 8, consists of 46 chromosomes (Figure 2.9). As mentioned

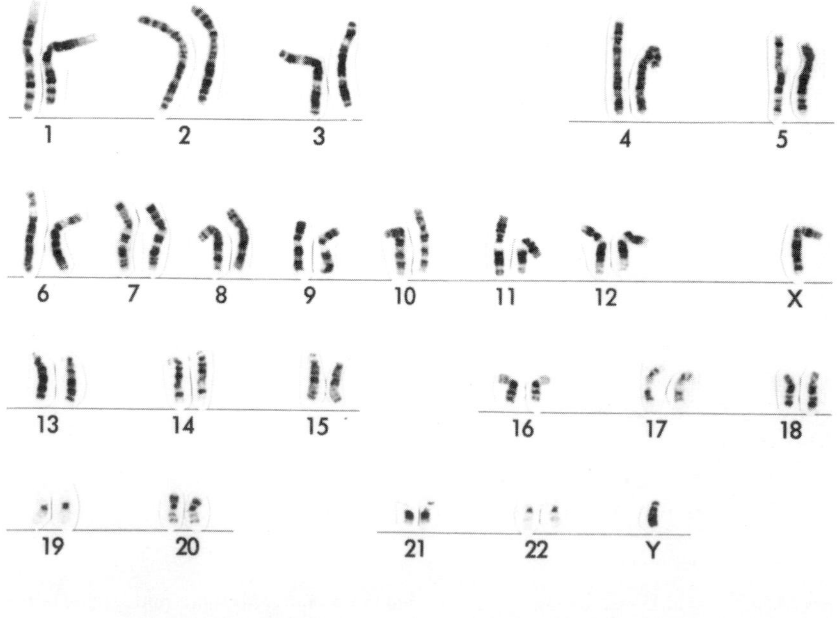

Figure 2.9. Karyotype of a normal human male, consisting of 22 pairs of autosomes, an X chromosome, and a Y chromosome.

above, the human is a diploid organism: 44 of these (the autosomes) occur in 22 homologous pairs, with each member of the pair containing the same genetic information. The remaining two chromosomes are the sex chromosomes; a female has two X chromosomes, and a male an X and a Y.

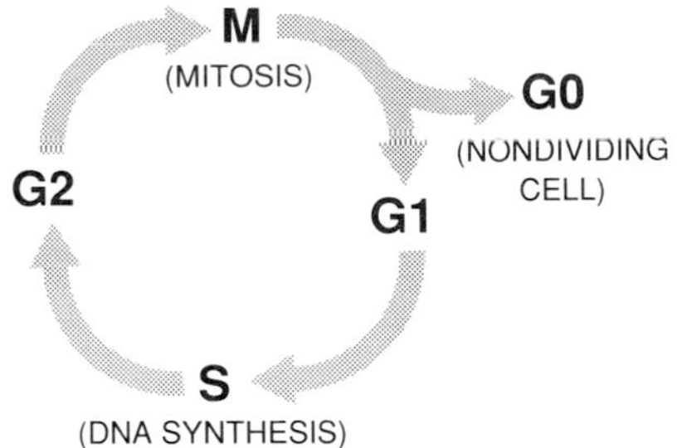

Figure 2.10. The cell cycle.

MITOSIS

There are two kinds of cell divisions: mitosis and meiosis. Mitotic division is the process whereby one cell divides to give rise to two that are genetically identical to the parent. It is mitosis that allows a single fertilized oocyte to give rise to a complete human being with its estimated 10^{14} cells, all (with a few exceptions) genetically identical to the original single cell. In mitosis, each daughter cell must receive the complete chromosome complement of 46 chromosomes.

Mitosis itself, the process of nuclear division, takes only a short time. However, it is part of a carefully programmed process, diagrammed in Figure 2.10, called the cell cycle. Just after division, the cell that is destined to divide again enters a stage called G1 whereas one that will not enters a resting phase called G0. A cell in G1 next moves into S phase, during which time DNA replication occurs, by the semiconservative mechanism described above wherein each DNA strand serves as a template for its own replication. The result is that each of the 46 chromosomes is duplicated into "sister chromatids," held together by a central constriction called the contromere. At the end of S phase, another gap phase (G2) begins, which then leads into actual mitosis (M).

In mitosis (Fig. 2.11) the sister chromatids and the centromere become clearly visible and line up along the plane of eventual cleavage. The centromeres of all 46 chromosomes then divide, so that one sister chromatid from each ends up in the daughter cell, completing the cell cycle.

MEIOSIS AND GAMETOGENESIS

Meiosis, the variety of cell division that is used to generate the male and female gametes (sperm and oocytes, respectively) is different in crucial ways from mitosis. A little reflection suggests this must be so: if sperm and egg cells contained the full complement ("diploid") set of 46 chromosomes, the fertilized oocyte would have 92 chromosomes, including three X's and a Y!

Meiosis, the special reduction process that is carried out in gametogenesis to generate sperm and egg cells, each bearing 23 chromosomes (the "haploid" state), is diagrammed in Figure 2.12. There are actually two divisions, meiosis I and meiosis II. In meiosis I, each chromosome replicates into sister chromatids, just as in mitosis. Unlike mitosis, however, the homologous chromosomes then align in pairs (a process called synapsis) and separate to *opposite* poles, with their sister chromatids still together. In meiosis II, the sister chromatids then separate, resulting in 23 chromosomes per gamete.

CROSSING OVER

An extremely important feature of meiosis I is that during synapsis, when homologous chromosomes are paired together, crossovers occur (Fig. 2.13). The practical result of this is that the chromosome retained in a gamete at the end of meiosis may be a patchwork of *both*

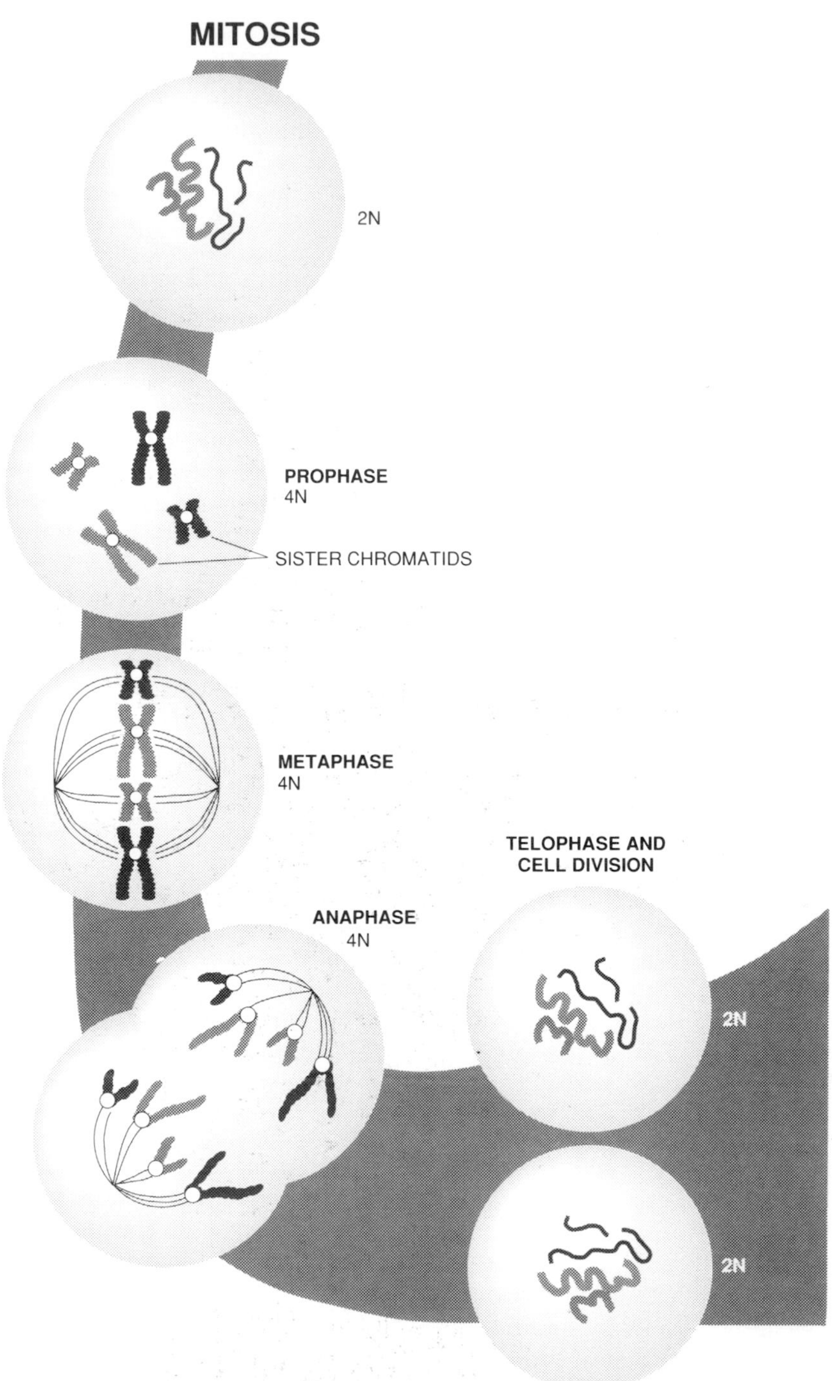

Figure 2.11. **Mitosis.** For simplicity only four chromosomes, consisting of two pairs of autosomes, are shown. The "ploidy" of the cell is shown at each stage: 2N represents the diploid state. After formation of sister chromatids but before cell division, the cell contains an amount of DNA corresponding to 4N.

homologous parental chromosomes. Genes that are close together on a chromosome, however (such as *A* and *B* in Fig. 2.13), are likely to be passed along together, whereas a crossover (or "recombination") is more likely to occur between genes that are far apart on a chromosome. On the average, about 30–40 crossovers (or 1–2 per chromosome) occur during a meiotic division.

Besides increasing enormously the potential genetic diversity of gametes, crossing over provides a quantitative estimate of the distance separating two genes on the same chromosome (called "syntenic" genes). As we shall see in Chapter 9, this has provided a powerful means of mapping genes.

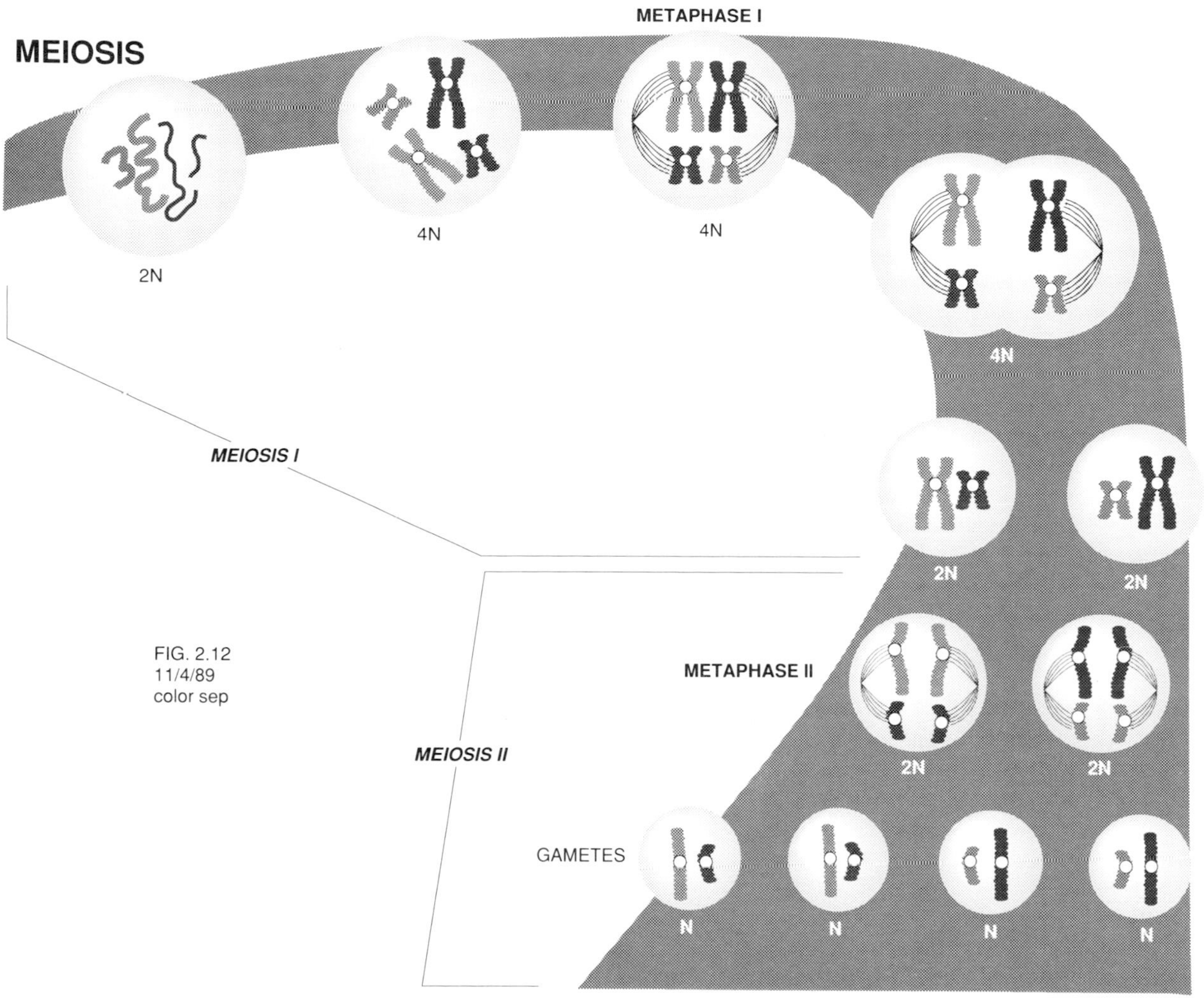

MEIOSIS
METAPHASE I
2N
4N
4N
4N
MEIOSIS I
2N
2N
FIG. 2.12
11/4/89
color sep
METAPHASE II
MEIOSIS II
2N
2N
GAMETES
N
N
N
N

Figure 2.12. Meiosis. Again, only two pairs of autosomes are shown. Note that after meiosis I each cell only retains *one* of the homologous pair. Meiosis II then leads to sister chromatid separation. For simplicity, no crossing over is shown.

MUTATION

Until now we have considered the DNA making up the human genome as unchanging and error-free. Were this the case, however, evolution would be impossible. On the other hand, mutations in DNA sequence, which must be possible to allow gradual selective change of organisms, must not be too frequent because the vast majority will be

SYNAPSIS
CROSSING OVER
CHROMOSOMES AFTER CROSSING OVER
A B A B a b a b
C C c c

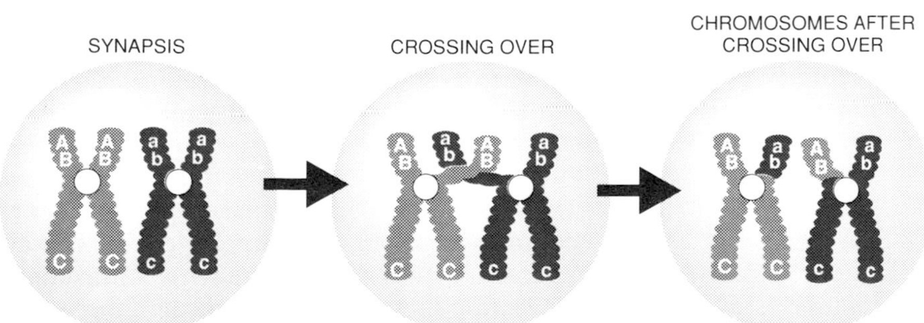

Figure 2.13. Crossing over in meiosis I.

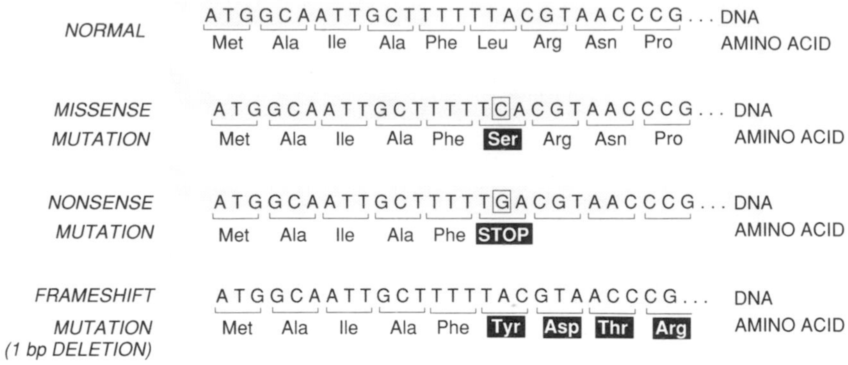

NORMAL	ATG GCA ATT GCT TTT TTA CGT AAC CCG...	DNA
	Met Ala Ile Ala Phe Leu Arg Asn Pro	AMINO ACID
MISSENSE MUTATION	ATG GCA ATT GCT TTT TCA CGT AAC CCG...	DNA
	Met Ala Ile Ala Phe **Ser** Arg Asn Pro	AMINO ACID
NONSENSE MUTATION	ATG GCA ATT GCT TTT TGA CGT AAC CCG...	DNA
	Met Ala Ile Ala Phe **STOP**	AMINO ACID
FRAMESHIFT MUTATION (1 bp DELETION)	ATG GCA ATT GCT TTT TAC GTA ACC CG...	DNA
	Met Ala Ile Ala Phe **Tyr** **Asp** **Thr** **Arg**	AMINO ACID

Figure 2.14. Examples of mutation. The "sense" strand DNA sequence of a coding region is shown, together with the encoded amino acid sequence. Three different mutations affecting the second nucleotide of a leucine codon are shown.

deleterious. As pointed out, many mutations are corrected using the undamaged DNA strand as a template to correct the damaged one. However, if damage occurs to both strands, or if it occurs just before or during DNA replication, the resulting alteration in DNA sequence becomes permanent for all the future progeny of that cell.

Considerable effort has been expended to attempt to determine the background mutation rate in humans. A new mutation in a given gene appears at a frequency of about one in a million as that gene is passed from parent to child. Because there are estimated to be about 50,000–100,000 genes in humans, this indicates that a surprising 5–10% of all newborns carry a new mutation. Fortunately, most of these are silent, because the balancing gene on the homologous chromosome is normal, so that their presence is not apparent. New mutations can take various forms at the molecular level. As we shall see throughout this text, the identification of an increasing number of mutations at the DNA level has borne out the principle that "whatever can go wrong, eventually will" (Murphy's law of the genome?). A few examples are shown in Figure 2.14. The simplest change is a substitution of one nucleotide for another, called a "point mutation." If this occurs in a coding region and changes the triplet codon to that for a different amino acid (a "missense mutation"), then the resultant protein will be structurally different. If the amino acid substitution occurs in a functionally important domain or alters the structure or stability of the protein, altered function will result. A particularly disruptive point mutation is one that converts the normal codon to UAA, UGA, or UAG, creating a premature stop codon. This is known as a "nonsense mutation."

If it does not represent a multiple of 3, insertion or deletion of a small number of nucleotides into a coding region will alter the reading frame of translation from that point onward, leading to a completely abnormal carboxy terminus of the protein. Such mutations are called "frameshifts."

Several other varieties of mutation alter transcription of a gene, but we will delay a discussion of these until Chapter 5, when a more complete description of gene anatomy is given. First, we will delve into the effects of mutation in creating human disease and the inheritance patterns that can result.

SUGGESTED READINGS

History of Molecular Biology

Judson HF: *The Eighth Day of Creation: Makers of the Revolution in Biology.* New York, Simon & Schuster, 1979.

Watson JD: *The Double Helix.* New York, Athenum, 1968.

General Reference Texts

Alberts B, Bray D, Lewis J, Raff M, Roberts K, Watson JD: *Molecular Biology of the Cell.* New York, Garland, 1983.

Darnell J, Lodish H, Baltimore D: *Molecular Cell Biology.* Scientific American Books, New York, WH Freeman, 1986.

Watson JD, Tooze J, Kurtz DT: *Recombinant DNA. A Short Course.* Scientific American Books, New York, WH Freeman, 1983.

Watson JD, Hopkins NH, Roberts JW, Steitz JA, Weiner AM: *Molecular Biology of the Gene.* 4th Ed. Menlo Park, CA, Benjamin/Cummings Publishing Co., 1986.

Classic Papers

Meselson M, Stahl FW: The replication of DNA in *E. coli.* Proc Natl Acad Sci USA 44:671–682, 1958.

Nirenberg MW, Matthaei JH: The dependence of cell-free protein synthesis in *E. coli* upon naturally occurring or synthetic polyribonucleotides. Proc Natl Acad Sci USA 47:1588–1602, 1961.

Watson JD, Crick FHC: A structure for deoxyribose nucleic acid. Nature 171:737–738, 1953.

2/ Study Questions

1/ Draw a schematic diagram of a methionine codon (ATG) in double-stranded DNA. Label the following structures:

a. 5′ ends
b. 3′ ends
c. Phosphodiester backbones
d. 2′ carbons
e. The "bases"
f. The chemical bonds responsible for Chargaff's base-pairing rules

2/ During normal spermatogenesis in man, spermatogonia serve both as self-renewing stem cells as well as a source of cells that can mature into primary spermatocytes. Primary spermatocytes enter meiosis, giving rise after meiosis I to secondary spermatocytes, which in turn give rise to spermatids following meiosis II. Spermatids mature into spermatozoa without further cell divisions. For each type of cell and cell cycle stage in the following table, provide the total number of DNA base pairs per cell, the number of chromosomes per cell, and the number of chromatids per cell. Designate the "ploidy" (haploid, diploid) for each.

	DNA (bp)	Chromosomes	Chromatids	Ploidy
Spermatogonia at G1				
Spermatogonia at G2				
Primary spermatocyte				
Secondary spermatocyte after meiosis I				
Spermatid after meiosis II				

3/ During DNA replication (or RNA transcription), the appropriate nucleotide triphosphate is used to add a base to a preexisting DNA (or RNA) strand. To which end, 5′ or 3′, is the new nucleotide added? What determines which nucleotide, A, G, C, or T (U for RNA), is added? What would happen if a synthetic *3′-deoxy* nucleotide were added to a growing nucleic acid strand?

4/ It is a truism that each of us is the beneficiary of genetic information inherited from both parents, four grandparents, eight great grandparents, etc. What is the chance that a child might carry information from only two of his/her four grandparents? For example, what is the chance that a child would have no genetic information from his/her grandmothers and has information only from his/her grandfathers? (Assume that no crossing over occurs.) What would the sex of this child be?

5/ The following sequence of amino acids represents part of a protein. What kind of mutation is most likely represented by each of the following amino acid sequences?

Normal	Glu-Cys-Met-Phe-Trp-Asp
Mutant A	Glu-Cys-Ile-Phe-Trp-Asp
Mutant B	Glu-Val-Cys-Ser-Gly-Thr
Mutant C	Glu-Cys-Met-Phe
Mutant D	Glu-Met-Tyr-Val-Leu-Gly

3

Mendelian Inheritance

"Those characteristics that are transmitted entire, or almost unchanged by hybridization, and therefore constitute the characters of the hybrid, are termed dominant, and those that become latent in the process, recessive."

—Gregor Mendel, 1865

In order to understand Mendelian inheritance, several essential terms must first be defined. A genetic **locus** is a specific position or location on a chromosome. Frequently, locus is used to refer to a specific gene. **Alleles** are alternative forms of a gene at a given locus. If both alleles at a locus are identical, the individual is **homozygous** at that locus; if they are different, he or she is **heterozygous.** Such individuals are called **homozygotes** or **heterozygotes,** respectively. An individual with two different mutant alleles at a given locus is a **compound heterozygote,** whereas an individual with one mutant allele at each of two different loci is a **double heterozygote.**

The **genotype** is the genetic constitution or composition of an individual. More specifically, it can refer to the alleles at a specific genetic locus. The **phenotype** is the observed result of the interaction of the genotype with environmental factors; more specifically, the observable expression of a particular gene or genes. The meaning of genotype and phenotype may be illustrated by a musical analogy. Figure 3.1 is a portion of the score of Mozart's Concerto in A Major for Piano and Orchestra, K. 488. The musical notation contains all of the necessary information or instructions for the notes to be played by each instrument and the temporal relationships of the various parts. This is the genotype. The phenotype is the sound we hear, which is strongly influenced by the environment, including the soloist, the conductor, the orchestra, and the hall in which it is performed, or the quality of the recording.

We define Mendelian diseases as diseases that are the result of a **single mutant gene** that has a large effect on phenotype and that are inherited in simple patterns similar to or identical with those described

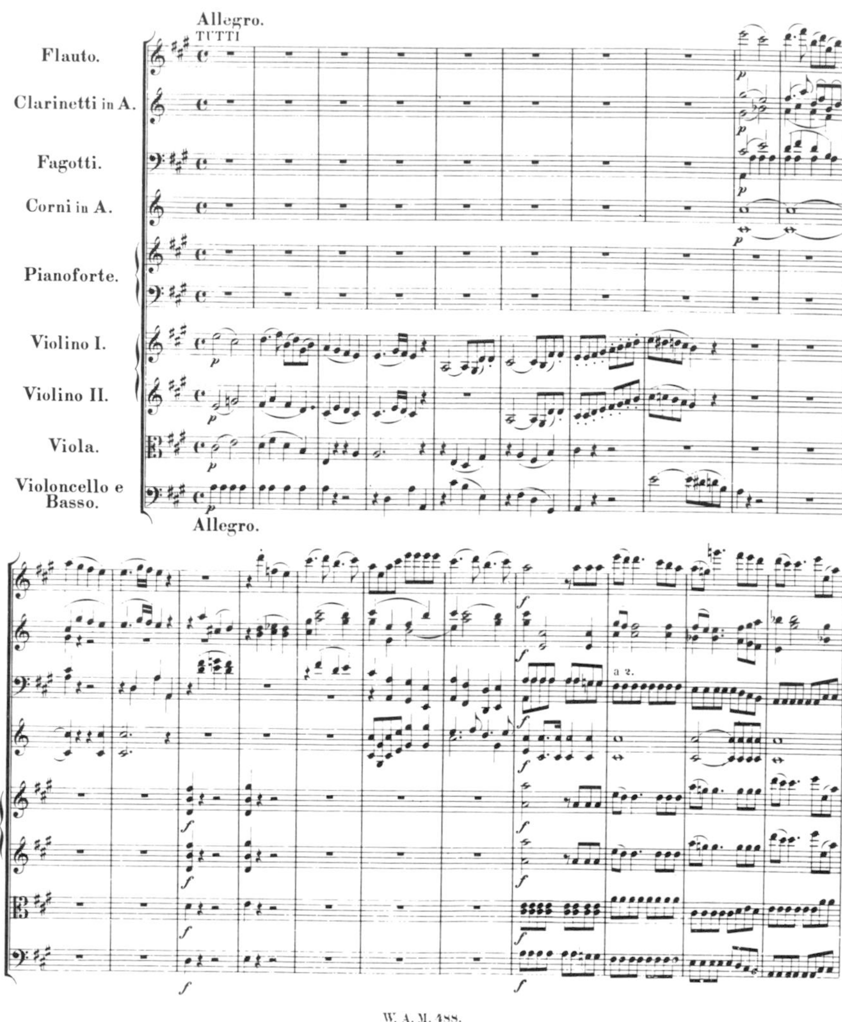

Figure 3.1. The first page of the orchestral score of the Concerto in A Major for Piano and Orchestra, K. 488 by Wolfgang Amadeus Mozart. (From Mozart WA: *Piano Concertos Nos. 23–27 in Full Score.* New York, Dover Publications, 1978, p. 1.)

by Mendel for certain discrete characteristics in garden peas. Mendelian diseases are **autosomal** if they are encoded by genes on one of the 22 pairs of autosomes, or non-sex chromosomes, and **X-linked** if encoded by a mutant gene on the X chromosome. Following Mendel, we define as **dominant** those conditions that are expressed in heterozygotes, i.e., individuals who have one copy of the mutant allele and one copy of the normal, or wild-type, allele, and **recessive** those conditions that are clinically manifest only in individuals homozygous for the mutant allele, i.e., carrying a double dose of the abnormal gene. It should be stressed that dominance and recessivity refer to traits, or phenotypes, and not to genes. Although we sometimes speak of dominant and recessive genes, this is a shorthand and should be understood to refer to traits. By now nearly 4000 human phenotypes known or presumed to be inherited in a Mendelian fashion have been catalogued (1). More than half are autosomal dominant traits, 36% are autosomal recessive, and less than 10% are X-linked. Of these 4000 traits, approximately 3000 are associated with human diseases.

The pattern of inheritance of most Mendelian traits has been deduced from observing the segregation or transmission of these traits within families. This information is expressed in the form of a pedigree, derived from the French expression "pied de grue" or crane's foot, from the branching pattern of the diagram. The standard symbols used for drawing a human pedigree are shown in Figure 3.2. The proband or index case, also called propositus or proposita, is indicated by an *arrow*. The position of individuals within the pedigree is indicated by *Roman numerals* for the generation and *Arabic numerals* for an individual within a single generation. For pedigrees in physician records or hospital charts, it is useful to note the individuals' age next to, but not inside, the symbol.

AUTOSOMAL DOMINANT INHERITANCE

Autosomal dominant diseases include many of the serious and more common genetic disorders of adult life including familial hypercholesterolemia, colonic polyposis, polycystic kidney disease, Huntington disease, and neurofibromatosis. The pedigree of a family with familial hypercholesterolemia is shown in Figure 3.3. This condition is characterized by an increased level of cholesterol in blood and by premature atherosclerotic cardiovascular disease with myocardial infarctions or heart attacks early in life. Although both men and women are affected, affected males tend to have coronary artery disease about a decade earlier than do women, just as is true for the general population without hypercholesterolemia. The basic defect in this condition has been defined as a deficiency in low density lipoprotein receptors on the cell surface (see Chapter 7). W. H. (II-4 in the pedigree in Figure 3.3) is a 33-year-old white advertising executive. At the age of 25 years he began to experience recurrent chest pain on exertion and, at age 30, suffered a myocardial infarction. Coronary arteriography revealed extensive coronary artery disease and he underwent coronary artery bypass surgery. Physical examination revealed evidence of cholesterol deposits in extensor tendons, and laboratory evaluation indicated significant hypercholesterolemia. A family history revealed that his father had died at age 52 years of his second myocardial infarction and that a paternal uncle (I-1) had also died of a myocardial infarction at age 46 years. The patient's 50-year-old sister was asymptomatic but was found to have hypercholesterolemia. W. H.'s three children were entirely healthy and normal on physical examination, but all had significant hypercholesterolemia.

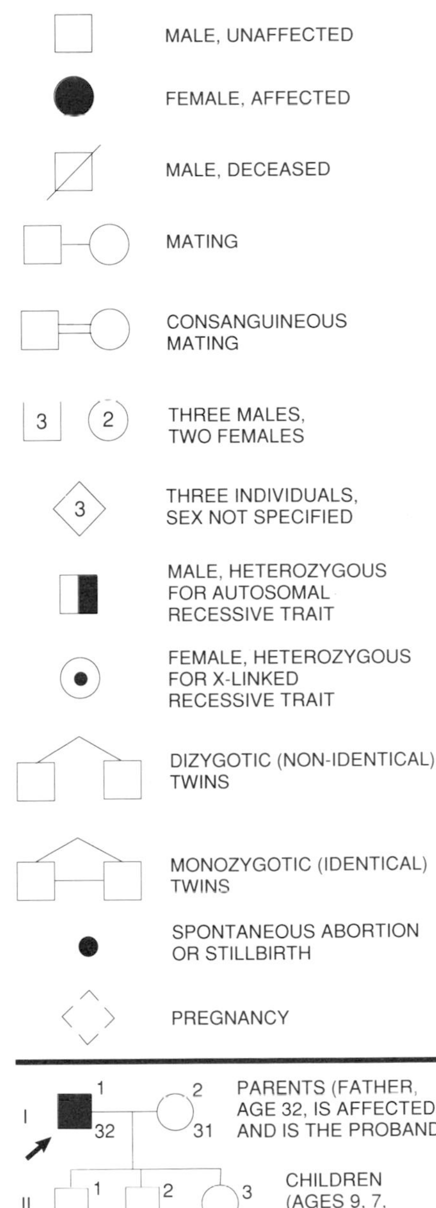

Figure 3.2. Standard pedigree symbols.

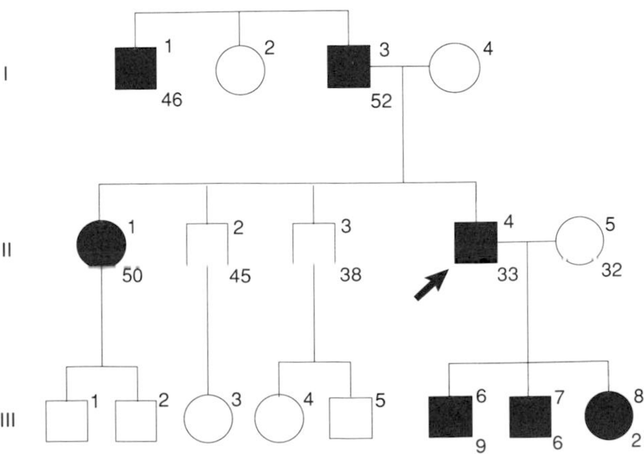

Figure 3.3. Pedigree of a family with autosomal dominant familial hypercholesterolemia. Affected individuals are indicated by the *solid red symbols*.

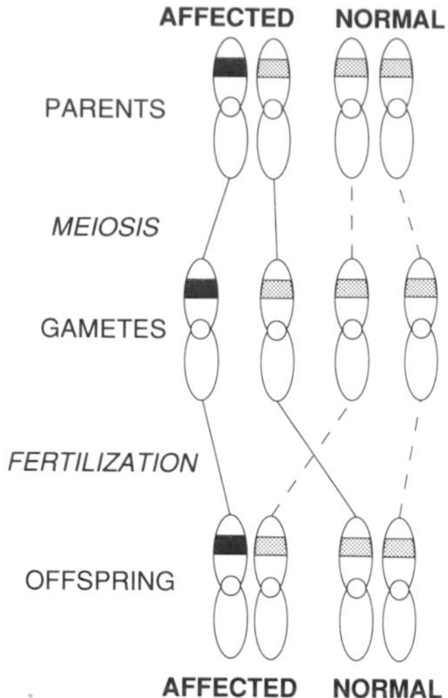

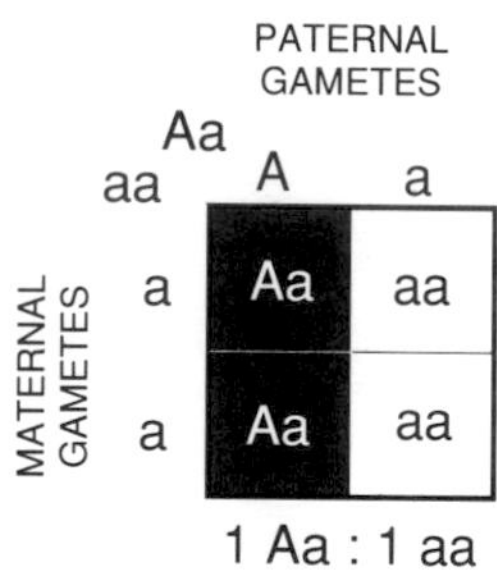

A = MUTANT, a = NORMAL

Figure 3.4. Autosomal dominant inheritance. The mating diagram *(top)* and Punnett square *(bottom)* show the outcome of a mating between a heterozygous affected individual and a homozygous normal individual. The mutant allele in the mating diagram is indicated in *red,* and affected offspring in the Punnett square are indicated in *red.*

As seen in this pedigree, the characteristic pattern of inheritance is *vertical;* that is, the disorder is passed from one generation to the next in a vertical fashion. Both males and females are affected and can transmit the trait with equal probability, although the severity of manifestations can be affected by the sex of the individual. Each affected individual has one affected parent. Note that in pedigrees of dominantly inherited conditions, the unaffected spouse is often omitted.

The pattern of inheritance of autosomal dominant traits is best understood by observing the segregation of chromosomes bearing the mutant and normal alleles during meiosis (Fig. 3.4). Assuming for simplicity that there is only one normal allele and one mutant allele, there are three possible genotypes: homozygous normal, homozygous affected, and heterozygous. Because both males and females may have any of the three genotypes, there are six possible mating types; however, because both males and females may transmit the abnormal gene with equal probability, sex differences will be ignored. Because homozygous affected individuals are very rare, the usual mating in dominantly inherited diseases is that between a homozygous normal individual and a heterozygous affected individual. Each gamete produced by these individuals will contain only one allele of the pair so that the possible gametes produced are shown in the mating diagram in the *top panel* of Figure 3.4. On the *bottom* is a Punnett square, an alternative method for showing the gametes produced and their possible combinations at fertilization. *Each* offspring of such a mating has a 50% probability of inheriting the chromosome bearing the mutant allele and a 50% probability of inheriting the chromosome bearing the normal allele. Thus, *on average,* approximately half of the offspring of affected individuals will themselves be affected. An unaffected child, inheriting the chromosome bearing the normal allele, can have only normal offspring. In the pedigree shown in Figure 3.3, two offspring of four born to the affected parent I-3 are themselves affected, i.e., the expected 50%. Within any given sibship (set of siblings), however, the 50% prediction may not be met; all three children of W. H. (III-6, III-7, and III-8) are affected with familial hypercholesterolemia.

To understand this divergence from expectation, it is appropriate at this point to introduce some basic principles of probability (2, 3). The **additivity principle** states that if two events are mutually exclusive, the probability of obtaining *one or the other* is the *sum* of their separate probabilities.

$$\Pr(A \text{ or } B) = \Pr(A) + \Pr(B)$$

For example, the probability of throwing a two *or* a three on a single roll of one die (of a pair of dice) is $\frac{1}{6} + \frac{1}{6}$, or $\frac{1}{3}$.

The **independence principle** states that the probability of the *joint* occurrence of two or more *independent* events is the *product* of their separate probabilities.

$$\Pr(A \text{ and } B) = \Pr(A) \cdot \Pr(B)$$

The probability of throwing box cars (two sixes) on a single roll of a pair of dice is $\frac{1}{6} \times \frac{1}{6}$, or $\frac{1}{36}$.

The probability of the joint occurrence of two *nonindependent* events is the *product* of the probability of one event times the probability of the second event *given* that the first event has occurred. This is known as **conditional probability** and will be discussed more extensively in Chapter 11 when we consider the use of Bayes theorem in genetic counseling. Note that Pr(B|A) means the probability of B given A.

$$\Pr(\text{A and B}) = \Pr(\text{A}) \cdot \Pr(\text{B}|\text{A})$$

Returning to the pedigree in Figure 3.3, the outcome in generation III can be understood by considering that each offspring represents an independent event with a 50% probability of being affected. The probability of all three children being affected is thus the product of these independent probabilities (independence principle) or (½)(½)(½) = ⅛. The probability that all three children would have been unaffected would similarly be ⅛. The probability that two of the three children would have been affected is ⅜, because there are three mutually exclusive birth orders in which two of three children could have been affected (additivity principle): A, A, N; A, N, A; or N, A, A, where N = normal and A = affected. Similarly, there is a ⅜th probability that only one of three children would have been affected. A general expression for computing the probability that there would be any specific number (k) affected children in a set of n children is given by the binomial formula (2–4).

In summary, the typical pedigree pattern for an autosomal dominant trait or disease is quite striking, showing vertical inheritance, involvement of both sexes with equal probability and with approximately half of the offspring of an affected parent being affected, but none of the offspring of an unaffected parent. This pattern of inheritance of a rare disease or trait through three generations virtually defines that trait as being inherited in an autosomal dominant fashion.

There are a number of special characteristics of autosomal dominant inheritance that may be thought of as exceptions to the rule that all affected individuals have an affected parent. In these situations, patients with an autosomal dominant disease appear to be sporadic cases, that is, they have apparently unaffected parents. First, a sporadic case may arise as a result of a new **mutation** or change in the genetic material. The more severe a disorder is with respect to fertility, the more likely it is that patients with this disease are the result of a new mutation in one of the gametes that formed them. If an autosomal dominant disorder generally causes death before reproductive age or severely impairs the ability to reproduce, then cases of such a disease would arise only as the result of a new mutation. Approximately 80% of cases of achondroplasia, a common form of short-limbed dwarfism (Fig. 3.5), which sig-

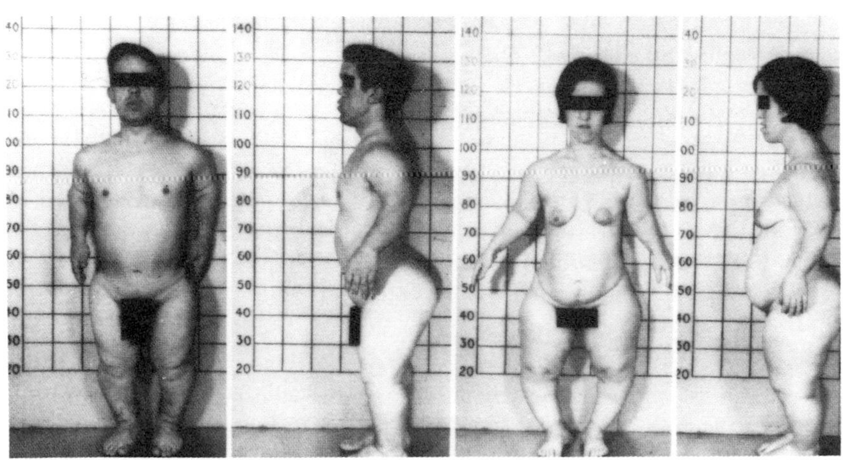

Figure 3.5. A man and a woman with achondroplasia. Note the short stature, relatively large head, short extremities especially in the proximal portion, and lordotic curvature of the spine. (From McKusick VA: *Heritable Disorders of Connective Tissue.* 4th Ed. St Louis, CV Mosby, 1972, p. 758.)

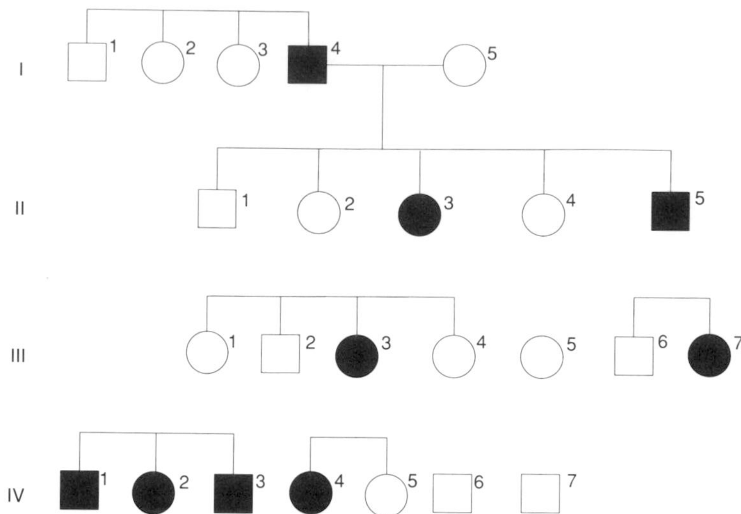

Figure 3.6. Pedigree of a family with autosomal dominant erythermalgia illustrating nonpenetrance. Note that individual III-1 is clinically unaffected but is an obligate heterozygote for the mutant allele.

nificantly reduces reproductive fitness, represent new spontaneous mutations. There is evidence that increased paternal age may increase the risk of mutation at some loci.

A second situation in which an affected child appears to have a normal parent can result from **decreased penetrance.** Penetrance is an all-or-none phenomenon that refers to the clinical expression, or lack of it, of the mutant gene. In a sense, penetrance is an artifact of our ability to recognize the expression or phenotype of a mutant gene. When the definition of expression is clinical disease, an individual carrying a mutant gene may not express the disease and thus the condition is nonpenetrant. We define penetrance quantitatively by determining the proportion of obligate gene carriers (heterozygotes) for a mutant allele who express the phenotype. Figure 3.6 shows the pedigree of a family with hereditary erythermalgia, an unusual disease characterized by red, hot, painful feet and occasionally hands. It is clear from this pedigree that the disease is inherited as an autosomal dominant trait in this family. Individuals I-4, II-3, II-5, III-1, III-3, III-7, and IV-1 through IV-4 are heterozygotes for the mutant allele. All are affected except III-1. This woman is an *obligate* heterozygote because she has an affected mother and three affected children; but she herself gave no history of, nor showed any signs of, this disease. In this pedigree, 9 of 10 obligate heterozygotes manifested the disease, suggesting a penetrance of approximately 90%. If a disease is described as being 90% penetrant, it means that there is a probability of 90% that an individual carrying the mutant allele will express observable disease. The expression itself, however, is all-or-none.

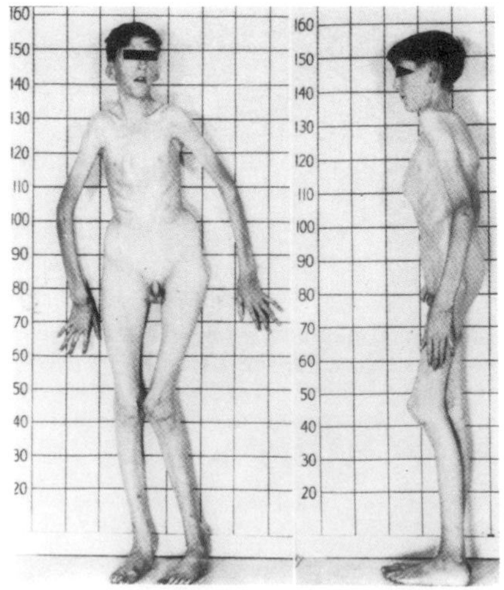

Figure 3.7. A 17-year-old boy with the Marfan syndrome. Note the long thin extremities, thin spider-like fingers (arachnodactyly), flat feet, and deformities of the breastbone and spine. (From McKusick VA: *Heritable Disorders of Connective Tissue.* 4th Ed. St. Louis, CV Mosby, 1972, p. 67.)

Variable expressivity, a frequent characteristic of autosomal dominant traits, is often confused with penetrance. The expressivity of a trait, however, refers to the nature and severity of the phenotype. Mutant genes with pleiotropic effects, i.e., affecting several organ systems and functions, frequently show variable expressivity. The Marfan syndrome is a good example (Fig. 3.7). This disorder affects the connective tissues of the body and primarily affects the skeletal system (long, thin extremities and fingers, lax joints, bony deformities of the spine and sternum), the eye (severe nearsightedness and dislocation of the lens), and the heart (valvular incompetence, widening of the root of the aorta, and sometimes dissection of the aorta and sudden death). An individual affected with the Marfan syndrome may have only one or all three major systems involved, and the nature of the manifestations may vary widely. Furthermore, as shown in the pedigree in Figure 3.8, this variability can occur among affected individuals within the same family who necessarily carry the same mutant allele. The cause of the variability must be either in environmental influences or in the effects of other genes that modify the expression of the mutant gene for the Marfan syndrome.

An even more striking example of variable expressivity is seen in neurofibromatosis 1 or von Recklinghausen disease (Fig. 3.9). This autosomal dominant condition is characterized by brownish spots on the skin called café au lait spots, benign hamartomatous nodules on the iris of the eye (Lisch nodules), and cutaneous and subcutaneous neurofibromas, fleshy benign tumors often arising along the course of nerves. The characteristic neurofibromas usually appear about the time of puberty and may increase during a lifetime to number in the thousands. In addition, this disease has protean manifestations affecting almost every system in the body. Highly vascular plexiform neurofibromas, which infiltrate surrounding tissues, can cause serious growth abnormalities and deformities. Manifestations of this disease can range from the mere presence of café au lait spots and Lisch nodules to cosmetically disfiguring cutaneous neurofibromas, to severe deformities

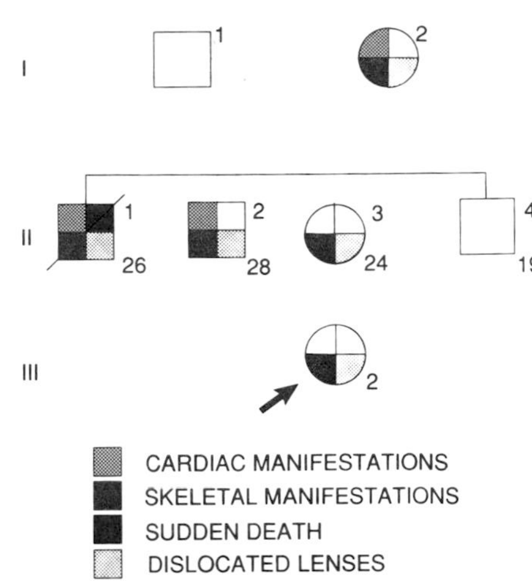

Figure 3.8. Pedigree of autsomal dominant Marfan syndrome illustrating variable expressivity. The proband and her mother both had skeletal manifestations and dislocated lenses but no clinical evidence of heart disease, whereas the proband's uncle (II-1) had severe cardiac manifestation and died suddenly at age 26 years.

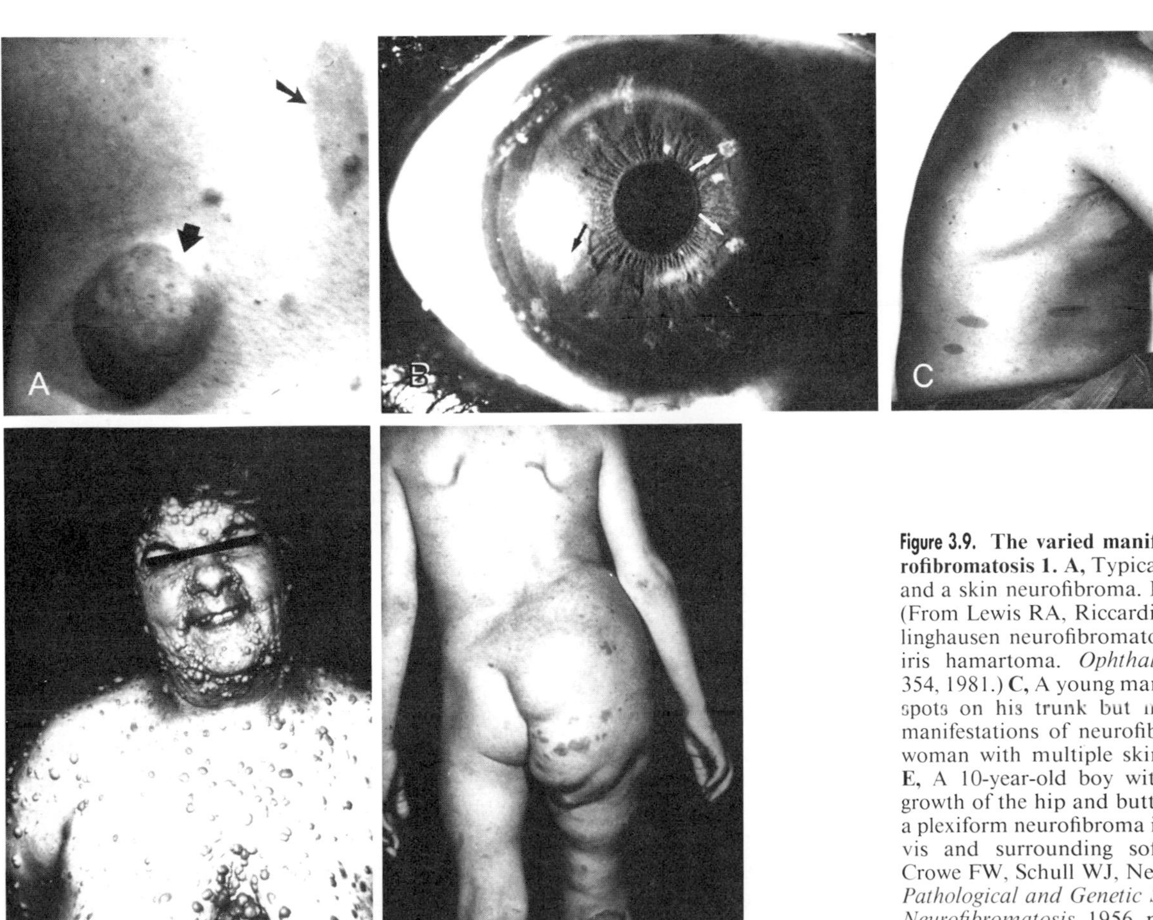

Figure 3.9. The varied manifestations of neurofibromatosis 1. A, Typical café au lait spot and a skin neurofibroma. **B,** Lisch nodules. (From Lewis RA, Riccardi VM: Von Recklinghausen neurofibromatosis: Incidence of iris hamartoma. *Ophthalmology* 88:348–354, 1981.) **C,** A young man with café au lait spots on his trunk but no other obvious manifestations of neurofibromatosis. **D,** A woman with multiple skin neurofibromas. **E,** A 10-year-old boy with massive overgrowth of the hip and buttock secondary to a plexiform neurofibroma involving the pelvis and surrounding soft tissue. (From Crowe FW, Schull WJ, Neel JV: *A Clinical, Pathological and Genetic Study of Multiple Neurofibromatosis.* 1956, p. 34. Courtesy of Charles C Thomas, Publisher, Springfield, IL.)

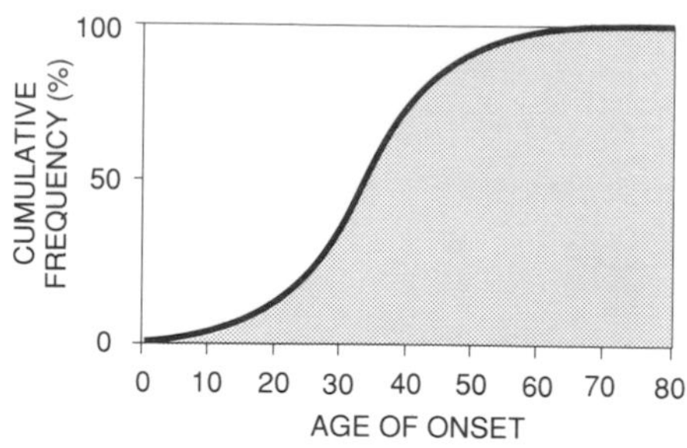

Figure 3.10. Age of onset of Huntington disease. Fifty percent of the patients in this study had onset of the disease by age 35 years. (From Conneally PM, Wallace MR, Gusella JF, Wexler NS: Huntington disease: Estimation of heterozygote status using linked genetic markers. Genet Epidemiol 1:81–88, 1984.)

and functional impairment in a few less fortunate patients. There is no way to predict how severe the manifestations will be in any affected individual nor is there any evidence that the severity "breeds true" in any given family.

A number of important autosomal dominant diseases are not present at birth but have manifestations only later in life *(delayed onset).* Polycystic kidney disease is characterized by bilateral enlargement of the kidneys by multiple cysts, blood in the urine, high blood pressure, abdominal pain, and progressive renal failure. Symptoms generally do not occur until the fourth decade of life or even later in many patients. The characteristic cysts in the kidney are not usually detectable by ultrasound or radiologic techniques until the second decade. Familial polyposis of the colon is characterized by the development of hundreds to thousands of adenomatous polyps of the large intestine with a virtually 100% probability of malignant degeneration causing cancer of the colon. The polyps usually do not appear until the second decade of life and malignant change is generally seen in the third and fourth decades. Even more striking is Huntington disease, a degenerative neurologic disorder characterized by abnormal movements (chorea) and progressive loss of mental function (dementia). As shown in Figure 3.10, the average age of onset of this condition is about 35 years. Therefore, it is possible that an individual carrying the gene could have children and die from unrelated causes (for example, a motor vehicle accident) before reaching an age at which the disease is manifest. Thus, it would appear that the disease had skipped a generation or that an affected offspring had an unaffected parent, but this would simply reflect the delayed age of onset of this particular dominantly inherited disease. It should be noted that such late age of onset also allows the gene to spread within the population since individuals do not become ill until they have already borne children and passed the mutant gene on to the next generation. The examples described above also emphasize that "genetic" is not synonymous with "congenital" (present at birth); genetic diseases clearly need not be congenital.

Finally, another source of apparent sporadic cases of an autosomal dominant disease is found in cases where the putative father is not the actual biological father of the affected child. In one large study in a predominantly Caucasian population, the frequency was approximately 5%.

The majority of inherited human diseases also show **genetic heterogeneity.** Genetic heterogeneity means that different mutations can cause an identical or similar phenotype. We further distinguish **allelic heterogeneity,** which refers to different mutations at the same locus, from **locus heterogeneity,** which refers to mutations at different loci. A good example of genetic heterogeneity is the group of Ehlers-Danlos syndromes (Table 3.1). These are disorders of connective tissue characterized by hyperelastic skin, loose joints, and variable degrees of weakness of blood vessels. At least half a dozen different Ehlers-Danlos syndromes are known that are inherited in an autosomal dominant fashion, but appear to be genetically distinct in that each form appears to breed true in a given family. Note, this is in contrast to the Marfan syndrome, mentioned above, in which there is great variability in expressivity among affected members within a single family. Ehlers-Danlos syndromes type I and II (and possibly III) are thought to represent examples of allelic heterogeneity. In addition, there are some forms of Ehlers-Danlos syndrome inherited in an autosomal recessive

Table 3.1. Ehlers-Danlos Syndromes[a]

Type	Clinical Features	Inheritance	Biochemical Disorder	Ultrastructural Findings
I Gravis	Soft, velvety skin; marked skin hyperextensibility, fragility, and easy bruisability; "cigarette paper" scars; large- and small-joint hypermobility; frequent venous varicosities; hernia. Prematurity due to ruptured fetal membranes is common.	AD[b]	Not known	Large collagen fibrils, many irregular in shape.
II Mitis	Soft skin, moderate skin hyperextensibility, and easy bruisability; moderate joint hypermobility; varicose veins and hernia do occur but are less common than in type I. Prematurity is rare.	AD	Not known	Large collagen fibrils, many irregular in shape.
III Benign familial hypermobility	Skin is soft but otherwise minimally affected; joint mobility is markedly increased and affects large and small joints; dislocation is common.	AD	Not known	Large collagen fibrils, many irregular in shape.
IV Ecchymotic or arterial	Skin is thin or translucent or both; veins are readily visible over the trunk, arms, legs, and abdomen. Repeated ecchymosis with minimal trauma. Skin is not hyperextensible, and joints (except the small joints in the hands) are usually of normal mobility. Bowel rupture (usually affecting the colon) and arterial rupture are frequent and often lead to death.	AD AR	Decreased or absent synthesis of type III collagen. Altered secretion of type III collagen.	Thin dermis, small fibers, often engorged cells in dermis, fibrils of variable size.
V X-linked	Similar to EDS II; muscle hemorrhage may be more extensive.	XR	Not known	Not known
VI Ocular	Soft, velvety, hyperextensible skin; hypermobile joints; scoliosis, scarring less severe than in EDS I; some patients have ocular fragility and keratoconus.	AR	Lysyl hydroxylase deficiency	Small collagen bundles; fibrils normal or similar to those in EDS I
VII Arthrochalasis multiplex congenita	Soft skin; scars near normal. Marked joint hyperextensibility, congenital hip dislocation.	AD	Amino acid substitution at the NH_2-terminal cleavage site of pro-α2	Not known
		AR	NH_2-terminal protease deficiency	
VIII Periodontal form	Marked skin fragility with abnormal, atrophic pigmented scars, minimal skin extensibility and moderate joint laxity. Aesthenic habitus, generalized periodontitis.	AD	Not known	Not known

[a]From Byers PH, Holbrook KA, Barsh GS: Ehlers-Danlos syndrome. In Emery AEH, Rimoin DL (eds): *Principles and Practice of Medical Genetics.* Edinburgh, Churchill Livingstone, 1983, p. 837.
[b]AD, autosomal dominant; AR, autosomal recessive; XR, X-linked recessive.

(type VI) or even X-linked fashion (type V). This indicates that mutations at different loci can cause a similar clinical phenotype, and these forms of the disease illustrate locus heterogeneity. Recent progress in understanding the molecular basis of several of the osteogenesis imperfecta syndromes, characterized by brittle bones that may spontaneously fracture before birth or fracture with minimal trauma later in life, has revealed another clear example of both allelic and locus heterogeneity.

For most relatively rare autosomal dominant diseases, affected individuals are heterozygotes. However, when the gene is sufficiently common, matings between heterozygous affected parents resulting in homozygous affected offspring are seen. In most cases, affected homozygotes are much more severely affected than are heterozygotes. This is best illustrated by familial hypercholesterolemia, in which homozygotes have much higher elevations of cholesterol and develop atherosclerotic cardiovascular disease in their teens. In contrast, putative homozygotes for Huntington disease have been described in large families living in Venezuela. In this case, homozygous affected individuals appear to be no more severely affected than heterozygous individuals.

AUTOSOMAL RECESSIVE INHERITANCE

Autosomal recessive diseases are characterized by clinical manifestations only in individuals homozygous for the mutant gene. The characteristic pedigree pattern (Fig. 3.11) is *horizontal* rather than vertical in that affected individuals tend to be limited to a single sibship and the disease is not found in multiple generations. Males and females are affected with equal probability. The usual mating (Fig. 3.12) is that between two individuals who are clinically normal but heterozygous for the mutant allele. There is a 1 in 4 chance that each offspring will be homozygous for the mutant allele and affected; a 1 in 4 chance that he or she will be homozygous for the normal or wild-type allele and clinically normal; and 2 chances in 4 that he or she will be heterozygous for the mutant allele and a clinically normal carrier like each parent.

The probability that two individuals heterozygous for the same mutant allele will mate depends upon the frequency of heterozygotes in the population and this in turn is a function of the mutant allele frequency. A more detailed discussion of gene frequencies will be presented in Chapter 4. It is intuitively apparent, however, that if the mutant allele is rare in the population, then the probability will be very low that any two individuals carrying this same mutant allele will marry. This probability would be increased if they were related and had inherited the same mutant allele from a common ancestor. Thus, **consanguinity,** or the mating between close relatives, is found more frequently among parents of children with rare autosomal recessive diseases. On the other hand, if the mutant gene is common in a population,

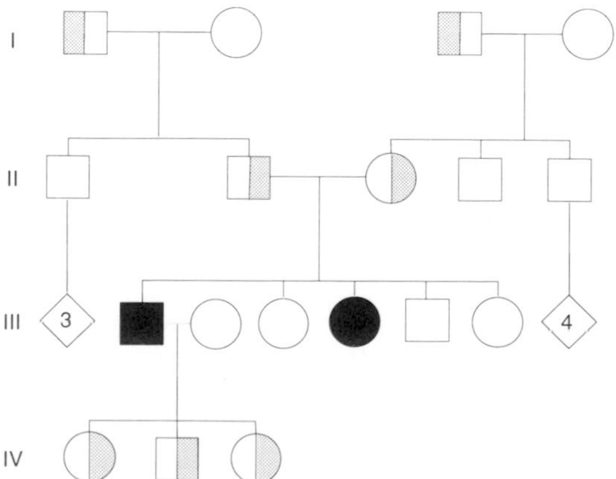

Figure 3.11. Pedigree of an autosomal recessive trait. Affected individuals, indicated by *solid red symbols,* are found in only one generation. Note that both parents of an affected child are obligate heterozygotes (designated by *half-shaded red symbols*), as are all of the offspring of a mating between an affected individual and a homozygous normal individual.

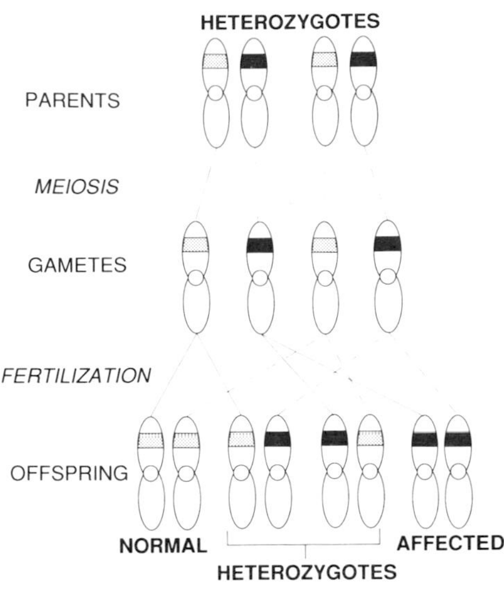

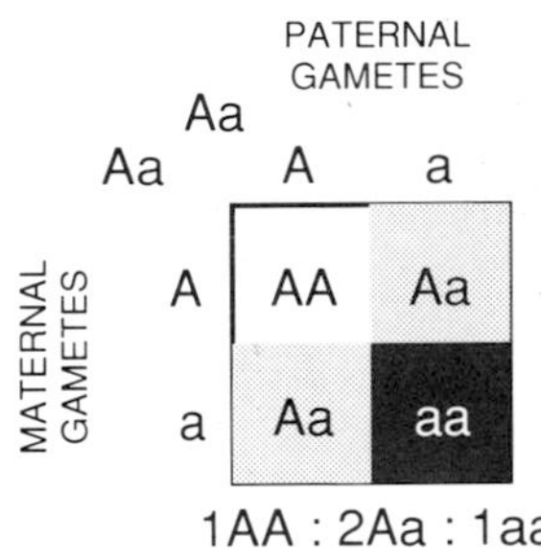

A = NORMAL, a = MUTANT

Figure 3.12. Autosomal recessive inheritance. The mating diagram and Punnett square illustrate the outcome of a mating of two individuals who are clinically normal but are heterozygous for the mutant allele. As in Figure 3.4, the mutant allele is indicated in *red* and affected individuals are indicated by the *solid red box*. Heterozygous carriers are indicated by the *light red boxes*.

such as cystic fibrosis in the white population, Tay-Sachs disease among Ashkenazi (Central and Eastern European) Jews, or sickle cell anemia among blacks, the mating of heterozygotes would be more common and parental consanguinity would not be expected to be found as frequently.

Because the risk is only 1 in 4 that a child will be affected if both parents are carriers and because most American families are small (two to three children), most affected individuals with autosomal recessive diseases will appear to be sporadic cases. That is, there will be only one affected member in the family. If two or more children are affected, the disease is more likely to be recognized as a genetic disorder. Nevertheless, it should be kept in mind that most autosomal recessive diseases will appear as sporadic cases and it is important that their genetic etiology not be overlooked because of the lack of a positive family history.

This point is illustrated in Figure 3.13. If one were able to ascertain all three-child families in which both parents were carriers of the same mutant allele, nearly half (42%) of these families would have no affected children. Because, in practice, we recognize matings between heterozygous carriers only by the presence of an affected child, such families would not be ascertained in the absence of a screening program for detecting heterozygous carriers. Another 42% of three-child families of

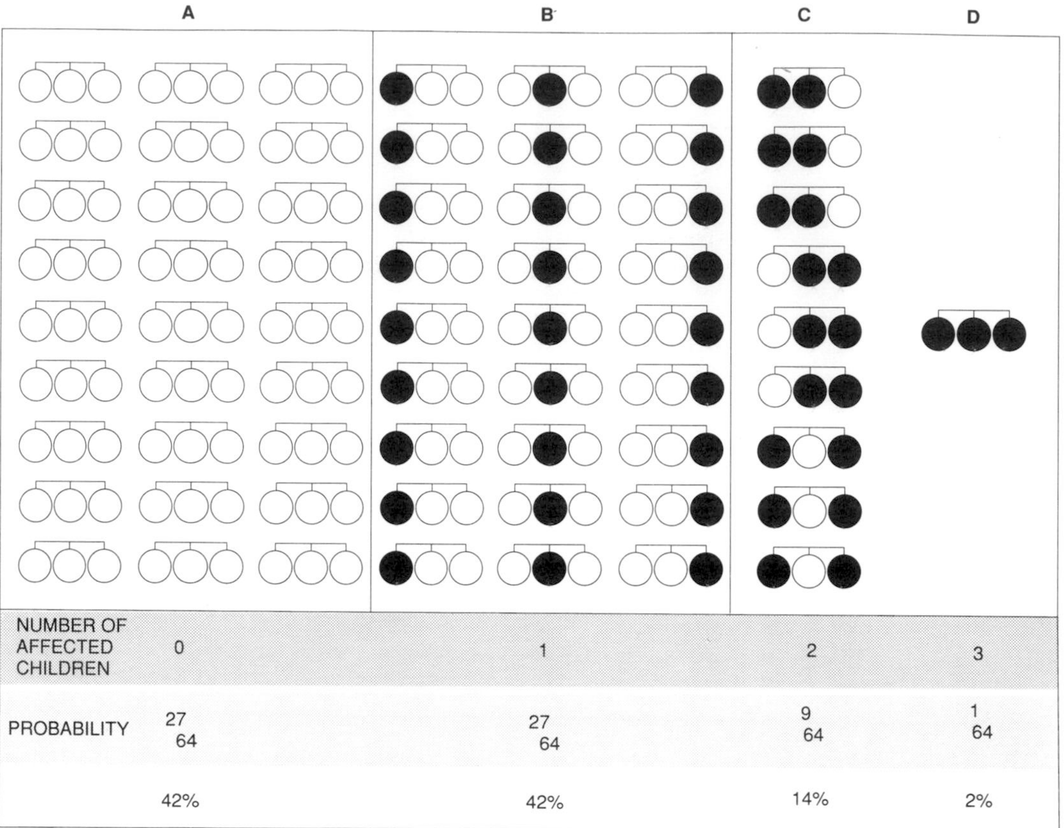

Figure 3.13. The probability of 0, 1, 2, or 3 of 3 children being affected in a mating between heterozygotes for an autosomal recessive trait. In this diagram, *circles* represent offspring of either sex; *red symbols* indicate affected individuals. The probabilities can be calculated using the binomial formula. Note that for families with three offspring, nearly half of the matings (42%) will result in no affected offspring and nearly half will result in a single affected offspring. (From Li CC: *Human Genetics.* New York, McGraw-Hill, 1961.)

this sort would have a single affected child; whereas 14% would have two affected children and only 2% of such families would have all three offspring affected. Even among the families ascertained because they have at least one affected offspring, nearly $\frac{3}{4}$ ($\frac{27}{37}$ or 73%) would have a single affected child and thus the disease would appear to be sporadic in these families.

How then do we recognize autosomal recessive traits? Obviously the appearance of multiple affected siblings within large sibships and the presence of parental consanguinity suggest the presence of a rare recessive disease. Stronger evidence, however, is the demonstration of a partial defect in obligate heterozygotes. Tay-Sachs disease (or G_{M2} gangliosidosis) is a degenerative neurological disorder in which there is virtual absence of the activity of a lysosomal enzyme, hexosaminidase A, in affected children. The clinically normal parents of a child with Tay-Sachs disease usually have approximately half the normal amount of this enzyme, confirming the autosomal recessive nature of the disease that was suggested by pedigree analysis. Such heterozygote detection techniques also allow for efficient screening programs in populations in which carriers are frequent, as is the case for Tay-Sachs disease among Ashkenazi Jews (approximately 3%) and sickle cell anemia among blacks (8%).

Sickle cell anemia also demonstrates that it is traits, not genes, that are dominant or recessive. Sickle cell anemia is an autosomal recessive disease in that it occurs only in individuals homozygous for the mutant β^S globin gene. Expression of the mutant β^S gene, however, is readily detected in heterozygous carriers, i.e., individuals with sickle cell trait, who are clinically normal. Thus, sickle cell trait is an autosomal dominant trait.

All of the offspring of an individual homozygous for a mutant allele causing an autosomal recessive disease are obligate heterozygous carriers, assuming that the mating is between a homozygous affected and a homozygous normal individual (Fig. 3.11, generation IV, and Fig. 3.14*A*). However, when a homozygous affected individual marries a heterozygous carrier, there is a 50% probability that any offspring will also be homozygous for the mutant allele, resulting in a pattern of inheritance that resembles autosomal dominant but is known as quasi-dominance (Fig. 3.14*B*) Such a mating is unlikely by chance, but is made more likely if the homozygous affected individual marries a close relative such as a first cousin or if the mutant allele is common.

The mating of two individuals homozygous for the same mutant allele results in all of the offspring being homozygous affected. The pedigree shown in Figure 3.15 shows an example of this latter type of mating involving individuals with autosomal recessive congenital deafness. All the offspring of individuals I-3 and I-4 and of II-10 and II-11 are congenitally deaf like their parents. However, none of the offspring (IV-1 through IV-6) of individuals III-7 and III-9 are deaf. The simple explanation for this apparent paradox is that each of these parents (III-7 and III-9) is homozygous for a different nonallelic mutant gene causing congenital deafness. Therefore, all six of their offspring are double heterozygotes, i.e., are heterozygous for two different, nonallelic mutant genes causing deafness. Because they are not homozygous for either one, they are normal in hearing. This pedigree is an example of locus heterogeneity, i.e., mutations at different loci causing the same phenotype, congenital deafness.

X-LINKED INHERITANCE

X-linked diseases are caused by mutant genes on the X chromosome. X-linked mutant genes are fully expressed in males, who have only a single X chromosome, i.e., are **hemizygous** for X-linked genes. All somatic cells in human females contain two X chromosomes; however, only one X chromosome is genetically active. One of the two X chromosomes is randomly and permanently inactivated early in embryonic development, a process called lyonization (see Chapter 8 for discussion). Because of this random X-inactivation, X-linked traits are variably expressed in women who are heterozygous for an X-linked mutant gene. A disease encoded by a mutant X-linked gene may or may not be expressed clinically in a heterozygous female. Diseases that are rarely expressed clinically in heterozygous females are called **X-linked recessive.**

Typical X-linked recessive disorders are hemophilia A and Duchenne muscular dystrophy. The former is the result of a deficiency of an essential clotting factor, factor VIII, and is characterized by soft

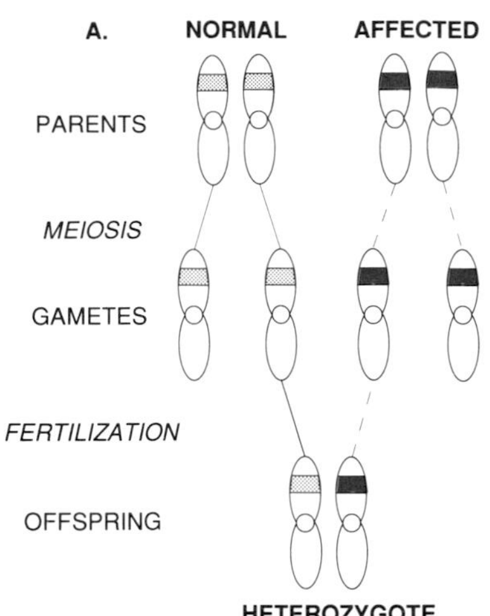

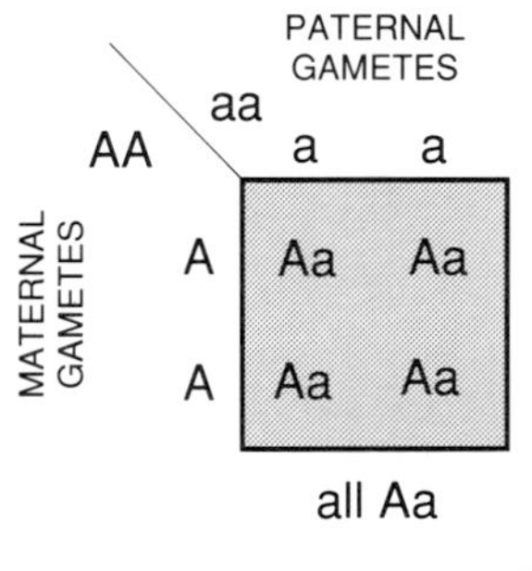

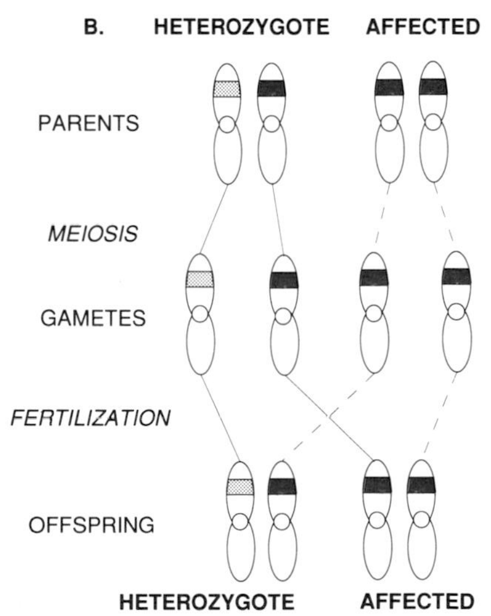

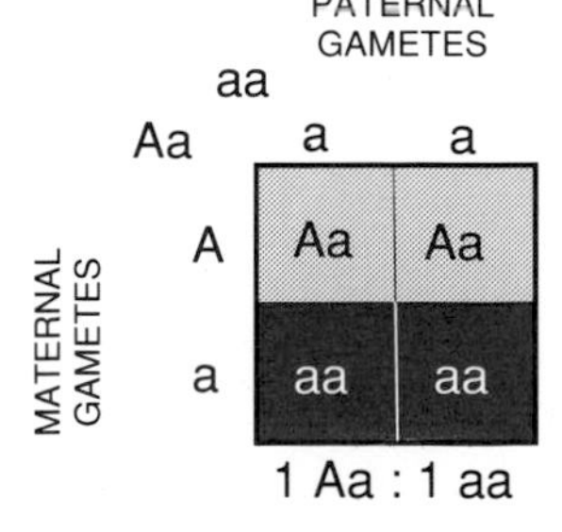

Figure 3.14. Mating diagram and Punnett square illustrating the outcome of a mating between a homozygous affected individual and a homozygous normal indivdiual (*A*) and between a homozygous affected individual and a clinically normal heterozygous individual (*B*). Note that all of the offspring in **A** are obligate heterozygotes, and that there is a 50% probability that each offspring in **B** will be homozygous affected.

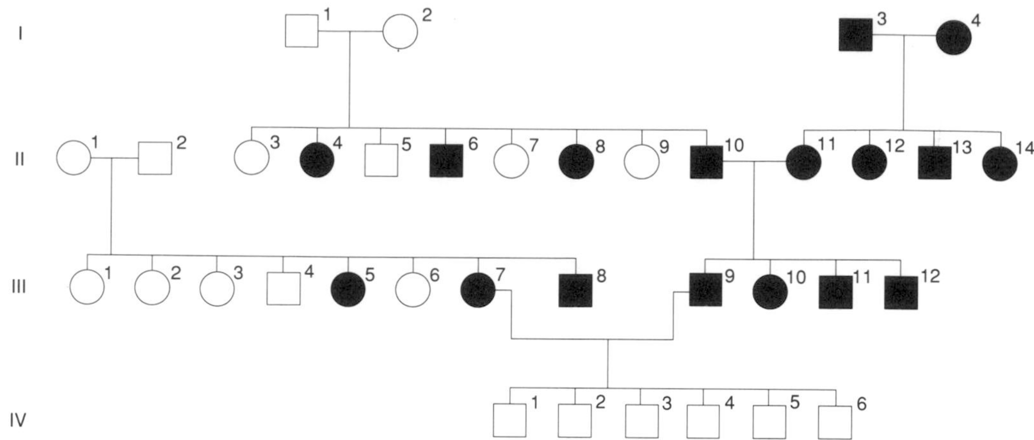

Figure 3.15. Pedigree of a family with autosomal recessive congenital deafness. All of the individuals in generation IV have normal hearing and are presumably double heterozygotes for two nonallelic mutant genes. (From Li CC: *Human Genetics.* New York, McGraw-Hill, 1961.)

tissue bleeding, often into joints. Duchenne muscular dystrophy is a form of muscular dystrophy that has its onset in boys under the age of 5 years and causes progressive muscle weakness, usually terminating in death in the 20s from respiratory complications. A characteristic pedigree for Duchenne muscular dystrophy is shown in Figure 3.16. Only males are affected, but the disease is transmitted by healthy females who are heterozygous carriers. Thus, one can trace the disease among male relatives on the mother's side of the family.

The pattern of inheritance of X-linked recessive traits is so characteristic that it has been recognized since antiquity. The Talmud makes reference to hemophilia and provides dispensation from circumcision in families with this bleeding disorder. Another example is the legend of the water drinker's curse from 18th century Nova Scotia. On a hot summer day, a gypsy stopped at a farmhouse seeking water for his thirsty young son. The farmer's wife refused them water and sent them away, whereupon the gypsy placed a curse upon her: "May your sons be afflicted with a terrible craving for water and may the curse be revisited upon the sons of your daughters, for generation upon generation." And

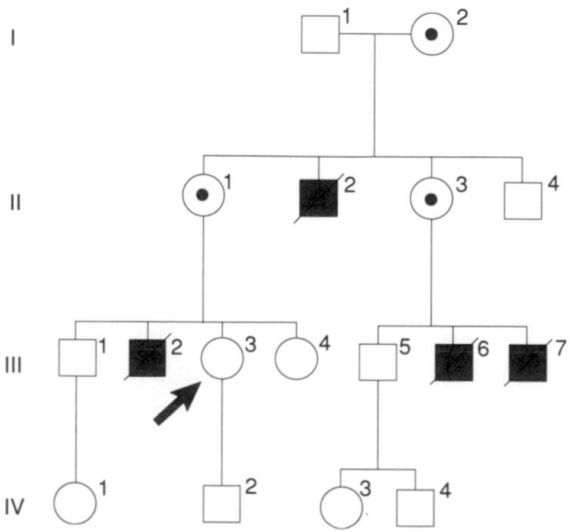

Figure 3.16. Pedigree of a family with X-linked recessive Duchenne muscular dystrophy. Obligate heterozygotes are indicated by the *red dot inside the circle.*

so it came to pass. The disease traced to early settlers in this area is nephrogenic diabetes insipidus, which is caused by an insensitivity of the kidney to antidiuretic hormone, resulting in the passage of large volumes of dilute urine, dehydration, and thirst.

X-linked inheritance can be best understood by paying attention to the X chromosome and remembering that these conditions are X-linked and not "sex-linked." The ususal mating is that between a heterozygous carrier woman and a normal man (Fig. 3.17*A*). Each son has a 50% chance of receiving the X chromosome bearing the mutant gene and of being affected. Daughters have the same 50% chance of inheriting the mutant gene, but will inherit a normal X chromosome from the father and will generally be clinically unaffected, although they will have a 50% chance of being a carrier. A second typical mating (Fig. 3.17*B*) is that between an affected man and a homozygous normal woman, as for example in hemophilia. In such a mating, all the sons are normal because they receive from the affected father his Y chromosome rather than the X chromosome, and they receive a normal X chromosome from the mother. However, all the daughters are *obligate* carriers because they receive an X chromosome carrying the mutant gene from their father. Thus, there is no transmission of an X-linked recessive trait from a father to his son; this lack of male-to-male transmission is a hallmark of X-linked inheritance.

The pedigree, shown in Figure 3.18, of a family with an inherited chronic renal disease, focal glomerular sclerosis, was felt by the physicians caring for these patients to represent "sex-linked inheritance." A consideration of the points made above, however, indicates that this cannot represent X-linked inheritance because there is male-to-male transmission. This pedigree illustrates that the designation sex-linked inheritance can be misleading and should not be used. In this family, the trait is likely to be autosomal dominant, possibly sex-limited or sex-influenced, i.e., being expressed in males more than, or rather than, in females even though the mutant gene is on an autosome rather than the X chromosome. A common sex-influenced autosomal dominant trait is male pattern baldness, which affects males predominantly and is transmitted from generation to generation, often in a male-to-male fashion.

Apparent male-to-male transmission of an X-linked trait can occur when the gene is sufficiently common, as for example the gene for deficiency of the enzyme glucose-6-phosphate dehydrogenase (G6PD) in black and Mediterranean populations (see Chapter 7). In United States blacks, approximately 18% of women are heterozygous carriers of G6PD A^- deficiency and approximately 10% of black men are hemizygous deficient. Thus, the apparent transmission of G6PD deficiency from father (II-4) to son (III-1), shown in Figure 3.19, is in fact due to the transmission of the gene on an X chromosome from the heterozygous carrier mother (II-3) and is independent of the fact that the father is also affected. It should be noted that when an X-linked gene occurs in such high frequency, homozygous affected females may also be seen with reasonable frequency.

Rarely, women or girls are observed to express diseases thought to be inherited as X-linked recessive traits. There are several reasons for this. First, as noted above, the mutant allele may be sufficiently common so that homozygous females are observed with reasonable frequency. For example, deficiency of G6PD (Gd A^-) occurs in approximately 1% of black women. Such women are homozygous for the mutant allele, inheriting one copy from an affected father and the other

Figure 3.17. X-linked recessive inheritance. The mating diagram and Punnett square illustrate the outcome of a mating between a clinically normal female heterozygous for the mutant allele (shown in *red*) and a normal male (**A**) and between a homozygous normal female and a hemizygous affected male (**B**). The Y chromosome is indicated in *black*. Note that there can be no male-to-male transmission of the mutant allele on the X chromosome, but that all of the daughters of an affected male are obligate heterozygotes.

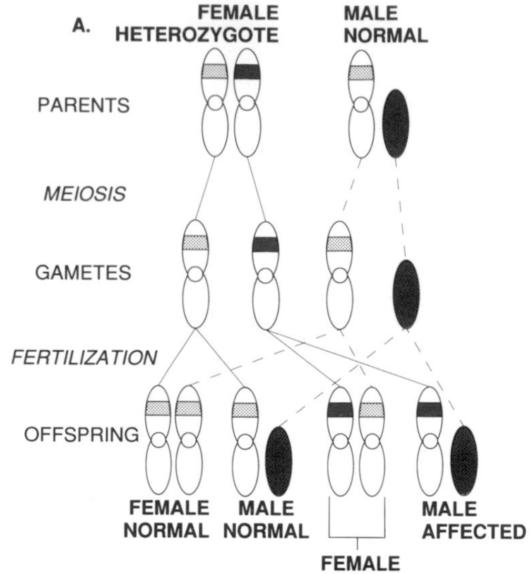

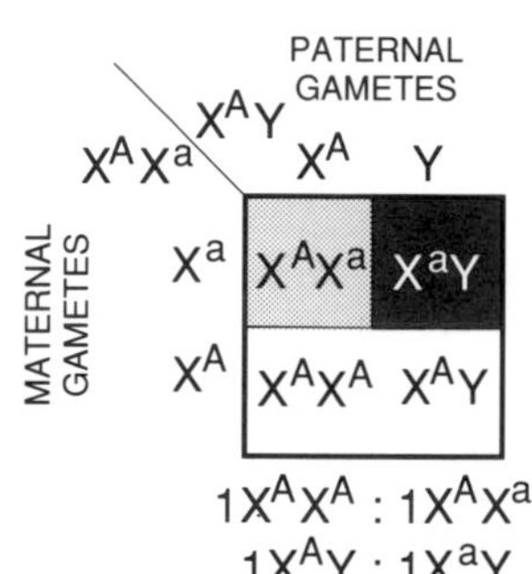

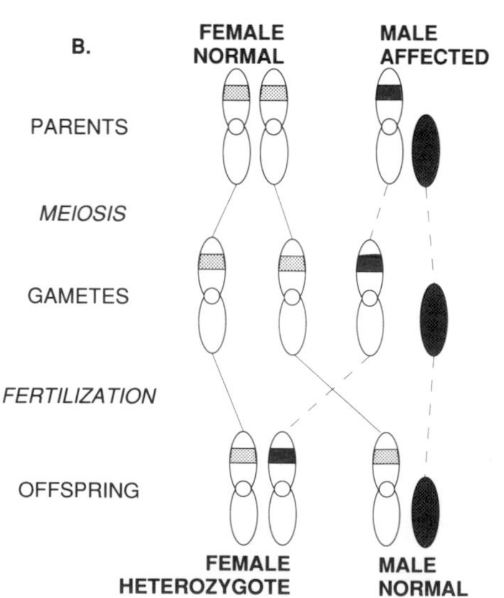

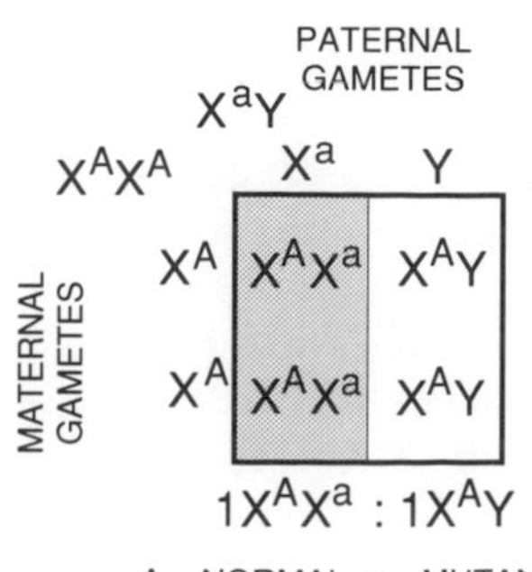

A = NORMAL, a = MUTANT

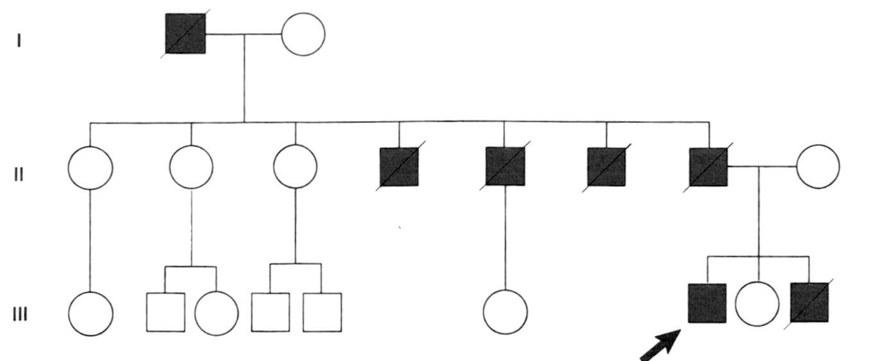

Figure 3.18. **Pedigree of a family with focal glomerular sclerosis.** Note the male-to-male transmission that rules out X-linked inheritance. This pedigree is most consistent with autosomal dominant inheritance despite the fact that only males are affected in this family.

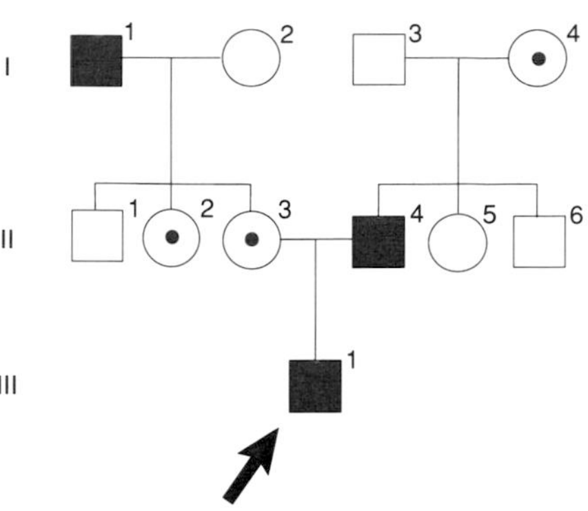

Figure 3.19. **Pedigree of a family with X-linked recessive glucose-6-phosphate dehydrogenase deficiency.** Despite the apparent male-to-male transmission, III-1 must have received the mutant allele from his mother (II-3) who is an obligate heterozygote.

from a carrier mother. Second, a female will occasionally express even a rare X-linked gene such as hemophilia because she is hemizygous for the X chromosome. This can occur in the Turner syndrome in which there are 45 rather than 46 chromosomes and only one X chromosome (to be described in Chapter 8). Third, rare chromosomal rearrangements involving exchange of material (translocations) between the X chromosome and an autosome and resulting in deletion of X-chromosomal material can result in expression of X-linked diseases such as Duchenne muscular dystrophy in females. These accidents of nature were critical in localizing the gene for this disease, as discussed in Chapter 9. Fourth, because of differences in the degree of lyonization (discussed in Chapter 8), it is possible that a heterozygous female will express clinical manifestations of an X-linked "recessive" disease. Finally, a woman may appear to have an X-linked recessive disease such as Duchenne muscular dystrophy, but in fact have a similar clinical phenotype caused by homozygosity for a mutant autosomal gene. This is another example of locus heterogeneity in which a different mutant gene can cause a similar phenotype (5).

Figure 3.20 shows a typical pedigree for an **X-linked dominant** trait, hypophosphatemic (or vitamin D-resistant) rickets, characterized

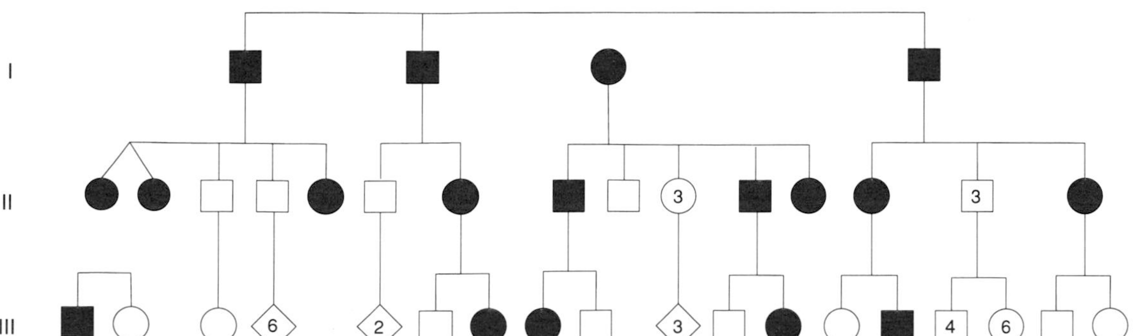

Figure 3.20. **Pedigree of a family with X-linked dominant hypophosphatemia rickets.** Note that all of the daughters of affected males are themselves affected and that the disease can be transmittted by both affected males and females but there is no male-to-male transmission. (After Williams TF et al.: In *The Metabolic Basis of Inherited Disease.* Stanbury JB, Wyngaarden JB, Fredrickson DS (eds), New York, McGraw-Hill, 1960. Permission granted by McGraw-Hill.)

by low blood and high urinary phosphate, short stature, and bony deformities. A characteristic of this pattern of inheritance is, once again, the absence of male-to-male transmission because the mutant gene is on the X chromosome. In this case, however, females are also affected and the ratio of affected females to males is approximately 2 to 1, reflecting the ratio of X chromosomes in females to males. Characteristically, the clinical expression of X-linked dominant diseases is more constant and more severe in hemizygous affected males than in heterozygous affected females, in whom the expression of the disease is often quite variable. All of the daughers of an affected man will be affected because all receive the X chromosome bearing a mutant gene from their father. All of the sons of an affected father, however, must be normal because they receive only the father's Y chromosome. Both daughters and sons of an affected woman have a 50% chance of receiving the X chromosome bearing the mutant allele and hence of being affected.

Recessively inherited disorders are often the result of enzymatic deficiencies; approximately 200 of 650 disorders inherited as autosomal or X-linked recessive traits are known enzyme deficiencies. This suggests that for most enzymes, 50% of normal activity is sufficient for normal function, or at least sufficient to prevent disease. In contrast, autosomal dominant diseases frequently represent abnormalities in noncatalytic proteins such as collagen or hemoglobin. For example, methemoglobinemia, characterized by methemoglobin in the blood and cyanosis, can result from an abnormal hemoglobin (Hb M), inherited as an autosomal dominant trait, or from a severe deficiency of the enzyme methemoglobin reductase, inherited as an autosomal recessive trait. In general, recessive diseases are more frequently severe and more frequently expressed in childhood; in contrast, autosomal dominant diseases may be mild in clinical severity, or, if severe, often have a later age of onset. However, multiple exceptions occur for all of the above generalizations and it is best to keep in mind Ralph Waldo Emerson's admonition, "A foolish consistency is the hobgoblin of little minds."

MITOCHONDRIAL INHERITANCE

Mendelian inheritance describes the transmission of genes encoded by chromosomes in the nucleus of cells. However, DNA is also found in mitochondria residing in the cytoplasm of cells. Although most mitochondrial proteins are encoded by nuclear genes, a few mitochondrial enzymes have been identified that are encoded solely by mitochondrial DNA. These include parts of the respiratory-enzyme complexes of the inner mitochrondrial membrane. Mitochondrial DNA, because of its cytoplasmic location, is maternally inherited. There is now evidence that certain human diseases characterized by structurally and functionally abnormal mitochondria, and often involving skeletal and cardiac muscle impairment, are inherited in a maternal fashion, which would be expected for mitochondrial genes (Fig. 3.21). Both males and females are affected but transmission is only by affected women. Furthermore, one might expect that all offspring of an affected woman should be affected. Proof of mitochondrial inheritance requires definition of the biochemical and/or molecular defect and mapping of the responsible gene to the mitochondrion. Certain muscle diseases and Leber's hereditary optic atrophy, a degenerative eye disease, are strongly suspected of being inherited in this fashion (6, 7).

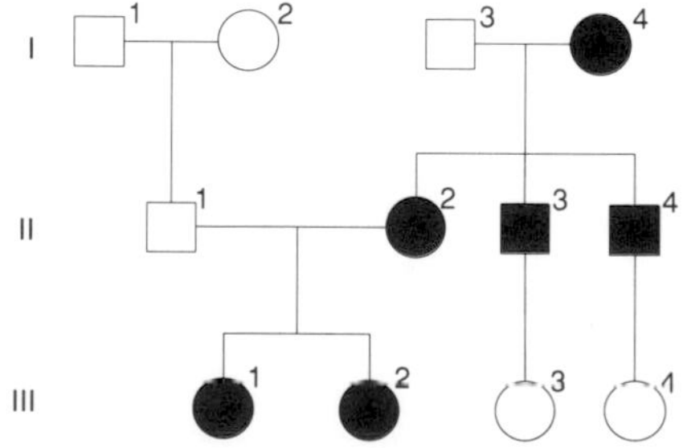

Figure 3.21. Pedigree of a family with a mitochondrial cytopathy manifesting muscle disease. Note the maternal transmission to both male and female offspring. (From Egger J, Wilson J: Mitochondrial inheritance in a mitochondrially-mediated disease. N Engl J Med 309:142–146, 1983.)

REFERENCES

1. McKusick VA: *Mendelian Inheritance in Man.* 8th Ed. Baltimore, John Hopkins University Press, 1988.
2. Murphy EA: *Probability in Medicine.* Baltimore, Johns Hopkins University Press, 1979, pp. 17–45, 86–103.
3. Ingelfinger JA, Mosteller F, Thibodeau LA, Ware JH: *Biostatistics in Clinical Medicine.* 2nd Ed. New York, Macmillan, 1987, pp. 1–15, 35–46.
4. McKusick VA: *Human Genetics.* 2nd Ed. Englewood Cliffs, NJ, Prentice-Hall, 1969.
5. Francke U, Darras BT, Hersh JH, Berg BO, Miller RG: Brother/sister pairs affected with early-onset, progressive muscular dystrophy: Molecular-studies reveal etiologic heterogeneity. Am J Hum Genet 45:63–72, 1989.
6. Merril CR, Harrington MG: The search for mitochondrial inheritance of human diseases. Trends Genet 1:140–144, 1985.
7. Wallace DC: Mitochondrial DNA mutations and neuromuscular disease. Trends Genet 5:9–13, 1989.

3/ Study Questions

1/ Both X-linked dominant and autosomal dominant traits are inherited vertically in families. What are four characteristics you might look for that would help you distinguish between X-linked dominant and autosomal dominant inheritance in a set of families all showing the same vertically inherited trait?

2/ Choose the term from the following list that best describes the situations labeled a through f below:

i. Allelic heterogeneity
ii. Pleiotrophy
iii. Variable expressivity
iv. Incomplete penetrance
v. Consanguinity
vi. Locus heterogeneity

a. A man shows no sign of myotonic dystrophy, an autosomal dominant muscle disease, although his father and two daughters have the disease.
b. Variegate porphyria, an autosomal dominant inborn error of porphyrin biosynthesis, can cause blistering skin photosensitivity, abdominal pain, peripheral neuropathy, and psychotic episodes.
c. A man with a few Lisch nodules and axillary freckles has a daughter with severe scoliosis and hundreds of subcutaneous neurofibromata.
d. A rare form of autosomal recessive growth hormone deficiency occurs only in certain small isolated villages in the Swiss Alps.
e. A nonsense mutation and a deletion in the ornithine transcarbamylase (OTC) gene both cause lethal neonatal hyperammonemia due to absence of OTC, an important hepatic enzyme in the urea cycle.
f. Retinitis pigmentosa, a form of retinal degeneration, occurs in autosomal and X-linked forms.

3/ True/ false:

a. For a disease to be considered a genetic lethal, it must cause the patient to die before he/she reaches puberty.
b. When an individual inherits a disease-causing mutant gene from a parent, the gene is present in utero and therefore is present at birth; therefore, all hereditary disease is congenital.
c. Whenever an autosomal dominant disease occurs in a child

born to two unaffected parents, the disease is the result of a new mutation.

d. It is unlikely that a patient has a genetic disorder if he/she is the only one in the family with the disease.

4/ A woman has cystic fibrosis. She is the only person in the family with this disease. What is the carrier risk for her mother, her father, her daughter, her daughter's son, her brother, her brother's child?

5/ A woman is a carrier of hemophilia, an X-linked disorder. What is her chance of having a son? Call this probability P1. What is her chance of having an affected child? Call this probability P2. What is her chance of having a child who is both male *and* affected? Is it P1 times P2? Why or why not?

*6/ A hematologist has collected data on 25 unrelated children with sickle cell anemia and their siblings. Of a total of 165 children in these 25 families, a total of 60 have sickle cell anemia. Because sickle cell anemia is an autosomal recessive disorder, the hematologist expected 25%, or 41 of the 165 children, to have the disease, and is puzzled that there seem to be too many affected children in the families. Can you help her out?

4

Population Genetics and Multifactorial Inheritance

"Almost all disorders in man are familial in that they are more likely to afflict someone with an affected relative than someone with an equivalent set of unaffected relatives."

—J. H. Edwards, 1969 (1)

In this chapter we will consider two topics that require a more quantitative approach to genetics: population genetics and multifactorial inheritance. Population genetics is the study of the distribution of genes in populations and of the factors that maintain or change the frequency of genes and genotypes from generation to generation. It is a central part of the discipline of human genetics and the study of evolution. In medical genetics, population genetic data are used primarily in genetic counseling and in planning genetic screening programs. Multifactorial inheritance deals with traits and diseases that are not inherited in a simple Mendelian fashion nor associated with chromosomal abnormalities, but in which there is considerable evidence that genetic factors play an important role in their causation. Examples include common diseases, such as hypertension and diabetes mellitus, and common birth defects, such as cleft lip and cleft palate. Multifactorial models provide a framework for understanding genetic predisposition to disease and for providing genetic counseling to patients and families with these conditions.

POPULATION GENETICS

For the medical geneticist, the most important concept in population genetics is the Hardy-Weinberg equilibrium. Independently described in 1908 by the English mathematician G. H. Hardy and the German physician W. Weinberg, it was derived to explain why dominant traits do not automatically replace recessive traits in the popula-

Table 4.1. Genotype Frequencies in Progeny

		Paternal Gametes	
		A (p)	a (q)
Maternal Gametes	A (p)	AA (p^2)	Aa (pq)
	a (q)	Aa (pq)	aa (q^2)

tion. Its utility for medical genetics, however, is in explaining why, in a large population with random mating, allele frequencies do not change from generation to generation and how, for any genetic locus, the genotype frequencies are determined by the relative frequencies of the alleles at that locus.

Hardy-Weinberg Equilibrium

Consider a single autosomal locus with two alleles (A and a), whose population frequencies in both sperm and eggs are p = frequency of allele A, and q = frequency of allele a. Because there are only two alleles, p + q = 1. Random mating (mating without regard to genotype) is mathematically equivalent to random mixing and union of sperm and eggs as shown in Table 4.1. The frequency of each genotype is shown in parentheses. The genotype frequencies in the progeny are thus:

genotype:	AA	Aa	aa
frequency:	p^2	2pq	q^2

In the next generation, each of the three paternal genotypes can mate with each of the three maternal genotypes as indicated in Table 4.2. The frequency of each mating type is in parentheses. The genotypes of the offspring for each mating type are shown in Table 4.3. Thus, the frequency of each genotype (AA, Aa, and aa) is stable over successive generations and the population is said to be in Hardy-Weinberg equilibrium.

APPLICATIONS OF THE HARDY-WEINBERG EQUILIBRIUM

The most important medical application of the Hardy-Weinberg equilibrium is the determination of allele frequency and heterozygote carrier frequency in a population for which the frequency of a trait is known. For example, cystic fibrosis occurs in approximately 1/2000 whites of Northern and Central European origin. Thus q^2, or the frequency of homozygous affected individuals, is 1/2000, and q, the frequency of the mutant allele, is $\sqrt{2000}$ = 1/45 or 0.022. The frequency

Table 4.2. Frequency of Mating Types

		Paternal Genotypes		
		AA (p^2)	Aa (2pq)	aa (q^2)
Maternal Genotypes	AA (p^2)	AA × AA (p^4)	AA × Aa ($2p^3q$)	AA × aa (p^2q^2)
	Aa (2pq)	Aa × AA ($2p^3q$)	Aa × Aa ($4p^2q^2$)	Aa × aa ($2pq^3$)
	aa (q^2)	aa × AA (p^2q^2)	aa × Aa ($2pq^3$)	aa × aa (q^4)

Table 4.3. Frequency of Different Genotypes in Offspring from Each Mating Type

		Offspring		
Mating Type	Frequency	AA	Aa	aa
AA × AA	p^4	p^4		
AA × Aa	$4p^3q$	$2p^3q$	$2p^3q$	
AA × aa	$2p^2q^2$		$2p^2q^2$	
Aa × Aa	$4p^2q^2$	p^2q^2	$2p^2q^2$	p^2q^2
Aa × aa	$4pq^3$		$2pq^3$	$2pq^3$
aa × aa	q^4			q^4

AA offspring = $p^4 + 2p^3q + p^2q^2 = p^2(p^2 + 2pq + q^2) = p^2(p + q)^2 = p^2(1)^2 = \mathbf{p^2}$.
Aa offspring = $2p^3q + 4p^2q^2 + 2pq^3 = 2pq(p^2 + 2pq + q^2) = 2pq(p + q)^2 = 2pq(1)^2 = \mathbf{2pq}$.
aa offspring = $p^2q^2 + 2pq^3 + q^4 = q^2(p^2 + 2pq + q^2) = q^2(p + q)^2 = q^2(1)^2 = \mathbf{q^2}$.

of the normal allele is $p = (1 - q) = 44/45$ or 0.978. The heterozygote carrier frequency is $2pq = 2 \times 44/45 \times 1/45 = 1/23$ or 0.044. Thus, more than 4% of whites are heterozygous for the cystic fibrosis allele, a fact of considerable importance in genetic counseling of families with cystic fibrosis.

For rare recessive traits ($q^2 \leqq 0.0001$), p approximates 1, so that the heterozygote carrier frequency (2pq) is approximately 2q, or twice the frequency of the mutant allele. It is clear that for any rare autosomal recessive disease the number of heterozygous carriers in the population (2pq) is much larger than the number of homozygous affected individuals (q^2), and, as shown in Table 4.4, this ratio (Aa/aa or $2pq/q^2$) increases as the disease frequency (q^2) decreases.

This relationship, in turn, has important implications for genetic screening programs. For example, the frequency of Tay-Sachs disease in the Ashkenazi Jewish population is approximately 1/3,600 or 0.0003; therefore, the frequency of the mutant allele (q) is approximately 0.017 and the frequency of heterozygous carriers (2pq) is 0.033. The frequency of matings between Ashkenazi heterozygotes, and thus of couples at risk of having a child with Tay-Sachs disease, is 2pq × 2pq or approximately 1/1,000. Assuming each couple has two children, one would have to screen approximately 2,000 couples in this population to avoid the birth of a child with Tay-Sachs disease. In contrast, the frequency of Tay-Sachs disease in the non-Ashkenazi population is approximately 1/360,000; thus, q = 0.0017 and 2pq = 0.003. The number of matings between non-Ashkenazi carriers of Tay-Sachs disease is approximately 1/100,000, so that one would have to screen 200,000 couples to avoid the birth of a single child with Tay-Sachs disease. Clearly, screening the Ashkenazi Jewish population is a far more cost-effective program than screening the entire population for this otherwise rare disease.

Table 4.4. Effect of Genotype Frequency on the Ratio of Heterozygotes to Homozygotes

Allele Frequency		Genotype Frequency			Ratio of Heterozygotes to Homozygotes
A (p)	a (q)	AA (p^2)	Aa (2pq)	aa (q^2)	Aa/aa ($2pq/q^2$)
0.999	0.001	0.998	0.002	0.000001	2000
0.997	0.003	0.994	0.006	0.00001	600
0.993	0.007	0.986	0.014	0.00005	280
0.990	0.010	0.980	0.020	0.0001	198
0.978	0.022	0.956	0.043	0.0005	86
0.968	0.032	0.936	0.062	0.001	62
0.929	0.071	0.864	0.132	0.005	26
0.900	0.100	0.810	0.180	0.010	18

For X-linked genes, estimation of allele frequencies is different from that for autosomal genes because males are hemizygous for X-linked genes, and thus the frequency of affected males is *equal* to the frequency of the mutant allele, q. For a rare X-linked recessive disease such as hemophilia A (where q, the disease frequency, is approximately 1/10,000 and $p \approx 1$), the frequency of heterozygous carriers is only twice the frequency of affected males ($2q = 1/5{,}000$). However, the ratio of affected males to homozygous affected females is very high because $q \gg q^2$ (1/10,000 versus 1/100 million for hemophilia). In contrast, for rare X-linked dominant diseases, the frequency of affected males is about half that of affected females, q:2q.

Factors That Alter Gene Frequencies

The Hardy-Weinberg principle is at best an approximation, because it is absolutely true only under certain very specific conditions, rarely met in human populations. Fortunately for medical geneticists, however, it "works" and allows estimation of clinically useful allele frequencies as described above. The Hardy-Weinberg equilibrium holds exactly only for large populations in which there is random mating and in which there is no selection, mutation, or migration. Deviation from any of these conditions can alter allele frequency in a population and lead to an increase or decrease in allele frequencies from one generation to another.

NONRANDOM MATING

In human populations, mating is seldom random. It is usually assortative in that members of a particular subpopulation are more likely to mate with other members of that same subpopulation, whether it is defined by racial, ethnic, religious, or other criteria. For example, congenitally deaf individuals marry congenitally deaf partners more often than would be expected by chance. A special form of nonrandom mating in the human population is **consanguinity,** or mating among close relatives. Although consanguinity (or inbreeding) does not change allele frequencies per se, it does increase the proportion of homozygotes in the next generation at the expense of heterozygotes, thereby exposing disadvantageous recessive phenotypes to selection. Such selection may in turn alter allele frequencies in subsequent generations. Consanguineous marriages not only have a greater risk of producing offspring homozygous for a deleterious recessive gene, but also offspring with increased susceptibility for polygenic or multifactorial diseases or birth defects. As discussed later in this chapter, the risk is proportional to the degree of relationship of the parents. The degree of consanguinity can be described by the **coefficient of relationship (r)** which is the probability that two persons have inherited a particular allele from a common ancestor. It also represents the proportion of all genes that are identical by descent from a common ancestor (Table 4.5).

Table 4.5. Coefficient of Relationship with Different Degrees of Relationship

Relationship	Degree	Coefficient of Relationship (r)
Parent-child	First	1/2
Siblings	First	1/2
Uncle-niece	Second	1/4
First cousins	Third	1/8
Second cousins	Fourth	1/16

As discussed in Chapter 3, consanguinity increases the probability of a mating between two individuals heterozygous for the same mutant allele. Therefore, one might expect an increased frequency of consanguinity among the parents of children with rare autosomal recessive disease. In fact, this is found, and the frequency of such consanguinity is inversely related to the frequency of the mutant allele; the more rare the disease, the more likely is parental consanguinity. This relationship can be approximated by the formula $k = c/16q$, where k is the frequency of consanguinity among parents of patients with autosomal recessive diseases, q is the frequency of the mutant allele in the population, and c is the frequency of first cousin marriages in the general population. In the general United States population the frequency of first cousin marriages is less than 0.1%; however, in certain isolates such as the Hutterites or the old-order Amish, the frequency of consanguineous matings is considerably higher. The relationship between the frequency of consanguinity and the frequency of a recessive disease is illustrated by comparing Tay-Sachs disease in the Ashkenazi and the non-Ashkenazi populations. In the latter, $q = 0.0017$ and k is approximately 4%, whereas in the Ashkenazi population, in which $q = 0.017$, k is less than 0.4%.

SMALL POPULATIONS

For political, religious, or geographic reasons, a small subgroup of the population may become physically and/or socially isolated from the rest of the population, forming a genetic isolate. The founder members of such an isolate may, by chance, be carriers of mutant alleles for certain recessive traits, so that the frequency of these alleles will be higher within the isolate than within the population at large. Furthermore, the actual frequency in such a small population will vary widely from one generation to the next, a phenomenon called ***genetic drift.*** By chance, one allele may fail to be passed on to the next generation and thus disappear from that line of descent, leaving only the alternative allele. Such a mechanism may account for the high frequency of certain rare diseases among genetic isolates. An example is the autosomal recessive Ellis-van Creveld syndrome, characterized by short-limbed dwarfism, polydactyly (extra fingers and toes), and congenital heart disease (Fig. 4.1), which has an allele frequency of $q = 0.07$ in the old-order Amish in Pennsylvania, but is extremely rare in the general population. Another example of such a possible "founder effect" is the high frequency of variegate porphyria, an autosomal dominant disease characterized by attacks of acute abdominal pain, weakness, and sun-induced skin problems, among the Afrikaner population in South Africa. This mutant allele is thought to have been introduced by Dutch settlers into a very small population in the Cape colony in the late 17th century and the disease now has a frequency of 1/400.

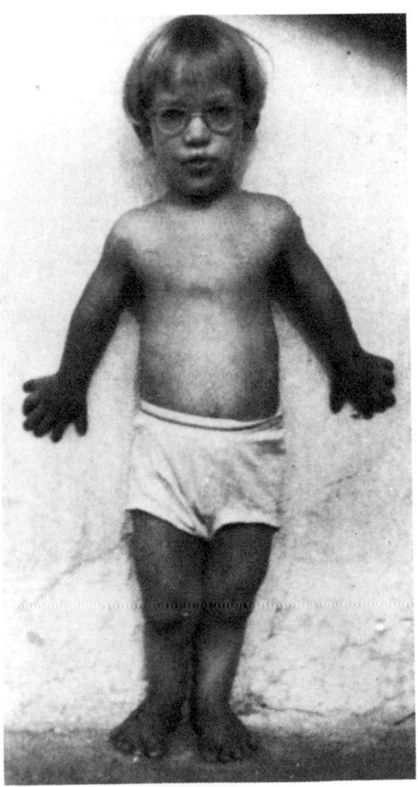

Figure 4.1. Child with Ellis-van Creveld syndrome. (From McKusick VA et al.: Trans Assoc Am Physicians 77:154, 1964.)

In contrast, the high frequency of autosomal recessive albinism among the Hopi Indians of Arizona ($q^2 = 1/220$ compared with 1/20,000 in the white population) probably has a different explanation. Albinism, with its decreased skin and eye pigmentation secondary to a deficiency of the enzyme tyrosinase, is associated with severe sun sensitivity and impairment of vision, characteristics which are highly disadvantageous in a desert environment. The high frequency of this gene in the Hopi population ($q = 0.067$) may be the result of cultural selection counterbalancing genetic selection. Hopi men farmed fields distant from the village, while the women remained in the village weaving. Albinos were excluded from this farming activity and remained in the village during the day. Because the Hopis were not strictly monogamous in the past, albino men had a greater opportunity to pass their genes to the next generation.

SELECTION

Selection represents the action of environmental factors on a particular phenotype, and hence its genotype, and may be positive or negative. It is the consequence of differences in the **biological fitness** (*f*) of individual phenotypes. Biological fitness is a measure of fertility and therefore of the contribution to the gene pool of the succeeding generation. Thus, selection may operate at any time from conception to the end of the reproductive period. A mutant allele may be a "genetic lethal" if it interferes with fertility, even though it causes no illness. Most deleterious dominant mutations have a fitness value between 0 (a genetic lethal) and 1 (the fitness of the normal allele). Mutant alleles encoding autosomal dominant traits are expressed in heterozygotes and thus exposed to direct selection; therefore, a change in selective forces can rapidly alter the allele frequency for a dominant mutation. In contrast, selection against mutant alleles encoding autosomal recessive diseases operates very slowly. As described above (Table 4.4), the frequency of heterozygous carriers of rare recessive disorders is much higher than the frequency of affected homozygotes; thus, the great majority of mutant alleles are carried by heterozygotes rather than homozygotes. For a lethal autosomal recessive disease with a frequency of approximately 1/15,000, restoring the biological fitness of the affected homozygote from 0 to 1 would lead to a doubling in the gene frequency only after 50 generations.

MUTATION

A mutation is a change in the genetic material. The **mutation rate** (μ) is the frequency of such change and is expressed as the number of mutations/locus/gamete/generation. Most information on human mutation rates comes from studies of rare autosomal dominant traits for which it is much easier to estimate mutation rates than for recessive traits. For rare autosomal dominant traits, the mutation rate is $\mu = \mathbf{n/2N}$, where n is the number of affected patients with unaffected parents and N is the total number of births. The denominator is 2N rather than N, because mutation of either allele at an autosomal locus could result in the mutant phenotype. Locus heterogeneity (mutations at different genetic loci resulting in a similar phenotype) and decreased penetrance in an affected parent may both lead to erroneously high estimates of mutation rate.

Estimates of mutation rates for a variety of autosomal dominant diseases have yielded rates that vary from 10^{-6} to as high as 10^{-4}. For most human genes, the best estimates for mutation rates lie between 10^{-6} and 10^{-5}/locus/gamete/generation. There is evidence that the frequency of mutations for certain autosomal dominant traits increases with increasing paternal age (2).

Two important genetic disorders are noteworthy for having extremely high calculated rates of mutation. One is von Recklinghausen neurofibromatosis (NF1) with an estimated rate of 10^{-4}. Although it has been suggested that this is because several different genetic loci may contribute to NF1, this explanation now appears unlikely (see Chapter 9). Duchenne muscular dystrophy is also thought to have a very high mutation rate of approximately 0.2 to 1.0 × 10^{-4}. In this case the high rate may be a reflection of the very large size of the gene (>2000 kilobases (kb)), perhaps presenting a large "target" for putative mutagenic agents.

At equilibrium, the birth frequency for a rare autosomal dominant trait with reduced fitness, such as achondroplasia, represents a balance between the introduction of new mutant alleles by mutation and their removal by negative selection. The more severe the reduction in biological fitness, the greater the proportion of patients whose disease is the result of new mutations. In the case of Huntington disease where the age of onset of clinical disease is late and biological fitness is only marginally impaired, new mutations account for few, if any, of the total cases of this disease.

Among the probable environmental causes of mutations in humans are ionizing radiation and chemical mutagens. Although there is good experimental evidence on the relationship between radiation dose and mutation rate in other mammals and in lower organisms, there are fewer data in human populations. Long-term studies on the genetic effects of radiation exposure due to nuclear bombings or radiation accidents have provided a major source of information on this topic. The assessment of possible mutagenic risk to humans from the tremendous number of both natural and synthetic chemicals known to be mutagenic in other biological systems is a major area of public health concern.

MIGRATION AND GENE FLOW

Migration of populations into new regions and intermarriage with indigenous populations can result in a change in allele frequencies in both populations, a phenomenon known as **gene flow.** This may account for the high frequency of the allele for blood group B in Asia, with a gradual decline as one moves westward across Europe. Another example is the flow of Caucasian genes into United States black populations. By comparing the allele frequencies of certain blood group genes in West African blacks, in whites, and in blacks in the United States, it has been estimated that approximately 25% of the total gene pool of United States blacks in northern cities is of Caucasian origin (2).

Polymorphism

The discussion up to this point has dealt primarily with rare mutant alleles at genetic loci where the vast majority of the population carries a single normal (or wild-type) allele. However, at many loci in humans, two or more alleles occur with appreciable frequency in the same population. A polymorphism is defined as the occurrence of two or more genetically determined alternative phenotypes in a population at such a frequency that the rarest could not be maintained by recurrent mutation alone. In practice, a genetic locus is considered polymorphic if the rare allele (or alleles) has (have) a frequency of at least 0.01, with the result that heterozygotes carrying this allele occur at a frequency greater than 2%. More than one-third of the human genetic loci that have been studied have been found to be polymorphic. Examples include the loci coding for common blood groups such as the ABO, MN, and Rh systems, for a variety of red blood cell enzymes and serum proteins, and for the cellular antigens encoded by the major histocompatibility locus (2, 3).

This extensive polymorphism allows for multiple combinations of alleles at different loci and hence tremendous genetic diversity in the population and genetic uniqueness of individuals. This genetic diversity is thought to account for differences in genetic susceptibility to a variety of diseases, as discussed later in this chapter. Polymorphisms, as markers of genetic diversity, are also valuable tools for mapping the human genome, as is discussed in detail in Chapter 9. DNA polymorphisms affecting restriction enzyme recognition sites (discussed in Chapter 5) are particularly valuable in this regard.

It is generally believed that most stable polymorphisms are the result of selection for advantageous mutant alleles, although the selective pressures responsible for such so-called balanced polymorphisms have in most cases remained elusive. The best understood example of selection resulting in a balanced polymorphism is that of the sickle cell allele. Individuals homozygous for this mutant allele are affected with sickle cell anemia, a severe hemolytic anemia, and often die before reproductive age. Nevertheless, the frequency of sickle cell anemia at birth in United States blacks is approximately 1/500, and in parts of equatorial Africa, up to 1/25 of the population are affected with this disease. Because the affected homozygote obviously has decreased fitness, the high frequency of the mutant allele must be the result of the increased fitness of individuals heterozygous for this allele. Sickle cell anemia is most frequent in regions of the world in which falciparum malaria (due to infection with *Plasmodium falciparum*) was common in the past (Fig. 4.2). In such regions, many people are ill with malaria and have reduced fertility. Heterozygous carriers of the sickle cell allele (individuals with sickle cell trait) are more resistant to malarial infection, apparently because their red cells, when parasitized by *P. falciparum,* are more effectively removed from the circulation than are parasitized red cells in normal individuals without sickle cell trait. Because the number of heterozygotes for an autosomal recessive trait is much greater than the number of affected homozygotes (Fig. 4.4), a relatively small selective

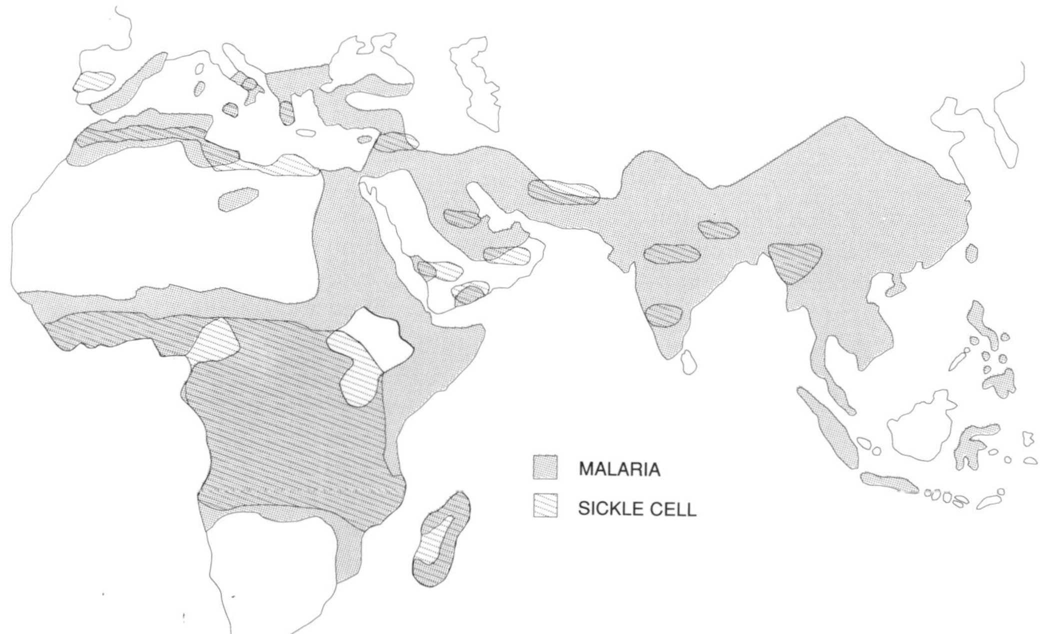

Figure 4.2. Geographic distribution of falciparum malaria prior to 1930 (*lightly shaded red area*) and of sickle cell anemia (*diagonal line pattern*). (Redrawn from Friedman MJ, Trager W: The biochemistry of resistance to malaria. Sci Am 244:154–164, 1981.)

advantage in the heterozygote can outweigh a large selective disadvantage in the homozygote. In the case of sickle cell anemia, it has been calculated that a 20% increase in fitness of sickle cell trait individuals could balance an 85% decrease in the fitness of individuals with sickle cell anemia (2). One might expect that, with the control of malaria in many parts of the world, the frequency of this allele should decline. The thalassemias, a group of autosomal recessive hemolytic anemias discussed in Chapter 6, and G6PD deficiency are also found in the same geographic distribution as is sickle cell anemia, and resistance to malaria may also be the positive selective force accounting for the high frequency of these diseases (2).

MULTIFACTORIAL INHERITANCE AND QUANTITATIVE TRAITS

Although many human diseases are inherited as simple Mendelian traits or are associated with chromosomal abnormalities, most of the common diseases of adult life (e.g., diabetes mellitus, hypertension, schizophrenia) and most common congenital malformations (e.g., cleft lip, cleft palate, neural tube defects) are not. Yet there is considerable evidence that genetic factors are important in their etiology. This genetic predisposition to disease is thought to reflect the cumulative effect of genetic variation at several and possibly multiple loci, each with a small effect on phenotype. We define as **polygenic** those traits or diseases caused by the impact of many different genes, each having only a small individual impact on phenotype, and as **multifactorial** those traits resulting from the interplay of multiple environmental factors with multiple genes. In practice, the terms are often used interchangeably. Polygenic traits are usually quantitative rather than qualitative in nature and are distributed continuously in the population, often in a more or less normal (Gaussian) frequency distribution, e.g., height and blood pressure.

To understand the normal distribution of quantitative traits, consider the hypothetical example of two independent genetic loci, A and B, which affect systolic blood pressure. Each has two alleles, A and a, and B and b, occurring in the population with equal frequency ($p = q = 0.5$). Assuming that the population is in Hardy-Weinberg equilibrium, the three genotypes at each locus (AA, Aa, aa and BB, Bb, bb) will occur in the ratio of $p^2{:}2pq{:}q^2 = (\frac{1}{4}){:}(\frac{1}{2}){:}(\frac{1}{4})$. The frequencies for the two-locus genotypes are obtained by multiplication of the separate probabilities for the single locus genotypes (independence principle) as shown in Table 4.6. Assume that the allele designated by the capital letter (A

Table 4.6. Frequency Distribution of Systolic Blood Pressure Determined by a Two-Locus Two-Allele Model[a]

	AA 1/4	Aa 1/2	aa 1/4
BB 1/4	1/16 *(40)*	2/16 *(30)*	1/16 *(20)*
Bb 1/2	2/16 *(30)*	4/16 *(20)*	1/16 *(10)*
bb 1/4	1/16 *(20)*	2/16 *(10)*	1/16 *(0)*

[a] The numbers in parentheses indicate the increment (in mm Hg pressure) to the systolic blood pressure above a basal level of 100 mm Hg contributed by each genotype.

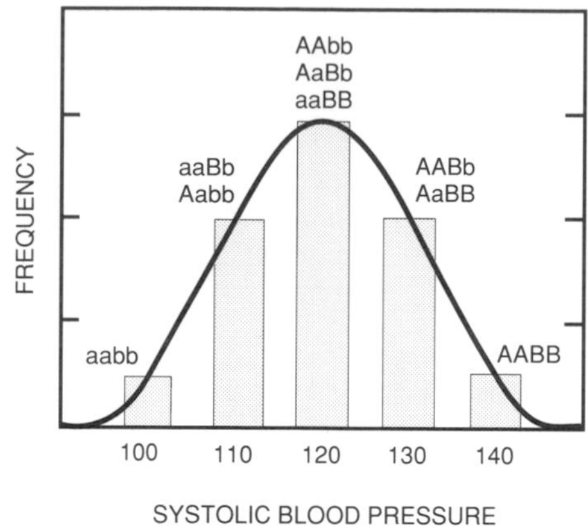

Figure 4.3. Frequency distribution of systolic blood pressure determined by a two-locus two-allele model. See text for explanation.

or B) contributes one unit (an increment of 10 mm Hg pressure) to the hypothetical quantitative trait of interest (systolic blood pressure above a basal level of 100 mm Hg) and that the allele designated by the lower case letter (a or b) contributes zero units (Table 4.6). The population distribution of the trait, shown in Figure 4.3, approximates a normal distribution.

The larger the number of individual genetic loci contributing to a trait and/or the more polymorphic the loci (that is, the more different alleles at any given locus) the more likely that the distribution of the trait will be a smooth normal curve. The effects of environmental factors may further modify the shape of the frequency distribution.

As suggested in Figure 4.3, an apparently continuous unimodal distribution of a quantitative trait may, in fact, represent the summation of several discrete phenotypes. This is illustrated by studies on red cell acid phosphatase activity. Six different phenotypes, distinguishable by differences in the electrophoretic mobility of the enzyme and determined by three alleles at a single autosomal locus occur in the British population. The six phenotypes represent the three homozygous genotypes, AA, BB, and CC, and the three heterozygous genotypes, BA, CA, and CB. Each type is associated with a characteristic range of enzyme activity. Although there is considerable variation in the amount of acid phosphatase activity between individuals with the same acid phosphatase genotype, significant differences in the mean level of activity between types is apparent. Figure 4.4 shows the individual distributions of enzyme activity (*black curves*) of the five common acid phosphatase phenotypes (CC is relatively rare), as well as the general population distribution of acid phosphatase activity (*red curve*) in the British population. The apparently unimodal distribution in the whole population is a composite of the five separate but overlapping distributions (3).

POLYGENES AND RELATIONSHIP

Although each individual, except monozygotic (or identical) twins, is genetically unique, each is more like his/her relatives than he/she is like unrelated individuals. As discussed below, polygenic disorders run in families; therefore, it is important to define the genetic relationship between relatives. This relationship is shown in the pedigree in Figure 4.5. The *number* inside the symbol indicates the degree of relationship with the proband, indicated by the *arrow* and *solid symbol.* First degree relatives share ½ of their genes with the proband; second degree relatives share ¼ of their genes; and third degree relatives share ⅛ of their genes. Note that the fraction of genes shared is the same as the coefficient of relationship (r). Spouses and other relatives by marriage are presumably unrelated and do not share any greater genetic relationship with the proband than any individual picked at random from the population.

In humans, the best example of a "pure" polygenic trait is the fingertip ridge count. This is the total number of ridges on the 10 fingertips, counted according to specific rules. The fingertip ridge pattern is determined early in development and there is apparently minimal influence from environmental factors. Its polygenic character is suggested by its normal distribution in the population and by the fact that the degree of correlation of fingertip ridge count among relatives corresponds very closely to the number of genes they share in common (Table 4.7) (4).

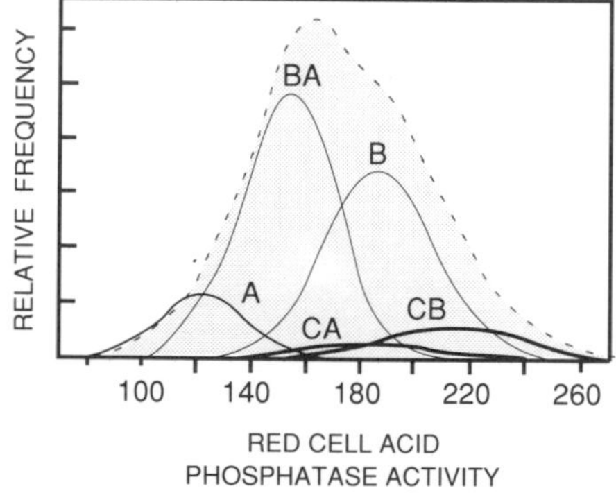

Figure 4.4. Distribution of red cell acid phosphatase activities in the general population *(broken red line)* and in individuals with the separate phenotypes. The *solid curves* are constructed from the data on the different phenotypes as found in the British population. (From Harris H: *The Principles of Human Biochemical Genetics.* 3rd Ed. Amsterdam, Elsevier/North-Holland, 1980, p. 186.)

Table 4.7. Correlation of Fingertip Ridge Counts among Relatives Compared with Expectations Based on the Proportion of Shared Genes[a]

Relationship	Observed Correlation	Expected Correlation
Monozygotic twins	0.95 ± 0.07	1.00
Dizygotic twins	0.49 ± 0.08	0.50
Siblings	0.50 ± 0.04	0.50
Parent-child	0.48 ± 0.04	0.50
Spouses	0.05 ± 0.07	0.00

[a]From Carter CO: Genetics of common disorders. Br Med Bull 25:52–57, 1969.

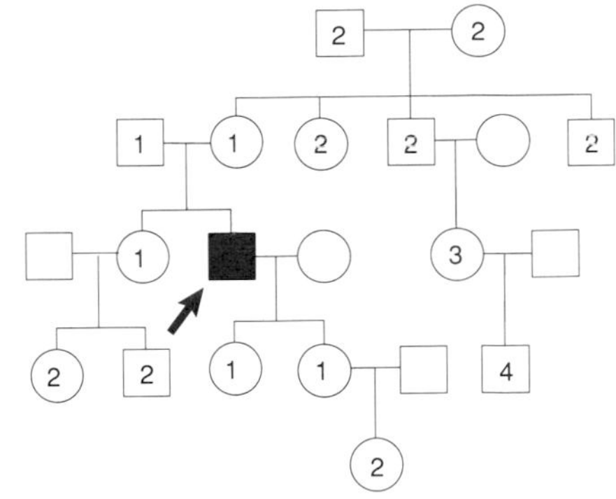

Figure 4.5. Pedigree showing degree of relationship. In this figure, the *numbers inside the symbols* indicate the degree of relationship to the proband *(red symbol).*

Evidence for Genetic Factors in Common Diseases and Malformations

The evidence that genetic factors are important in common diseases and malformations comes mainly from epidemiologic studies comparing the frequency of disease among genetically related individuals with that in the general population. First, certain malformations have a different frequency in different racial and ethnic groups. For example, talipes equinovarus (club foot) is six times more common in the Polynesian population than in the Caucasian population in Hawaii, in which it is three times as frequent as in the Chinese population of the Hawaiian Islands (5).

Second, there is a higher frequency of specific malformations among relatives of affected individuals (a "familial tendency") that is proportional to the degree of relatedness. This is illustrated in large-scale family studies on the frequency of cleft lip with or without cleft palate (Fig. 4.6) from both Europe and North America, where the frequency of this anomaly is approximately 1/1000 (Table 4.8). It is clear that the proportion of affected relatives is not consistent with either autosomal dominant or recessive inheritance. The sharp decline in frequency of affected second degree relatives compared with first degree relatives, and to a lesser extent, third degree relatives compared with second degree, is greater than would be predicted by autosomal dominant inheritance, in which the frequency is expected to decrease by ½ with each step. The similar proportion of affected siblings and children

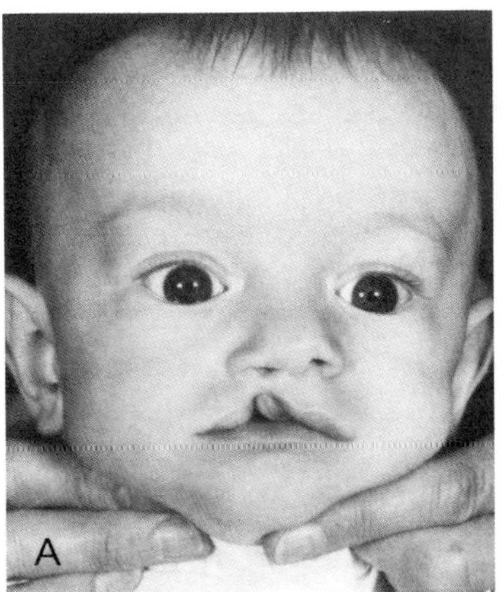

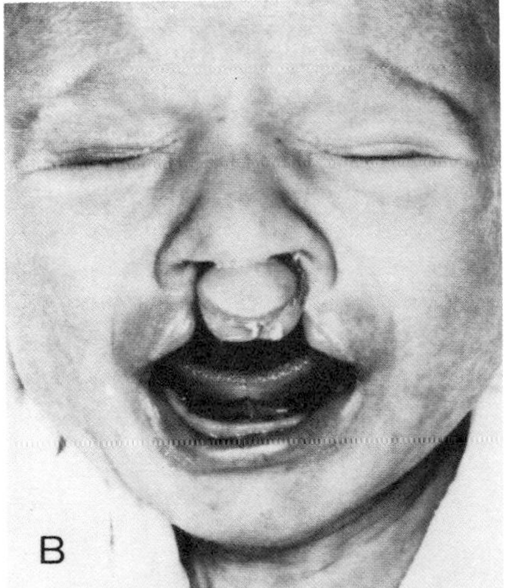

Figure 4.6. **A**, Child with unilateral cleft lip, **B**, Child with bilateral cleft lip and cleft palate. (From Ross RB, Johnson MC: *Cleft Lip and Palate.* Baltimore, Williams & Wilkins, 1972, pp. 131, 141.)

Table 4.8. Family Studies of the Incidence of Cleft Lip (±Cleft Palate)[a]

Relatives	Percentage of Relatives Affected	Incidence Relative to General Population
First degree		
Sibs	4.1	×40
Children	3.5	×35
Second degree		
Aunts and uncles	0.7	×7
Nephews and nieces	0.8	×8
Third degree		
First cousins	0.3	×3

[a]From Carter CO: Genetics of common disorders. Br Med Bull 25:52–57, 1969.

of affected probands is inconsistent with autosomal recessive inheritance.

It should be noted, however, that not everything that is familial is genetic; families also share common environments. The percentage of medical students with a parent who is a physician is certainly much higher than expected from the frequency of physicians in the general population; yet it would be difficult to argue that being a medical student is a genetically determined trait.

A third and more convincing line of evidence supporting the role of genetic factors in the causation of common diseases and malformations comes from twin studies. If a trait (or disease or malformation) is entirely genetic, 100% of monozygotic (MZ) or genetically identical twin pairs should be concordant for the trait (i.e., both have the trait or both do not have the trait); 50% of the dizygotic (DZ) or nonidentical twin pairs, who share 50% of their genes (but share a common environment), should be concordant. If a trait is entirely nongenetic, however, concordance among MZ and DZ twin pairs will be roughly equal and significantly less than 100%. Finally, if a trait is multifactorial with a significant genetic component, MZ twin pairs will be concordant less than 100% of the time, but significantly more frequently than DZ twin pairs. Data for several common diseases and malformations that show significant genetic components are listed in Table 4.9.

Discontinuous Traits (Disease) from Continuously Distributed Liability: The Threshold Model

From the data presented above, it is clear that there are important genetic factors in the causation of a number of common diseases and malformations. Because the concordance for a given disease among monozygotic twins is considerably less than 100%, however, it is also

Table 4.9. Concordance among Monozygotic and Dizygotic Twins for Common Malformations and Diseases

Trait	Concordance MZ	Concordance DZ
	%	%
Cleft lip ± cleft palate	40	4
Club foot	30	2
Pyloric stenosis	22	2
Congenital dislocation of hip	33	3
Schizophrenia	60	10
Insulin-dependent diabetes mellitus	50	10

clear that there are environmental triggers that must be present to bring out the disease. One model to account for these facts proposes a continuously distributed, genetically determined liability for a given disease. Some proportion of individuals above a certain threshold of genetic liability will develop the disease, especially if exposed to the appropriate environmental triggers (4, 6). Such a threshold model accounts for the presence of discontinuous traits or diseases from continuously distributed, genetically determined liability (Fig. 4.7). This model supposes that affected individuals fall at the extreme right end of the liability distribution. It follows, therefore, that first degree relatives of an affected individual, who share ½ of their genes with that individual, will have a distribution of genetic liability for that condition that is shifted considerably to the right of that for the general population (Fig. 4.8). Second degree relatives who share ¼ of their genes with the affected individual (their remaining genes can be considered to be drawn from the general population) will have a distribution of liability that is shifted closer to

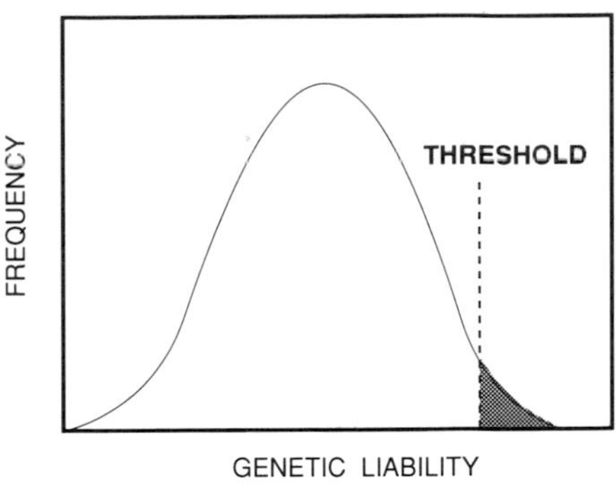

Figure 4.7. Threshold model of multifactorial inheritance. See text for details.

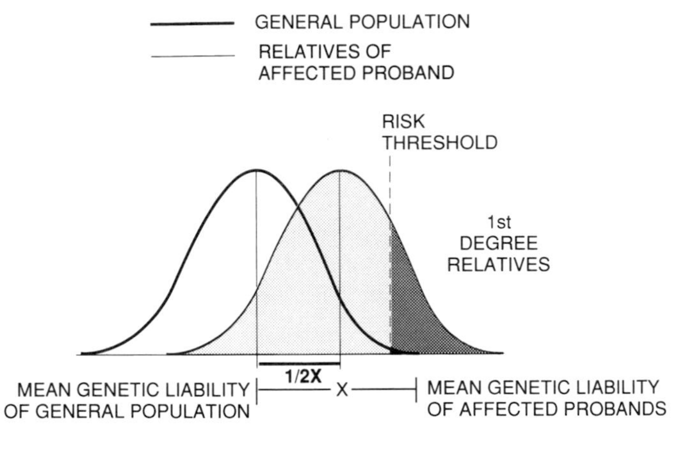

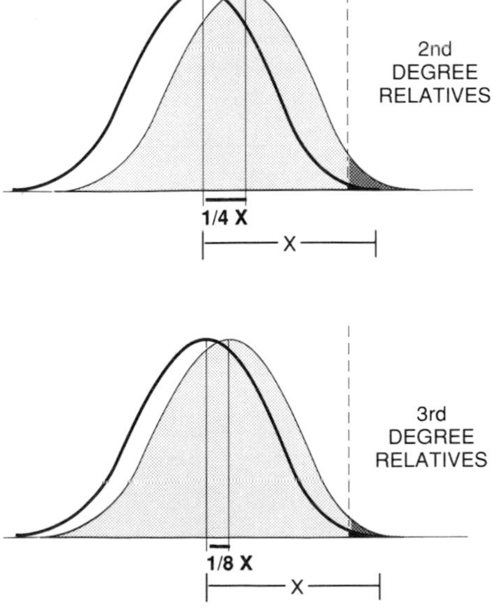

Figure 4.8. Multifactorial threshold model: distribution of genetically determined liability among relatives. The distribution of genetic liability in relatives of an affected proband is indicated by the *lightly shaded red area below* the *red curve. X* is the difference in mean genetic liability between affected probands and the general population. See text for details. (From Carter CO: Multifactorial genetic disease. Hosp Pract 5:45–59, 1970.)

the mean for the general population but still to the right of it. Third degree relatives who share only ⅛ of their genes with the proband will have a distribution of genetic liability that is much closer to the mean of the general population. In each case, the proportion of first, second, and third degree relatives who will fall above the threshold for a given genetically determined trait will be progressively smaller as the degree of relatedness to the affected proband decreases. Because of the geometric properties of the normal distribution, there should be a markedly increased risk to first degree relatives, moderately increased risks to second degree relatives, and only a slightly increased risk to third degree relatives (Fig. 4.9).

Predictions of the Multifactorial Threshold Model Regarding Recurrence Risks for Polygenic Disease or Malformations

The multifactorial threshold model makes a number of predictions about the recurrence risk of diseases or malformations in relatives of affected probands; these predictions are different from those of Mendelian inheritance.

1. Recurrence risks represent average risks and will vary among different families. The multifactorial threshold model assumes that affected individuals fall above a certain threshold in the population distribution of genetically determined liability, but that their exact position cannot be directly defined. The average recurrence risks predicted are derived from empiric data such as those shown in Tables 4.8 and 4.10, as opposed to being determined by specific models or patterns of inheritance, as is the case for Mendelian traits. The model also predicts that recurrence risks for relatives will decline sharply as the degree of relatedness decreases, as shown in Figures 4.8 and 4.9. That this is indeed the case is shown in Table 4.10 for the recurrence risk to first, second, and third degree relatives of individuals affected with several common congenital malformations.

2. The risk increases with the number of affected relatives. For an autosomal recessive disease such as cystic fibrosis, the recurrence risk for a sibling of an affected child is 25%, whether that family has previously had one, two, or several affected children. In contrast, the recurrence risk for a sibling of a child with cleft lip, with or without cleft palate, is approximately 4%; whereas that risk increases to more than 10% if there are two affected first degree relatives such as two siblings or a parent and a sibling. The presence of a second affected individual does not alter the risk per se; however, it suggests that the family is further to the right in the distribution of genetic liability. Therefore,

Table 4.10. Family Patterns in Some Common Congenital Malformations[a]

		Incidence Relative to General Population			
Malformation	Incidence in General Population	Monozygotic Twins	First Degree Relatives	Second Degree Relatives	Third Degree Relatives
Cleft lip (±cleft palate)	0.001	×400	×40	×7	×3
Club foot	0.001	×300	×25	×5	×2
Neural tube defects	0.002		×8		×2
Congenital dislocation of hip (females only)	0.002	×200	×25	×3	×2
Congenital pyloric stenosis (males only)	0.005	×80	×10	×5	×1.5

[a]From Carter CO: Genetics of common disorders. Br Med Bull 25:52–57, 1969 and Smith DW, Aase JM: Polygenic inheritance of certain common malformations. J Pediatr 76:653–659, 1970.

this family can be identified as having a higher than average recurrence risk.

3. The risk increases with the severity of the malformation or disease. The recurrence risk for a sibling of a child with unilateral cleft lip without cleft palate is approximately 2.5%, whereas the recurrence risk for a sibling of a child with bilateral cleft lip and cleft palate is approximately 6%. This reflects the assumption that the more severe the defect, the greater the underlying genetic liability, and, therefore, the placement of the severely affected individual further to the right on the distribution curve.

4. The differential risk to relatives of an affected proband increases as the frequency of the disease or malformation in the general population decreases. The higher the incidence of a malformation in the general population, the lower the genetic threshold is presumed to be, resulting in a smaller difference between the average genetic liability of the population at large and that of affected individuals. Therefore, there will be a smaller difference in average genetic liability between relatives of an affected proband and the general population; and the increase in risk with close relationship to a proband will be relatively less. Because the actual frequency of the malformation in the general population is higher, however, the absolute risk to relatives will be higher than for a rarer malformation. For cleft lip, with an overall incidence of 1/1000, the relative risks for first, second, and third degree relatives are, respectively, 40, 7, and 3 times that in the general population. For congenital pyloric stenosis (males only), with an overall frequency of 5/1000, the relative risk factors are 10, 5, and 1.5 for first, second, and third degree relatives (Table 4.10).

5. When the sex ratio of affected probands deviates significantly from unity, offspring of affected probands of the less frequently affected sex are at higher relative risk. Congenital pyloric stenosis, an obstruction to the stomach outlet caused by muscular hypertrophy, is five times more common in boys than in girls. This suggests that the threshold for genetic liability for girls is higher than for boys (Fig. 4.10). Therefore, an affected girl might be expected to have a higher degree of genetic liability, and her relatives should have higher recurrence risks than those of an affected boy. In fact, children of affected females are three times more likely to have this same malformation than children of affected males. However, male offspring are still at higher risk than are female offspring (Table 4.11). The opposite holds for congenital dislocation of the hip, which is six times more common in females than in males; the recurrence risk for offspring of affected males is higher than for affected females. This contrasts with autosomal dominant or recessive inheritance in which the sex of the affected proband has no bearing on the recurrence risk for other family members.

Although the above considerations do not prove the validity of the threshold model, and indeed other, nonthreshold models of multifactorial disease have been developed (1, 7, 8), the multifactorial threshold model provides a useful framework for providing genetic counseling for families with common congenital malformations and common diseases. In the absence of known Mendelian inheritance, such patients are all too often counseled erroneously, either being told that they have a high risk of recurrence (when they do not) or that they have no risk at all (when they do). For most multifactorial conditions, such as insulin-dependent diabetes mellitus, cleft lip, or congenital heart disease, the recurrence risk for children or siblings of an affected proband is approximately 5% or less (4–6).

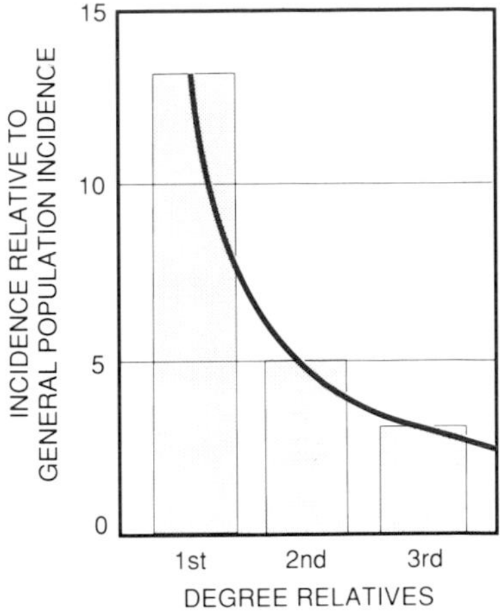

Figure 4.9. Multifactorial threshold model: predicted recurrence risks for relatives. (From Carter CO: Multifactorial genetic disease. Hosp Pract 5:45–59, 1970.)

Table 4.11. Proportion of Children Affected with Pyloric Stenosis[a]

Proband	Children: Sons	Children: Daughters
	%	
Father	5.5	2.4
Mother	19.4	7.3
Population incidence	0.5	0.1

[a]From Carter CO: Genetics of common disorders. Br Med Bull 25:52–57, 1969.

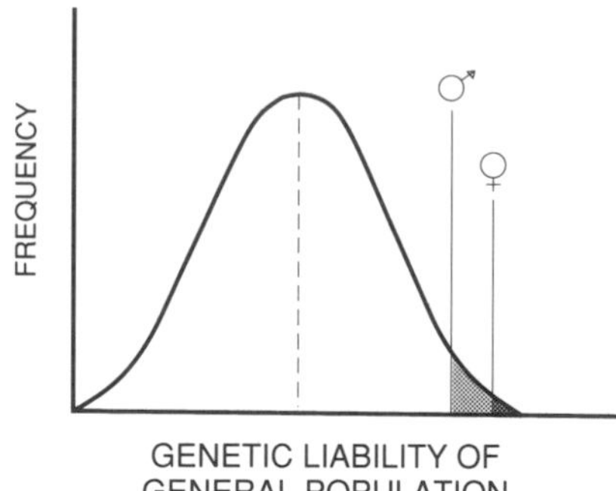

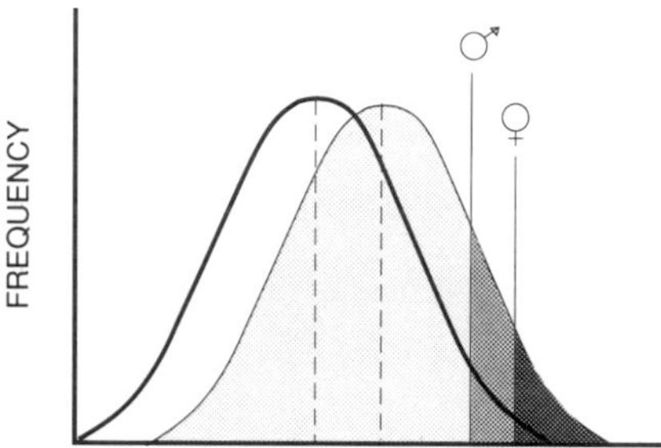

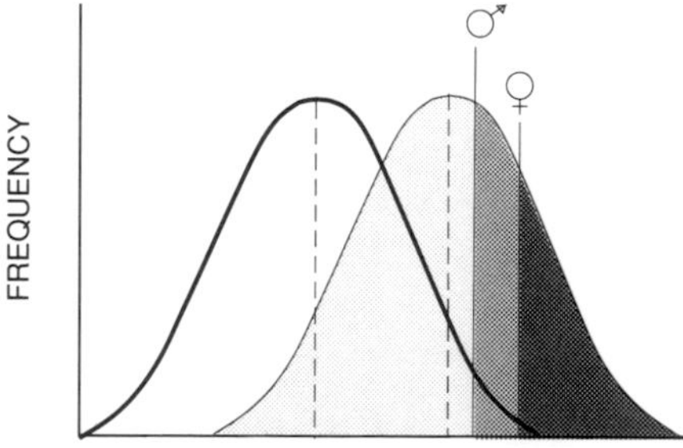

Figure 4.10. Multifactorial threshold model: explanation for sex differences in incidence of pyloric stenosis in probands and their relatives. The risk thresholds for males and females are indicated by the *solid vertical lines.* The distribution of genetic liability in relatives of male and female probands is indicated by the *red shaded areas below* the *red curve.* Affected individuals are indicated by the *darker red areas.* See text for details. (Redrawn from Thompson M: *Genetics in Medicine.* 4th Ed. Philadelphia, WB Saunders, 1986, p. 217.)

Implications of Multifactorial Inheritance

The multifactorial threshold model suggests that environmental triggers of disease are most likely to have a major impact on genetically predisposed individuals. Therefore, searching for environmental triggers of multifactorial diseases should be most fruitful when it is focused on those at highest genetic risk. Identification of these individuals should aid in identifying the environmental components in multifactorial illnesses. Correspondingly, medical intervention in the form of altering the environment of such individuals can then be focused on those at highest risk and thus most likely to benefit from such intervention.

Perhaps more important in the long run, it should be possible to identify genetic markers of liability to common diseases. Although the discussion above has assumed multiple genes, each with a small effect, it is possible that at least some non-Mendelian diseases may be the result of the effects of relatively few genes, some of which have rather large effects on phenotype. Thus, these diseases may be oligogenic rather than polygenic. The familial aggregation of insulin-dependent diabetes mellitus (type I, or juvenile-onset diabetes) is not consistent with simple Mendelian inheritance, and it was long considered that this disease was multifactorial. There is now evidence, however, that there may be only two major genes involved in susceptibility to this disease, one of which may be a part of the major histocompatibility locus (HLA) on chromosome 6 (9). This latter fact is useful in counseling diabetic families. Molecular genetic approaches offer the potential for a more refined definition of the major genes involved in susceptibility to this disease.

Another example of the potential of this approach is in the study of susceptibility to coronary artery disease, one of the most common disorders of humans. As is discussed in Chapter 7, monogenic abnormalities in lipoprotein metabolism are associated with a high risk of early atherosclerotic coronary artery disease; however, most patients with coronary artery disease do not have such monogenic diseases. It might be assumed that quantitative variation in the expression of a limited number of genes relevant to coronary artery disease (e.g., genes for lipoproteins) plays a role in determining genetic susceptibility. Intensive investigation seeking associations of polymorphisms in such genes with coronary artery disease shows promise of leading to a better understanding of the multifactorial genetic susceptibility to this common disease in the general population (10).

REFERENCES

1. Edwards JH: Familial predisposition in man. Br Med Bull 25:58–64, 1969.
2. Vogel F, Motulsky AG: *Human Genetics.* 2nd Ed, Berlin, Springer-Verlag, 1987.
3. Harris H: *The Principles of Human Biochemical Genetics.* 3rd Ed. Amsterdam, Elsevier/North-Holland, 1980.
4. Carter CO: Genetics of common disorders. Br Med Bull 25:52–57, 1969.
5. Smith DW, Aase JM: Polygenic inheritance of certain common malformations. J Pediatr 76:653–659, 1970.
6. Carter CO: Multifactorial genetic disease. Hosp Pract 5:45–59, 1970.
7. Kurnit DM, Layton WM, Matthyse S: Genetics, chance, and morphogenesis. Am J Hum Genet 41:979–995, 1987.
8. Kendler KS, Kidd KK: Recurrence risks in an oligogenic threshold model: The effect of alterations in allele frequency. Ann Hum Genet 50:83–91, 1986.
9. Todd JA, Bell JI, McDevitt HO: HLA-DQ_β gene contributes to susceptibility and resistance to insulin-dependent diabetes mellitus. Nature (Lond) 329:599–604, 1987.

10. Humphries SE: DNA polymorphisms of the apolipoprotein genes: Their use in the investigation of the genetic component of hyperlipidaemia and atherosclerosis. *Atherosclerosis* 72: 89–108, 1988.

SUGGESTED READINGS

Cavalli-Sforza LL, Bodmer WF: *The Genetics of Human Populations.* San Francisco, WH Freeman, 1971.

CIBA Foundation Symposium 130: *Molecular Approaches to Human Polygenic Diseases.* Chichester, England, John Wiley & Sons, 1987.

Emery AEH: *Methodology in Medical Genetics. An Introduction to Statistical Methods.* 2nd Ed. Edinburgh, Churchill Livingstone, 1986.

King RA, Rotter JI, Motulsky AG (eds): *The Genetic Basis of Common Disease.* New York, Oxford University Press, 1990.

McKusick VA: *Human Genetics.* 2nd Ed. Englewood Cliffs, NJ, Prentice-Hall, 1969.

Steinberg AG, Bearn AG, Motulsky AG, Childs B: *Genetics of Cardiovascular Disease.* Vol. 5 of Progress in Medical Genetics, New Series, Philadelphia, WB Saunders, 1983.

Williams RR: Nature, nurture, and family predisposition. N Engl J Med 318:769–771, 1988.

4/ Study Questions

1/ Two large tribes of equal size live on separate neighboring islands but are unaware of each other's existence. In tribe 1, the incidence of one form of autosomal recessive albinism is 1 in 10,000 whereas in tribe 2 the same disease is 100 times more common. Volcanic activity suddenly produces a land bridge and the two tribes quickly find each other and begin to mix and mate freely. (Assume no selective disadvantage to this form of albinism). Answer the following questions:

a. What were the allele frequencies for the normal and albinism alleles in each tribe prior to the appearance of the land bridge?
b. What were the allele frequencies for the normal and albinism alleles in the two tribes taken as a whole immediately after the tribes mixed? What was the frequency of the disease at that time?
c. What were the allele frequencies and disease frequency in the mixed tribe after one generation?

2/ In a population study, 5000 individuals were typed for the MN locus, an autosomal codominant trait. There were 2400 MM individuals, 2400 MN individuals, and 200 NN individuals. What are the allele frequencies for M and N alleles? Is this population in Hardy-Weinberg equilibrium?

3/ A Finnish woman is the mother of a child with Meckel syndrome (a rare autosomal recessive disorder occurring in 1/9000 births in her part of Finland). She is widowed and is now going to remarry. What is the risk of the disease in a pregnancy in her new marriage if her new husband is

a. an unrelated Finnish man from her geographic area?
b. her former husband's brother?
c. her own first cousin?

***4/** Gyrate atrophy of the retina is an autosomal recessive retinal disease with onset in late childhood and adolescence. Suppose the disease occurs with a frequency of 1 in 324 individuals in a particular population.
Nine couples with normal vision from this population split off and form a new genetic isolate by moving to a remote area to begin homesteading. What is the probability that the new isolate will not have the gene for gyrate atrophy in its gene pool? What is the chance that the gene will be about as common in the isolate as in the original population? More common?

5/ Every occurrence of a genetic lethal autosomal dominant disorder is a new mutation. Why?

6/ In the table below are shown concordance rates for three different disorders in monozygotic twins, dizygotic twins, and siblings. Comment on the probable roles played by heredity and environment for each disorder.

Disorder	Concordance		
	Monozygotic	Dizygotic	Siblings
	%	%	%
A	100	25	25
B	50	6	6
C	10	10	0.1

If heredity plays a major role in any of these disorders, can you form any hypotheses concerning the number of loci involved?

***7/** A particular clinical syndrome can be inherited either as an autosomal recessive trait or as a completely nonhereditary phenocopy with no known environmental cause. If the phenocopy form of the syndrome accounts for 80% of all cases of the disease, what would you expect the recurrence risk to be for a couple with one child with the disorder?

5

Molecular Genetics: Gene Organization, Regulation, and Manipulation

"Just as our present knowledge and practice of medicine relies on a sophisticated knowledge of human anatomy, physiology and biochemistry, so will dealing with disease in the future demand a detailed understanding of the molecular anatomy, physiology and biochemistry of the human genome. We shall have to have physicians who are as conversant with the molecular anatomy of chromosomes and genes as the cardiac surgeon is with the structure and workings of the heart and circulatory tree."

—Paul Berg, M.D.
Nobel Lecture, 1981

The flow of information from DNA to RNA to protein is described in general terms in Chapter 2. An understanding of the true nature of human genetic disease requires a more detailed grasp of the structure and function of human genes. This also requires us to delve more deeply into the techniques of genetic analysis, which are together and sometimes rather loosely referred to as "recombinant DNA technology."

GENERAL STRUCTURE OF GENES AND GENE FAMILIES

There are an estimated 10,000 to 100,000 genes dispersed throughout the 25 chromosomes of humans. The smallest of these genes may occupy no more than a few hundred base pairs of DNA, whereas the largest may be more than a million base pairs in length. As an example, in Figure 5.1 are shown the genes for adult human hemoglobin, about

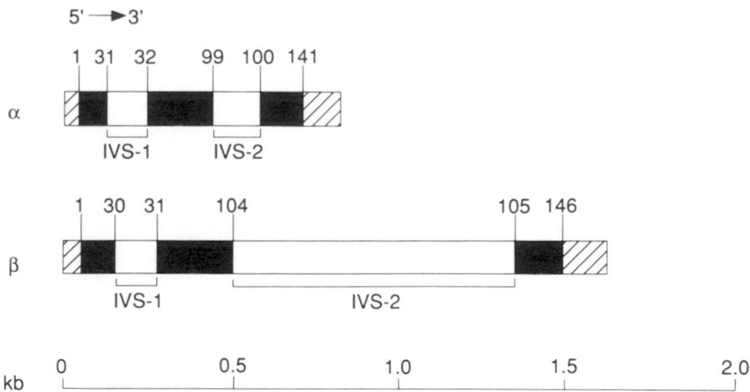

Figure 5.1. Structure of the human α- and β-hemoglobin genes. The *solid blocks* are the coding regions of the gene (the exons), which are divided into three blocks by the *open areas* (the introns or intervening sequences, IVS-1 and IVS-2). *Numbers* above the gene indicate the amino acid residues at the junctions. The *crosshatched* areas are transcribed into messenger RNA but not translated into protein and thus are often called the 5′- and 3′-untranslated regions.

which we will have much more to say in Chapter 6. Hemoglobin is a tetramer composed of two α-protein chains and two β-protein chains. The genes for these proteins are on different chromosomes, with α being on chromosome 16 and β on chromosome 11. The α gene is approximately 800 bp in length whereas the β gene is nearly twice this long. The protein products, however, are similar: α is 141 amino acids long, and β is 146.

A striking feature of most eukaryotic genes is the presence of "introns," which are stretches of DNA located within the gene, transcribed into RNA, but then spliced out before the RNA is translated into protein. These are shown as open areas in Figure 5.1. The *solid areas* of the gene diagram indicate regions that contain coding information; these are denoted as exons. Thus, in the α gene, exon 1 encodes amino acids 1–31, exon 2, amino acids 32–99, and exon 3, amino acids 100–141. There are also untranslated regions at either end of the gene, which are marked as *crosshatched* regions in Figure 5.1. The 5′-untranslated region represents a sequence that is transcribed into messenger RNA by RNA polymerase but is not translated. In general, translation does not begin until the first AUG that appears in the RNA, and sequences that are located 5′ to this therefore do not appear in the protein. The 3′-untranslated region represents a sequence that appears in the mRNA but occurs after the stop codon (UAG, UGA, or UAA, see Table 2.2) and therefore also does not get translated into protein.

Genes sometimes occur in clusters, with genes of similar function located near each other. In Figure 5.2 are shown the α- and β-globin gene clusters of humans. Located near the β-globin gene are four other functional genes, namely ϵ, $^{G}\gamma$, $^{A}\gamma$, and δ, which also code for hemoglobin proteins but are expressed at different times during development. Similarly, the α-globin genes (there are actually two, α2 and α1, with identical coding regions) are also part of a gene cluster. The ζ gene is an embryonic gene, and the gene marked θ1 remains to have its function determined. In the β-globin cluster, an additional gene marked ψβ1 is shown, and in the α-globin cluster, a ψζ and a ψα1 gene are indicated. These so-called "pseudogenes," designated by ψ, are DNA sequences that have some of the structures of expressed genes and were presumably once functional but have acquired one or more mutations during evolution that render them incapable of producing a protein product.

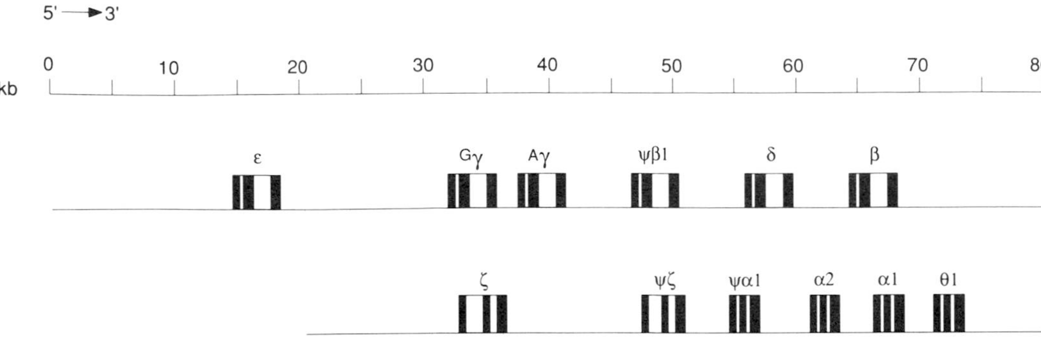

Figure 5.2. Map of the β-globin gene cluster on the short arm of chromosome 11 and the α-globin gene cluster on the short arm of chromosome 16. In each case the genes are arranged from 5′ to 3′ in order of their developmental activation. The ζ and ϵ genes are embryonic genes. $\psi\zeta$, $\psi\alpha 1$, and $\psi\beta 1$ are pseudogenes, which have acquired a number of inactivating mutations that prevent their giving rise to a functional globin chain. $\theta 1$ is a newly described globin-like gene whose function remains unknown. Hemoglobin F, the predominant hemoglobin in fetal life, consists of α and γ chains; the two α genes ($\alpha 2$ and $\alpha 1$) code for identical proteins and the two γ genes ($^G\gamma$ and $^A\gamma$) differ by a single amino acid at codon 136. In adulthood the major hemoglobin is $\alpha_2\beta_2$, with a minor contribution from $\alpha_2\gamma_2$. *Open blocks* within the genes indicate introns. Note that there is a large amount of "spacer" DNA between the genes, some of which contains repetitive sequences.

Note that in Figure 5.2 there are relatively long stretches of DNA in between the transcribed genes, so that in the 80 kb (1 kb = 1,000 bp) of DNA depicted around the β-globin genes, only about 12% is actually used for coding information. The nontranscribed DNA is termed "intergenic" DNA. Some of the sequences in intergenic DNA close to expressed genes are crucial for control of gene expression (as we shall see shortly), but a large amount of intergenic DNA seems to be rather dispensable and of no known function. Located within intergenic DNA, and sometimes also within introns, are repetitive sequences that occur dispersed throughout the genome in many thousands of copies and of no apparent known function. The most ubiquitous of these, the so-called *Alu* repetitive sequence, is about 300 bp in length and occurs approximately 500,000 times in the human genome. Since their dispersal into the genome millions of years ago, the *Alu* sequences have diverged, so that one *Alu* repeat is about 80% identical to another one. It is unusual to find a stretch of DNA longer than about 30 kb that does not contain at least one of these sequences.

THE TOOLS OF THE TRADE: RECOMBINANT DNA TECHNOLOGY

Before delving further into the anatomy of a typical human gene, it is necessary to describe some of the techniques that have permitted analysis of gene structure and function in such detail. It will be difficult to appreciate the full power of these techniques as they are initially presented; indeed, some of them may seem rather pointless. However, throughout the remainder of this textbook, it will be apparent that each of these techniques has at some time played a major role in defining the nature of a human genetic disease.

Restriction Enzymes

Restriction enzymes, also called restriction endonucleases because they cut within a DNA strand, are enzymes, purified from bacteria, which have the ability to cut double-stranded DNA at a specific nucleotide sequence. Examples are shown in Figure 5.3. The enzyme *Eco*RI,

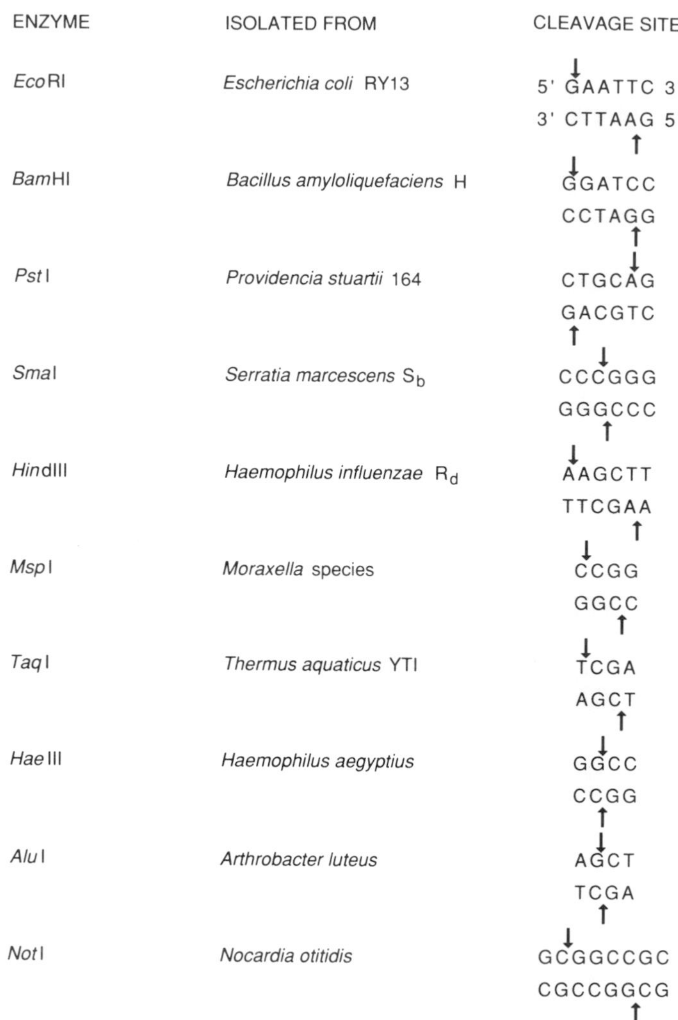

REPRESENTATIVE RESTRICTION ENZYMES

ENZYME	ISOLATED FROM	CLEAVAGE SITE
*Eco*RI	*Escherichia coli* RY13	5' G↓AATTC 3' 3' CTTAA↑G 5'
*Bam*HI	*Bacillus amyloliquefaciens* H	G↓GATCC CCTAG↑G
*Pst*I	*Providencia stuartii* 164	CTGCA↓G G↑ACGTC
*Sma*I	*Serratia marcescens* S_b	CCC↓GGG GGG↑CCC
*Hin*dIII	*Haemophilus influenzae* R_d	A↓AGCTT TTCGA↑A
*Msp*I	*Moraxella* species	C↓CGG GGC↑C
*Taq*I	*Thermus aquaticus* YTI	T↓CGA AGC↑T
*Hae*III	*Haemophilus aegyptius*	GG↓CC CC↑GG
*Alu*I	*Arthrobacter luteus*	AG↓CT TC↑GA
*Not*I	*Nocardia otitidis*	GC↓GGCCGC CGCCGG↑CG

Figure 5.3. Some representative restriction enzymes, the bacterial strain from which they were isolated, and the DNA sequences that they recognize. The *arrows* in the cleavage site indicate the actual location of the cut. Thus, some enzymes like *Eco*RI leave overhanging sticky ends, whereas others like *Sma*I generate blunt ends.

named because it was isolated from *Escherichia coli* strain RY13, will cleave DNA anywhere that it encounters the sequence GAATTC. The cleavage is such that an overhanging single-stranded end remains after cutting, as shown in Figure 5.3. These overhanging or "sticky" ends are often useful because they promote the religation of two fragments of DNA that have been cut with the same enzyme; ligation is accomplished by another enzyme called DNA ligase.

Not all restriction enzymes generate sticky ends; for example, the enzyme *Sma*I in Figure 5.3 generates a blunt end. Some restriction enzymes recognize sequences of 4 bp (*Alu*I and *Hae*III), and the enzyme *Not*I actually recognizes an 8-bp sequence and thus cuts rather rarely in genomic DNA.

Making Recombinants

Restriction enzymes allow the cleavage of a specific fragment of DNA, but to prepare this fragment in large quantity it is necessary to insert it into a "vector," which is a DNA segment capable of autonomous replication. The most commonly used vectors are bacterial plasmids (circular DNA molecules bearing antibiotic resistance genes) and bacteriophage (bacterial viruses). By inserting a specific DNA segment into one of these vectors, milligram amounts of DNA can be prepared that allow detailed analysis of gene structure. Figure 5.4 diagrams how restriction enzymes and the sticky ends they produce can be used to create recombinants.

Complementary DNA (cDNA)

Sometimes it is desirable to start with the RNA transcribed from the gene rather than the genomic DNA sequence itself. To take advantage of the recombinant DNA strategy, single-stranded RNA first must be converted to double-stranded DNA. This is accomplished by means of an enzyme called reverse transcriptase. This conversion of single-stranded mRNA to double-stranded DNA (so-called complementary DNA or cDNA) is diagrammed in Figure 5.5.

Molecular Hybridization

The detection of a specific desired sequence in this and many other situations is based on a molecular hybridization. Simply stated, hybridization is the ability of a single-stranded DNA to base-pair ("anneal") to its complementary single strand, while failing to anneal to an unrelated sequence. Thus, in Figure 5.4, the probe DNA is usually labeled with a radioisotope so that its fate can be followed. If a large number of independent clones are fixed to a nitrocellulose filter, for example, hybridization with labeled probe, followed by placing this sheet against x-ray film, will detect the specific clone bearing a homologous DNA sequence.

Where Do "Probes" Come From?

The strategy diagrammed in Figure 5.4 requires the availability of a reagent (the "probe") which is capable of recognizing the desired clone in a complex mixture of many different DNA sequences. If one is trying to clone a mutant β-globin gene, for example, this is not really a problem because the normal β-globin sequence can be used. However, if this is a gene that has never previously been cloned, designing the probe is a challenging task. If the gene is expressed at very high levels in a particular tissue, making cDNA clones from this tissue is likely to yield some that have the right insert. Red blood cells, for example, contain α and β globin as their major protein component; thus reticulocytes, which are young red blood cells still containing mRNA, were used successfully to obtain the first hemoglobin cDNAs. If no such abundantly expressing tissue is available, then one must know something about the gene. Often, limited amino acid sequencing of the protein product is performed. Using the genetic code (Table 2.2), a short single-stranded DNA molecule (14–30) nucleotides long, called an "oligonucleotide") can be chemically synthesized, which is predicted to match the sequence coding for this protein. Because of the degeneracy of the genetic code, it

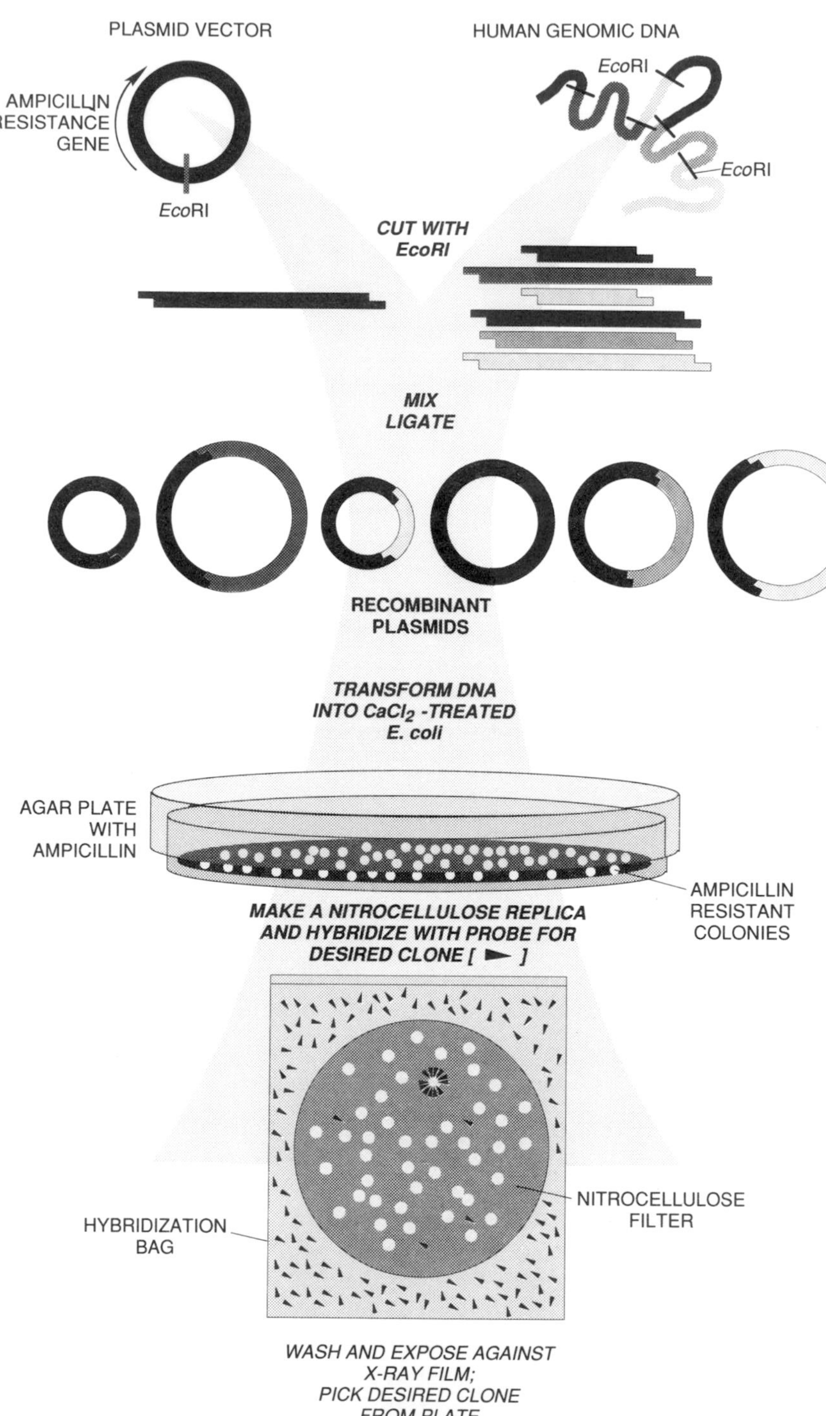

Figure 5.4. Diagram of the process of generating a specific recombinant DNA molecule. In this example, the vector, a bacterial plasmid carrying an ampicillin resistance gene, is cut with the restriction enzyme *Eco*RI, as is the genomic DNA, which contains within it the desired fragment. The sticky ends can be ligated together to generate a series of recombinant molecules, in which different genomic fragments have been inserted into the vector. This mixture is then transfected into ampicillin-sensitive *E. coli,* which have been treated with calcium chloride to promote their uptake of DNA. Only those bacteria that have taken up a plasmid will form colonies when plated on ampicillin. To identify the specific recombinant carrying the desired genomic fragment, one then can carry out a hybridization. In order to fix the colony DNA on an inert membrane, a nitrocellulose filter replica is made of the plate, and this is incubated in a hybridization bag with radiolabeled denatured "probe," which contains at least part of the DNA sequence of interest. The probe will selectively bind to DNA from the colony that harbors the desired plasmid and therefore can be identified by placing the filter against x-ray film.

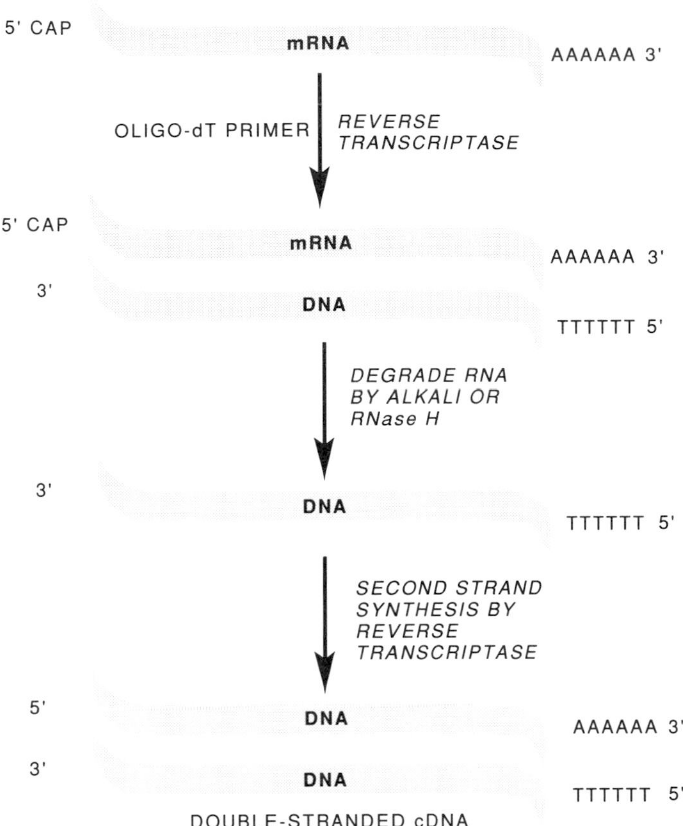

Figure 5.5. Steps involved in making a double-stranded cDNA from single-stranded messenger RNA. RNase H is an enzyme that will nick and degrade the RNA strand of an RNA-DNA heteroduplex.

usually is not possible to predict the exact sequence, so a mixture of oligonucleotides that covers all of the possibilities is often made. An example of this strategy is shown in Figure 5.6.

If no protein sequence is available but an antibody to the gene product can be obtained, the cDNA for the protein can often still be cloned. Vectors have been designed that allow one to clone cDNAs into the middle of the coding region of a bacterial gene such as the enzyme β-galactosidase. Those cDNAs that are present in the correct orientation and reading frame will give rise to hybrid protein molecules with amino-terminal β-galactosidase residues and a carboxy-terminal protein sequence derived from the cDNA. Sufficient amounts of this hybrid protein can be produced to allow detection of the desired clone by screening a large number of recombinants with a labeled antibody (Fig. 5.7).

CLONING FROM AMINO ACID SEQUENCE INFORMATION

AMINO ACID SEQUENCE: —Phe—Trp—Met—Asp—Cys—Arg—

OLIGONUCLEOTIDE: —TT(T/C)—TGG—ATG—GA(T/C)—TG(T/C)—CG—

Figure 5.6 Constructing a DNA probe from amino acid sequence information. If limited amino acid sequence is available on a protein, it is possible to construct a synthetic oligonucleotide that will hybridize with the gene encoding that protein, allowing cloning of the gene. Using the genetic code dictionary (see Table 2.2), the codons for each amino acid can be predicted; because of the degeneracy of the code, many amino acids have more than one codon, so in practice one synthesizes a mixture of oligonucleotides to cover all the possibilities. In the example above, a mixture of eight 17-mers should include the correct sequence and allow cloning of the gene.

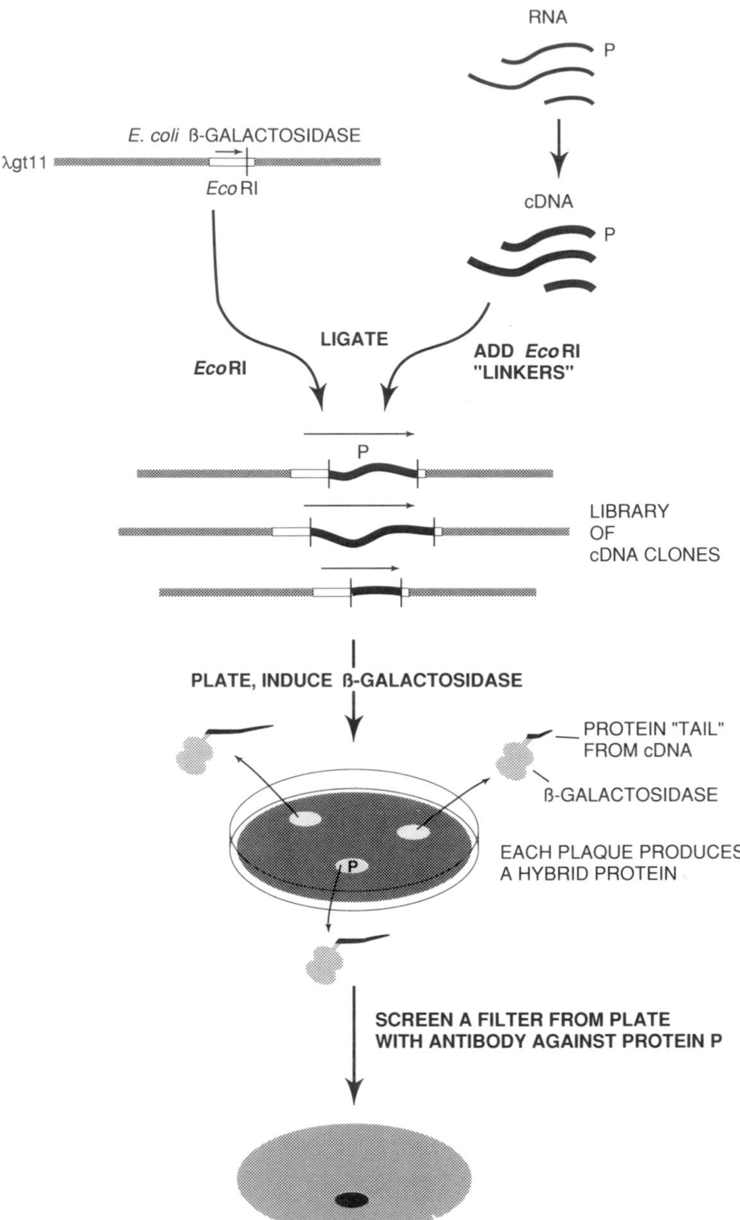

Figure 5.7. Cloning a cDNA for a gene when an antibody to the protein product is available. cDNA clones prepared from a tissue where the gene is expressed are inserted into a vector (λgt11) that contains the expressed protein *E. coli* β-galactosidase. The cloning site is placed at the end of the β-galactosidase coding region, so that a cDNA that is in the correct orientation and reading frame will be translated, generating a hybrid protein that contains β-galactosidase with an additional protein-coding region derived from the clone. A replica of these colonies can be made on a nitrocellulose filter, and then a labeled antibody against the protein of interest can be incubated with that filter. The binding of antibody indicates that this particular clone contains at least a part of the coding region of the cDNA for the protein recognized by that antibody. In this way, antibodies can be used to clone the relevant gene. For simplicity, only three clones are shown; in practice, several hundred thousand would be screened.

Southern Blotting

Once a DNA segment has been cloned, that segment can be used as a hybridization probe to identify variability among individuals. One such technique is the Southern blot, which derives its name from its originator and not from any geographic considerations. In this procedure, diagrammed in Figure 5.8, genomic DNA from an individual is

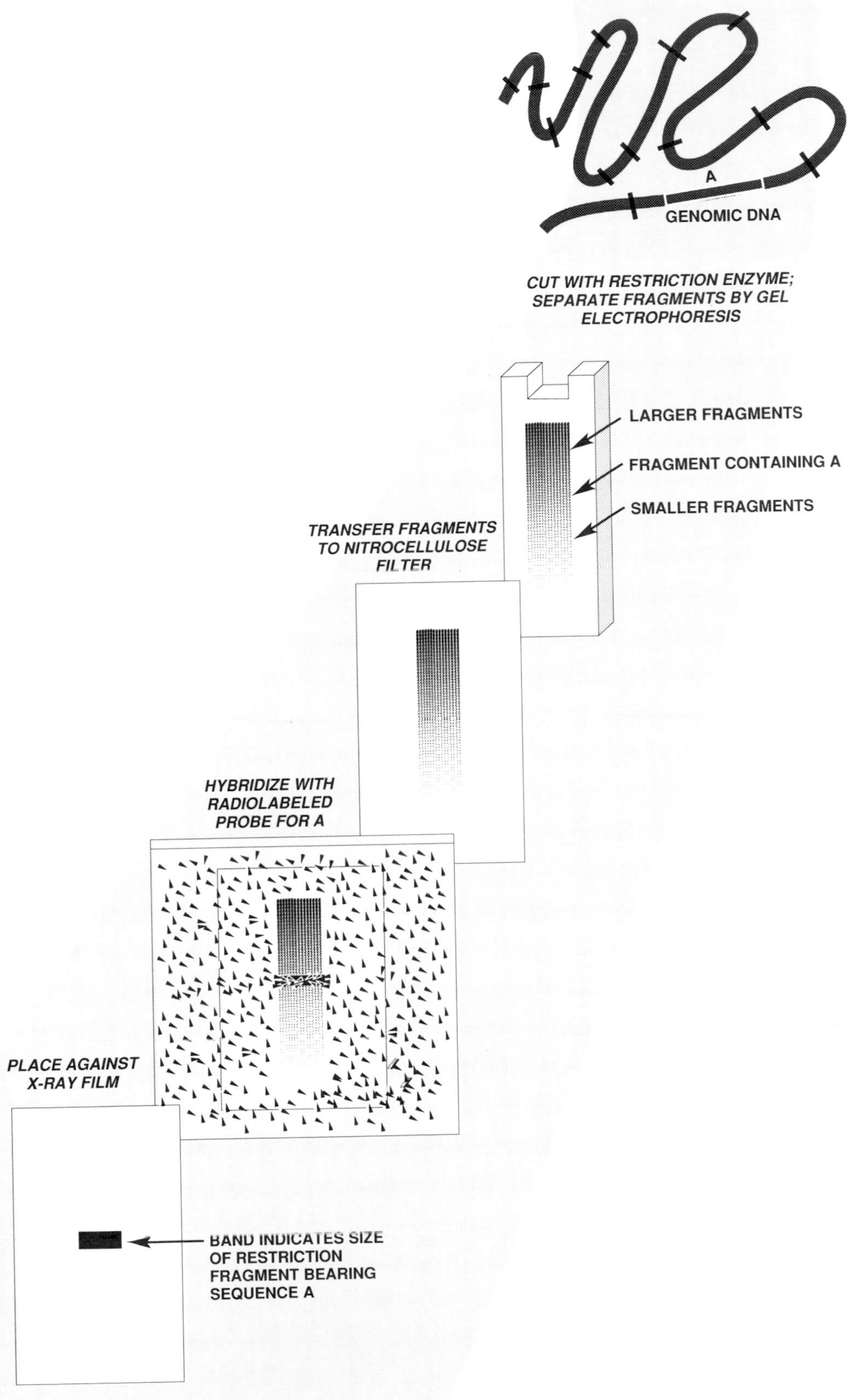

Figure 5.8. Southern blotting. This technique allows detection of a specific genomic fragment (here denoted as gene *A*) in a mixture of about a million such fragments.

digested with a restriction enzyme. The resulting myriad of fragments is separated by size on an electrophoretic gel and the DNA is then transferred to a nitrocellulose filter and hybridized with a labeled probe. Only those DNA fragments containing sequences homologous to the probe will be detected. Two sorts of mutational differences can be discovered when the result is compared to a normal pattern: (*a*) any rearrangement, such as a deletion or insertion, that is larger than 50–100 bp usually can be detected by a change in size of a fragment; and (*b*) a single base difference that creates or destroys a restriction site for the enzyme used to digest the DNA will result in an altered band size.

Restriction Fragment Length Polymorphisms

Another area in molecular genetics technology that has far-reaching consequences for human gene mapping (as we shall see in Chapter 9) is the concept of restriction fragment length polymorphisms (RFLPs). This phenomenon may at first seem like only a curiosity, but as we consider examples of the applications of molecular genetics to human disease, it will become clear that RFLPs provide the opportunity to follow human disease genes in families in ways that would otherwise be impossible.

As previously pointed out, the majority of human DNA is not involved in coding sequences and is therefore not subject to tight selection. Perhaps for this reason, differences in DNA sequence between individuals are not a rarity. Specifically, if one looks at the sequence of a noncoding autosomal region from 10 individual chromosomes, a nucleotide will be found approximately every 200 bp at which there is sequence variation. These variations usually take the form of simple base changes and are called DNA polymorphisms. Strictly speaking, in order for a nucleotide position to be called polymorphic in a given population of individuals, the most common sequence at that position should account for less than 99% of the sequences found in the total population.

DNA sequencing is, however, slow and impractical to do on a large scale (see below). But a subset of these sequence differences, namely those that destroy or create a recognition site for a restriction enzyme, can be readily detected using a simple Southern blot. Figure 5.9 shows an example of this situation. In this example, chromosome A

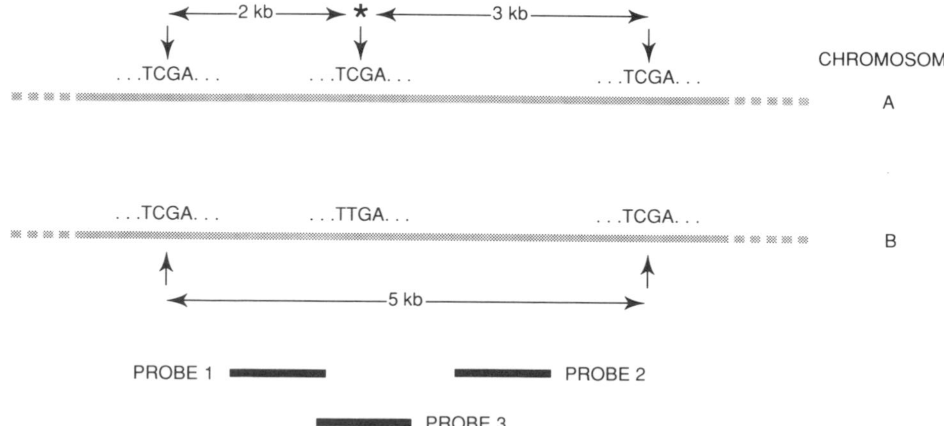

Figure 5.9. Restriction fragment length polymorphism (RFLP). Chromosomes A and B differ at a sequence marked by the *asterisk*, which results in the presence of a *TaqI* site for chromosome A but not for chromosome B; *TaqI* recognizes the sequence TCGA.

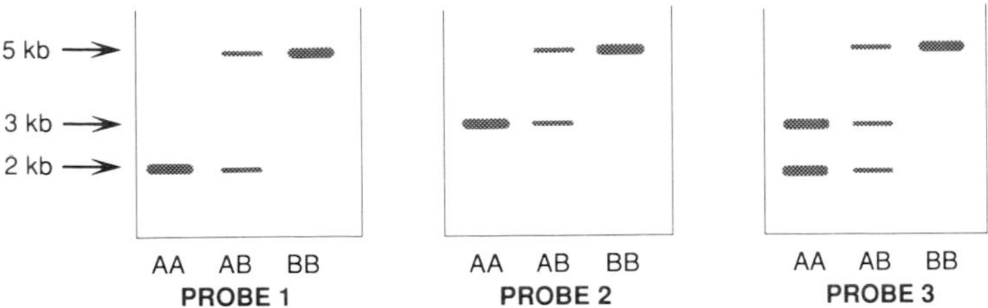

Figure 5.10. Southern blotting results of the *Taq*I polymorphism diagrammed in Figure 5.9, when probed with probe 1, 2, or 3. Note that the Southern blotting pattern depends on which probe was used because fragments are visualized only if they overlap the probe at least partially. AA is a homozygous individual for chromosome A, AB is a heterozygote, and BB is homozygous for chromosome B.

contains the sequence TCGA at the *asterisk,* whereas chromosome B carries TTGA. The restriction enzyme *Taq*I recognizes the sequence TCGA and therefore will cut the A chromosome at this position but not the B chromosome. The nearest flanking sites for *Taq*I are also shown in the figure; because most restriction sites are not polymorphic, in general the flanking sites are fixed and do not vary from one chromosome to the next. Therefore, the A chromosome when cut with *Taq*I would generate 2- and 3-kb fragments, whereas the B chromosome would generate a single 5-kb fragment. In order to visualize this difference, a Southern blot must be performed to detect these specific genomic fragments in the large background of other *Taq*I fragments generated from other places in the genome. Figure 5.10 shows the pattern that one would see, depending on whether probe 1, probe 2, or probe 3 was used. Note that the pattern differs as a function of which fragments are overlapped by the labeled probe. (A genomic fragment will be detected if even part of this DNA sequence is shared with the probe because these can then hybridize; it is not necessary for the entire probe sequence to overlap the genomic fragment.)

In the figure are shown the results that one would obtain for an individual who has two A chromosomes, one A and one B chromosome, or two B chromosomes.

There are four crucial things to remember in interpreting RFLP analysis. (*a*) The pattern observed on the blot depends on which probe is being used. This is clear from Figure 5.10. (*b*) In general, the base change detected by the restriction enzyme that leads to an RFLP is *not in itself responsible for disease,* but is a neutral change with no functional consequences. It can still be used, however, to mark a specific chromosome and follow its inheritance. On rare occasions, a mutation causing disease will actually alter a restriction site (sickle cell anemia is a case in point, which we will discuss in Chapter 6), but in general, this is not the case. (*c*) The inheritance of RFLP alleles strictly follows Mendelian expectation. Thus, for example, the offspring of an AA individual and a BB individual would all be AB. (*d*) In using RFLPs to follow the inheritance of a chromosome in a family, the most useful RFLPs (also called markers) will be those for which most individuals are heterozygous. While the reasons for this will not become fully clear until we consider some examples, it may be intuitively apparent that one cannot follow the inheritance of the two specific chromosomes from a homozygous AA individual.

The RFLPs we have considered so far are simple point polymorphisms that create or destroy a restriction site. A rarer but very useful type of polymorphism is diagrammed in Figure 5.11. These polymor-

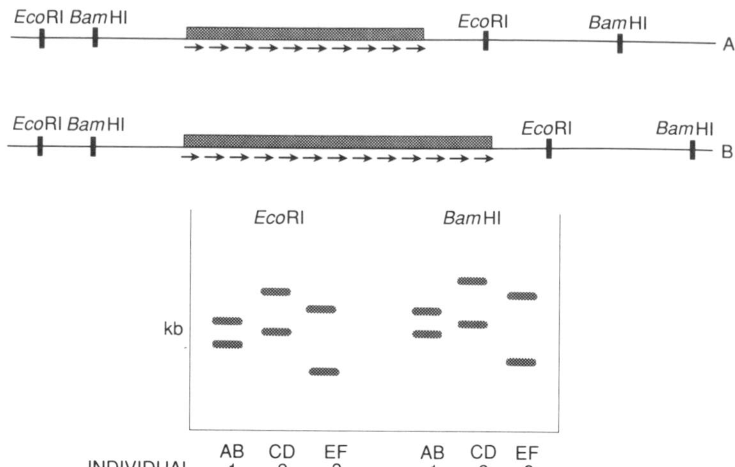

Figure 5.11. A variable number of tandem repeat (VNTR) polymorphism. The *boxed area* is a long array of a short tandemly repeated sequence. The number of the repeated elements varies from chromosome to chromosome, but is heritable. The different lengths can be visualized on a Southern blot, almost regardless of what restriction enzyme is used. An example of the results of analyzing three individuals with *Eco*RI and *Bam*HI demonstrates that all three are heterozygous, which is the major advantage of this sort of polymorphism.

phisms are called length polymorphisms or "variable number of tandem repeats" (VNTRs) and are created by the presence of short sequences arranged in a head-to-tail fashion and repeated multiple times in a tandem array. The function of such sequences, if any, remains unknown, but the number of repeated units within such an element (and hence, the total length of the element) frequently varies from one homologous chromosome to another. In this setting, any restriction enzyme that cuts outside the tandem repeat will generate a fragment whose length will reflect the size of the VNTR. The feature that makes these polymorphisms particularly useful is that a large number of alleles are possible because the total length of the repeat may take on a large number of different possibilities from chromosome to chromosome. In Figure 5.11 is shown an example of such a VNTR polymorphism. All three of the individuals shown are heterozygous. It turns out that the actual DNA sequences in these VNTR polymorphisms, which are scattered throughout the genome, are somewhat homologous to each other. Therefore, it is even possible to develop probes that detect many of these VNTR loci simultaneously. An example is shown in Figure 5.12, where a single probe has generated a very complex Southern blot pattern, which is obviously highly variable from one individual to the next. The variation is so extreme that the chances of seeing an identical pattern in two individuals who are not monozygotic twins is essentially zero. This allows the use of such probes to "fingerprint" specific individuals, which has found an important place in paternity testing and forensic medicine.

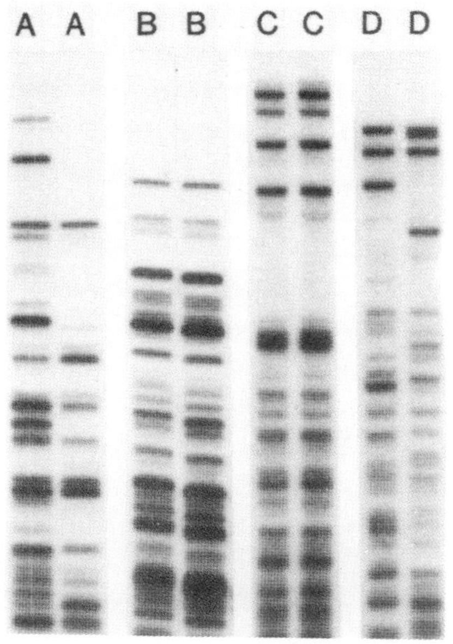

Figure 5.12. DNA fingerprint analysis using a single probe that detects a large number of VNTR polymorphisms located in widely scattered regions of the genome. Each pair of samples represents DNA from twins. Note the perfect match in B and C indicates that these are identical twins, whereas A and D are fraternal. Because the pattern detected by this probe is so variable from one individual to the next, it is quite useful in forensic medicine, where a perfect match of blood, skin, hair or semen DNA from the scene of a crime with DNA from a suspect can be used as strong evidence of guilt.

The usefulness of RFLPs may be clearer with the consideration of an example. As described in Chapter 3, hemophilia A is an X-linked recessive disorder due to a mutation in the gene for factor VIII. Defective factor VIII leads to an inability to form proper blood clots. The factor VIII gene has been cloned and is a very large gene approximately 200,000 bp in length (see Fig. 5.13). Most mutations in this gene that lead to hemophilia A turn out to be missense or nonsense mutations; they are therefore not easily detectable directly because Southern blot

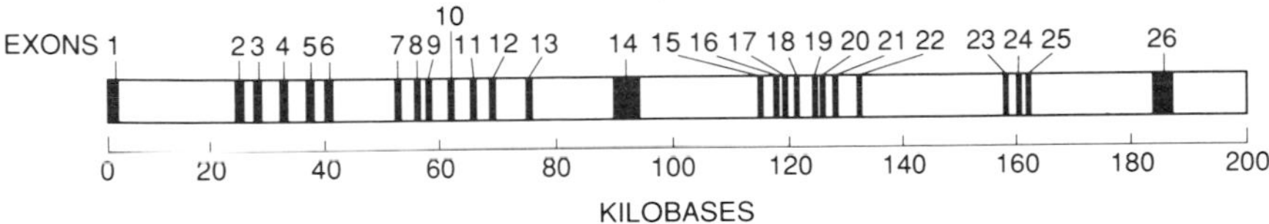

Figure 5.13. A map of the factor VIII gene on the X chromosome. Each exon is numbered, and the large size of the gene is apparent. Defects in the factor VIII gene, which produces a protein involved in blood clotting, result in hemophilia A. (From Lawn RM, Vehar GA: The molecular basis of hemophilia, Scientific American, (1986 Mar) 254:48–54)

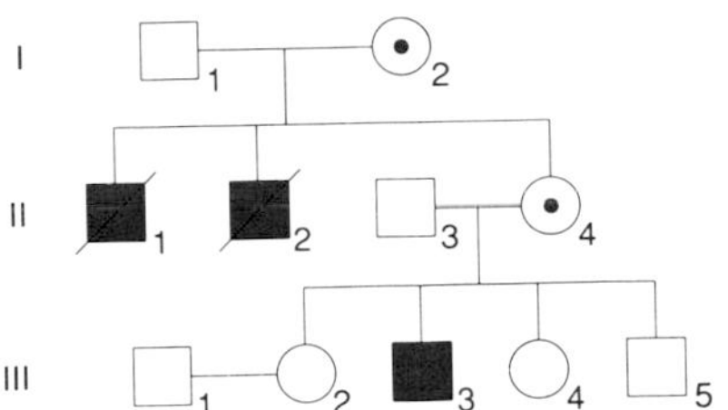

Figure 5.14. A typical pedigree of hemophilia A, demonstrating X-linked inheritance. Individual III-2 is at 50% risk of being a carrier based on the pedigree, but more precise information can be obtained using RFLP analysis.

patterns are unchanged. The sequencing of such a large region for each new mutation is quite impractical. In Figure 5.14 is shown a typical family in which hemophilia A is occurring. Note that there are affected males in generations II and III. Inspection of the pedigree indicates that I-2 and II-4 are obligate heterozygotes for hemophilia A. Individual III-2, whose risk of being a carrier is 50% based on the pedigree, wishes to be more sure of this risk before beginning a family. In general, carriers of hemophilia A are found to have approximately half normal protein levels of factor VIII in the blood, so this can sometimes be used to distinguish carriers from homozygous normal females. However, there is considerable overlap between the carrier and normal ranges, so that an unequivocal distinction is often not possible based on protein measurement. In a family such as this, a more accurate way to determine whether III-2 is a carrier is to use RFLPs. In Figure 5.15 is shown a restriction map of a region of an intron in the factor VIII gene that contains a polymorphism for the enzyme *Hin*dIII. If the polymorphic site is present and the probe indicated is used, a 3-kb fragment is generated, whereas if the polymorphic site is absent the fragment is 4 kb in length. To take advantage of this RFLP, DNA is obtained from white blood cells of all of the individuals of this family, and a Southern blot is per-

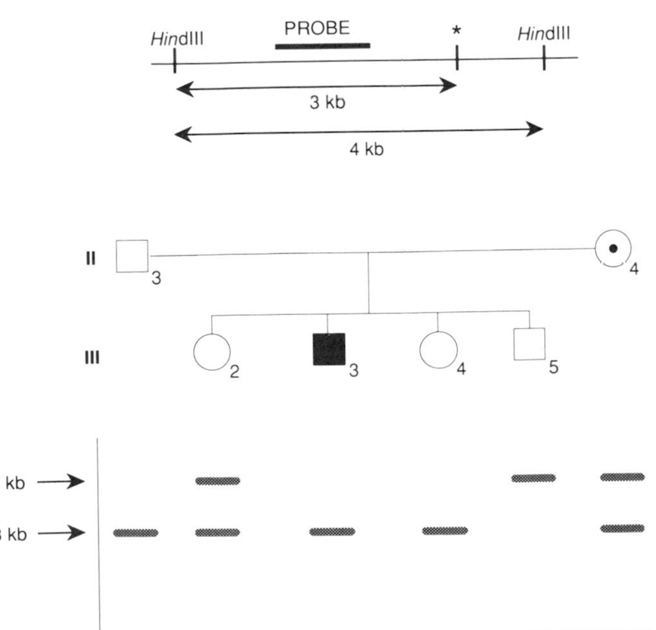

Figure 5.15. Diagram of an RFLP in an intron of the factor VIII gene, and the results of a Southern blot analysis on part of the family in Figure 5.14. The site marked with an *asterisk* is a polymorphic *Hin*dIII site. The results indicate that III-2 is *not* a carrier for hemophilia A.

formed with this intron probe. The results are shown in Figure 5.15. While this pattern may at first seem confusing, RFLP analyses are usually readily understood if one looks first at the affected individuals. Note that the affected male has only the 3-kb allele. This means that in this family the X chromosome carrying the hemophilia A mutation has a 3-kb allele for this particular RFLP. Note that this example illustrates an important point noted above; the *Hin*dIII RFLP itself (in an intron) is *not* the hemophilia mutation, but simply serves to mark the chromosome; other chromosomes with this same allele do not carry the hemophilia gene, as demonstrated by individual II-3.

To determine whether III-2 is a carrier is now relatively straightforward. Since she is a female she must have inherited an X chromosome from each parent. The father, who is XY, must have passed his 3-kb allele to her, and therefore the 4-kb allele must have come from her mother (II-4). But by looking at II-4's sons, it is clear that her hemophilia chromosome is the one with the 3-kb RFLP allele, whereas the 4-kb allele chromosome is normal. Therefore, III-2 inherited her mother's *normal* X chromosome and is not a carrier. Because this concept is so important, it is well worth studying this pedigree until the complete pattern of inheritance, both of the RFLP marker and of the hemophilia A gene, is clear. While in this example we have considered an X-linked recessive disease, RFLPs can also be very successfully used for autosomal dominant and autosomal recessive diseases, and we shall encounter many examples of this in later chapters.

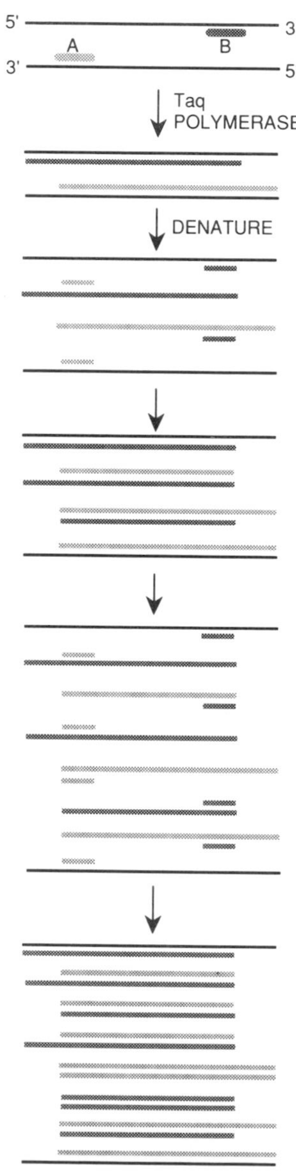

Figure 5.16. Diagram of the polymerase chain reaction. Repeated cycles of DNA synthesis using the A and B primers builds up an exponential amount of DNA located between these primers. Analysis of a large number of cycles (not shown) reveals that the major product after 20–30 cycles is DNA which begins precisely at the beginning of the A primer and ends precisely at the end of the B primer, as shown in the third and sixth duplexes of the last panel.

The Polymerase Chain Reaction (PCR)

A new development in DNA technology that has far-reaching consequences for diagnostics is the ability to amplify a short sequence of DNA from a complex mixture. This allows the analysis of a particular DNA fragment without first having to clone it, which greatly increases the speed of analysis. The principle of the method is diagrammed in Figure 5.16. It is necessary to synthesize two short "oligonucleotide" primers based upon the known sequence of the region. These primers, marked as A and B in Figure 5.15, can be chemically synthesized and are usually 20–35 nucleotides long. The primers are added to genomic DNA, which is then denatured to melt it into single-stranded DNA. Because the primers are present in great excess, each primer will "find" its complementary sequence in the genomic DNA and hybridize to it. An enzyme capable of withstanding temperatures as high as 95°C, called *Taq* polymerase, is also added, which synthesizes a DNA strand from the end of the annealed primer, using the genomic DNA as a template. The mixture is then denatured again, additional primers are annealed, and the polymerase reaction is carried out again. This entire process can be easily cycled, with each cycle requiring about 5 minutes, and as many as 30 or 40 cycles can be carried out without the need to add fresh enzyme or primers. As shown in the figure, the result of this is an exponential increase in the amount of DNA in the region between the two primers. The amount of this material doubles with each cycle; therefore, at the end of 30 cycles, this has been amplified 2^{30} times, or about 1 billion-fold. The practical consequence of this is that one can start with nanogram amounts of DNA, carry out the PCR, and then run the sample on a gel to visualize a specific band corresponding precisely to the distance between the A and B primers (including the length of the primers themselves).

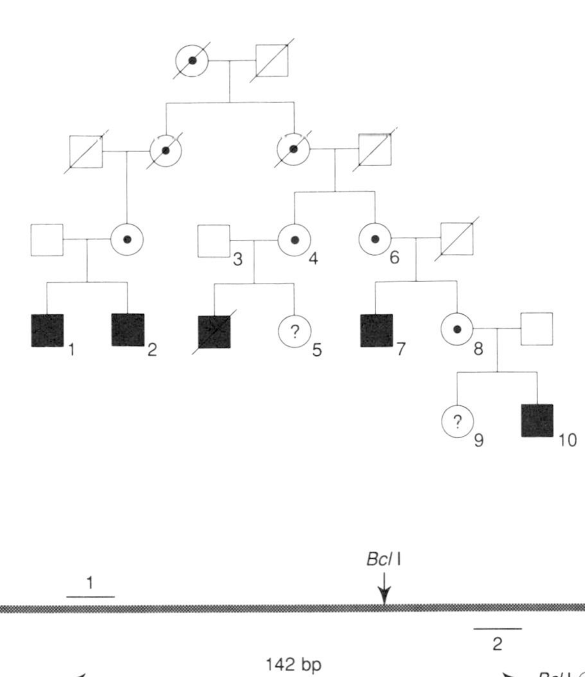

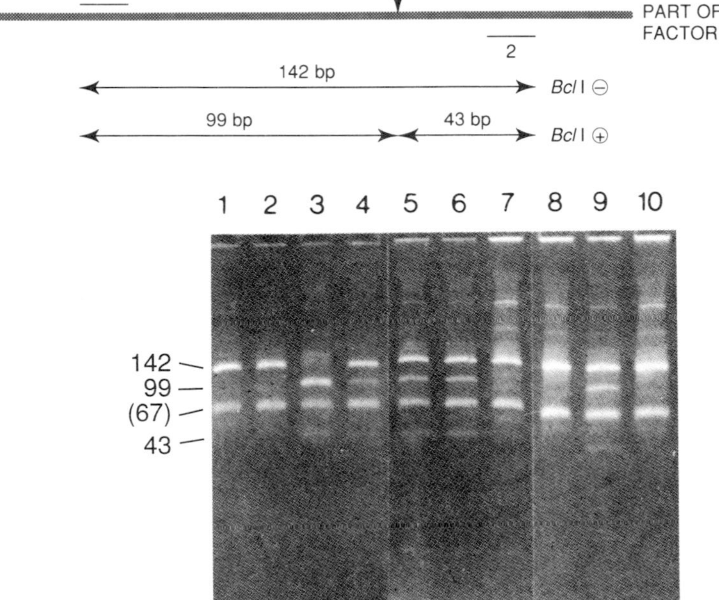

Figure 5.17. Another family with hemophilia A. Below the pedigree is a diagram of the region to be analyzed by PCR, showing the location of the primers and of the polymorphic *Bcl*I site. PCR with primers 1 and 2 gives a product of 142 bp, which when digested with *Bcl*I will give a 99-bp and a 43-bp product if the *Bcl*I site is present. The photograph shows the actual results of the analysis; the *numbers* above each lane correspond to the individual *numbers* on the pedigree. A constant band at 67 bp is of unknown origin and can be ignored for the purposes of this analysis. The hemophilia A gene is associated with the presence of the 142-bp band (i.e., lacking the *Bcl*I site) in all of the affected males. Careful inspection reveals that individual 5 must be a hemophilia carrier. The status of individual 9 cannot be determined because her mother is a homozygote for the polymorphism. (From Kogan SC, Doherty M, Gitschier J: An improved method for prenatal diagnosis of genetic diseases by analysis of amplified DNA sequences. Application to hemophilia A. N Engl J Med 317:985–990, 1987.)

This approach can be applied to the analysis of RFLPs quite readily. If the polymorphic restriction site is located between the primers, the amplified DNA can be cut with this enzyme and directly run on a gel to determine whether the site is present. An example is shown in Figure 5.17, which is an analysis of a family with hemophilia A. A *Bcl*I polymorphism in the factor VIII gene is being assessed in this family. A

PCR product of 142 bp is generated using primers 1 and 2; if the *Bcl*I site is present, digestion with this enzyme yields bands of 99 and 43 bp, whereas if it is absent the full 142 bp is seen. It can be readily appreciated that all of the males with hemophilia have the 142-bp band, indicating that the X chromosome carrying the hemophilia mutation lacks the *Bcl*I site. The advantage of the analysis shown in Figure 5.17 over that in Figure 5.14 is 2-fold. In the first place, PCR is much more rapid, with the results of the analysis available in a few hours rather than a few days. In the second place, only a tiny amount of genomic DNA is needed from each individual. Successful PCR has been carried out, for example, using DNA prepared from saliva specimens (which contain enough epithelial cells to provide sufficient DNA for PCR) or even from archived blocks of paraffin-embedded tissue stored in surgical pathology laboratories from patients long since deceased.

The use of PCR is not limited to detection of nucleotide changes that alter a restriction site. The ability to use PCR to generate an essentially pure sample of a single DNA fragment also makes it possible to carry out delicate hybridization experiments that allow the detection of single nucleotide differences of all sorts. In Figure 5.18 is diagrammed a method for doing this, applied to the detection of the mutation causing sickle cell anemia (see Chapter 6). In addition to the oligonucleotides synthesized to carry out PCR, one also generates "allele-specific oligonucleotides" (ASOs) for the internal part of the fragment, located over the site of the DNA sequence difference. The ASOs are usually 15–19 bp in length; careful hybridization experiments (primarily by controlling the temperature and salt concentration) will allow the "perfect match" ASO to hybridize efficiently to its target, whereas the ASO with a single nucleotide mismatch will not hybridize. In general, one synthesizes ASOs for both of the possible sequences of a given region and separately tests each probe on PCR-amplified material, labeling the ASO so that it is possible to tell whether it hybridized or not to the PCR-amplified DNA. An example, as applied to the same hemophilia family of Figure 5.17, is shown in Figure 5.19. One ASO has been synthesized to be a perfect match for the chromosome containing the *Bcl*I site (TGATCA is the recognition site for *Bcl*I). The other ASO matches the chromosome that does not have the *Bcl*I site, which has TGAACA instead. Genomic DNA from the family has been amplified by PCR, and then small amounts of this DNA have been applied to nitrocellulose in elliptical slots. The upper strip has been hybridized with the labeled *Bcl*I+ ASO, and the lower strip with the labeled *Bcl*I− ASO. After washing off the excess ASO probes, the filter is placed against x-ray film. The results completely agree with the gel analysis shown in Figure 5.17. Note, however, that this ASO method did not depend on the presence of a restriction site at the location of the nucleotide difference between the chromosomes, but could have been applied to detect *any* difference. One must, however, know sequence information about a particular region in order to carry out PCR, since the oligonucleotide primers and the ASOs depend upon this information.

Northern Blotting

Cloned DNA probes can also be used to analyze whether or not a gene is being transcribed ("expressed"). Messenger RNA is prepared from the tissue of interest and separated on a gel by size. The RNA can then be transferred to a filter and hybridized with a DNA probe. (This

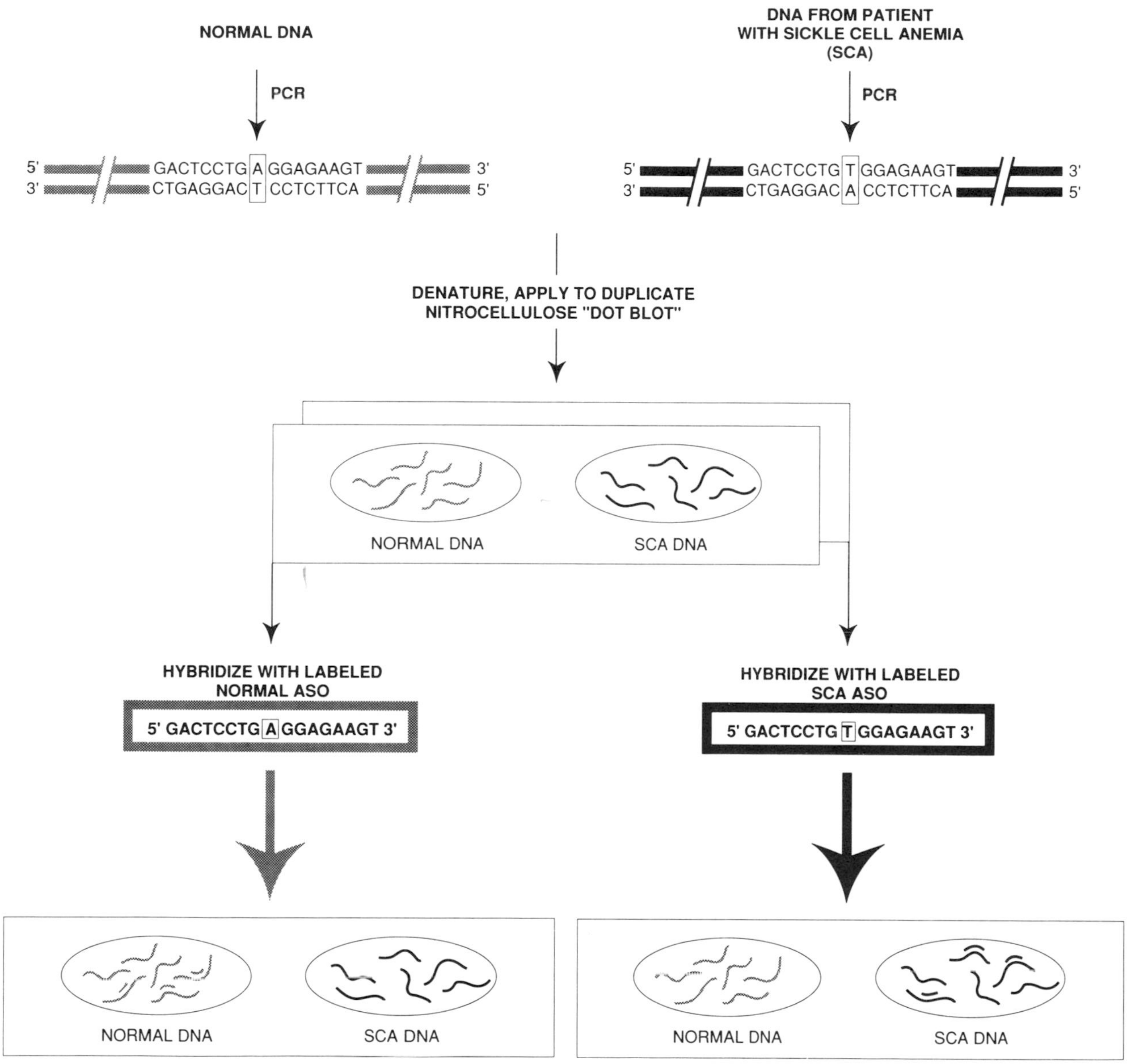

NORMAL DNA

PCR

5' GACTCCTG A GGAGAAGT 3'
3' CTGAGGAC T CCTCTTCA 5'

DNA FROM PATIENT WITH SICKLE CELL ANEMIA (SCA)

PCR

5' GACTCCTG T GGAGAAGT 3'
3' CTGAGGAC A CCTCTTCA 5'

DENATURE, APPLY TO DUPLICATE NITROCELLULOSE "DOT BLOT"

NORMAL DNA SCA DNA

HYBRIDIZE WITH LABELED NORMAL ASO

5' GACTCCTG A GGAGAAGT 3'

HYBRIDIZE WITH LABELED SCA ASO

5' GACTCCTG T GGAGAAGT 3'

NORMAL DNA SCA DNA

NORMAL DNA SCA DNA

Figure 5.18. Detection of single base differences in DNA using allele-specific oligonucleotides (ASOs). In this example, the ASOs are designed to detect the difference between normal DNA and DNA containing the mutation causing sickle cell anemia. This disease is caused by an A to T change in the β-globin gene (see Chapter 6). Under careful hybridization conditions, the labeled "perfect-match" ASO will stick to the target DNA, but a single-mismatch ASO will not; this allows a clear distinction of the two DNA samples.

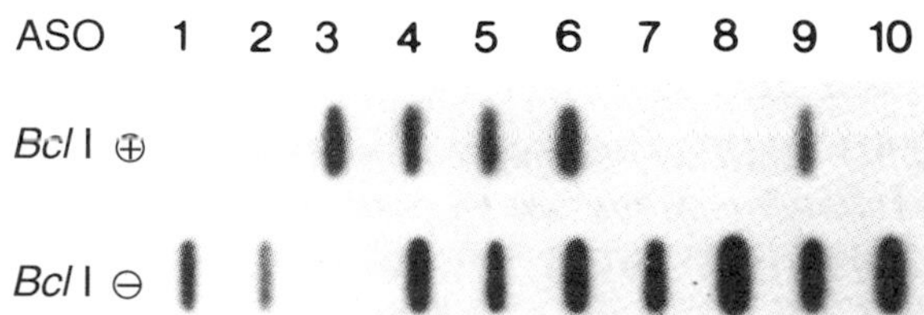

Figure 5.19. Analysis of the pedigree in Figure 5.17 using ASO testing of PCR-amplified DNA. The results are the same as the gel analysis in Figure 5.17. (From Kogan SC, Doherty M, Gitschier J: An improved method for prenatal diagnosis of genetic diseases by analysis of amplified DNA sequences. Application to hemophilia A. New Engl J Med 317:985–990, 1987.)

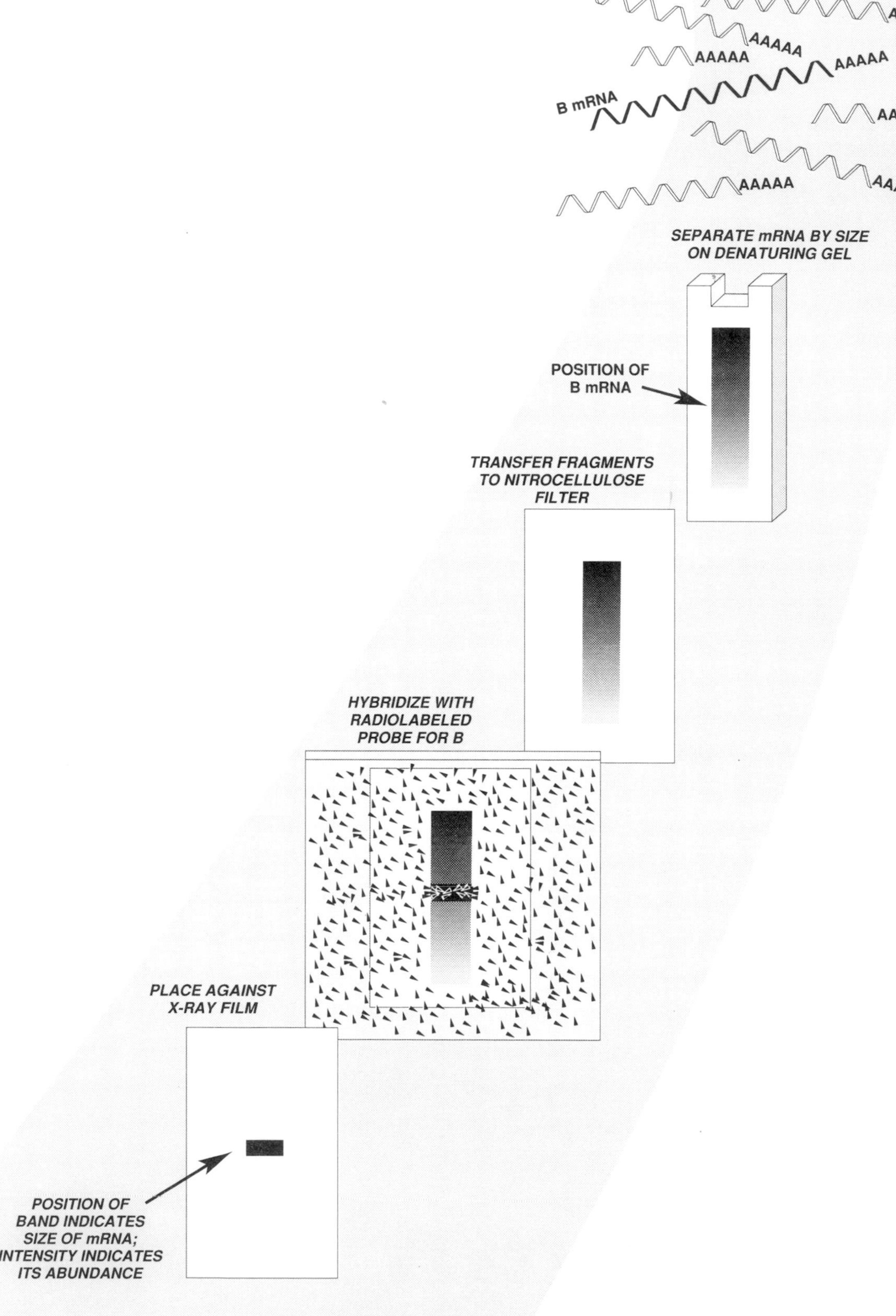

Figure 5.20. Northern blotting. A specific RNA molecule (here denoted as *B*) can be detected in a complex mixture by this procedure. The size of the RNA can be determined by how far it has migrated in the gel, and its abundance by the intensity of the band.

is called a "Northern blot" (Fig. 5.20).) As it happens, DNA-RNA hybrids are even more stable than DNA-DNA hybrids. The resulting band identified by the probe indicates the size of the mRNA, and the intensity of the band is a rough indication of its abundance. In searching for mutation, this approach can uncover mRNAs of abnormal size as well as alterations in the level of expression.

The exact nucleotide sequence of a cloned fragment of DNA can also readily be determined. In one procedure, the Sanger method (Fig. 5.21), an enzymatic approach is used, whereas in the other method (the Maxam-Gilbert method), a chemical degradation process is employed.

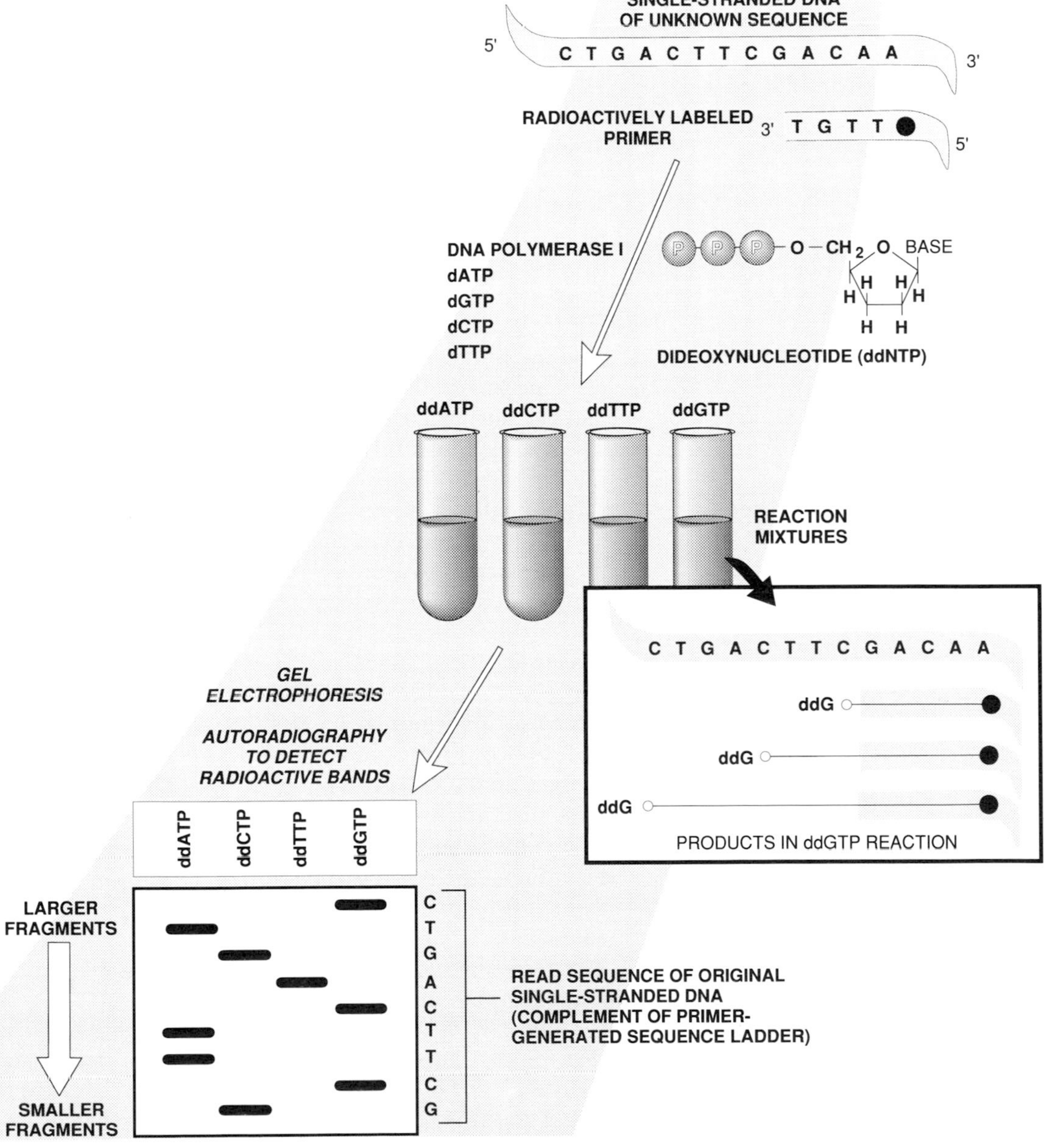

Figure 5.21. The DNA sequencing method developed by Sanger. Using a primer homologous to one end of a DNA strand to be sequenced, the complementary strand is synthesized using DNA polymerase. Small amounts of a dideoxynucleotide (ddATP, ddCTP, ddTTP, ddGTP) are included in four separate such reactions; when a dideoxynucleotide is incorporated into a growing chain, synthesis of that molecule stops. Separation of the resultant labeled fragments in *four lanes* of a polyacrylamide gel, followed by exposure to x-ray film, allows the sequence to be read off directly.

In both procedures, the result is a ladder of bands from which the DNA sequence can be directly read. A region of approximately 300 bp can routinely be sequenced in a single set of reactions, and recent progress in automation has raised the theoretical possibility of sequencing the entire human genome in the next 10–20 years (see Chapter 12).

Gene Transfer

The sequence of a gene is extremely useful, as it predicts precisely the amino acid sequence of the resulting protein. However, it is not possible to look at the sequence of a gene or its flanking regions and predict how that gene will be regulated or in what tissues it will be expressed. To obtain this information, it is highly desirable to have a system for gene transfer, where a gene can be sequenced, altered in any way desirable by removing certain sequences or changing others, and then placed back into cells and its expression into mRNA and protein studied. When the gene is to be put back into cells that grow in culture flasks, the method of gene transfer is often to create a precipitate of the DNA along with calcium phosphate. Such precipitates are taken up by many types of cells, and the DNA finds its way into the nucleus and is expressed. In a small proportion of such transfected cells, the foreign DNA actually becomes covalently integrated into a chromosome at a random site. For cells that do not seem to take up such precipitates, a new method called electroporation has been applied. In this approach, cells are suspended in a buffer containing the DNA to be transferred, and the suspension is subjected to a short, high voltage, electric pulse. The pulse apparently punches holes in the cytoplasmic and nuclear membranes of the cells so that some of the DNA enters the nucleus and subsequently is expressed.

An exciting recent development has been the transfer of genes into mouse oocytes just after fertilization, using a very fine pipette to inject the purified DNA under direct vision. The oocyte is then reimplanted into a different mouse and normal embryogenesis of the injected egg proceeds. About 10–30% of the mouse progeny are found to have covalently integrated several copies of the injected DNA into their germline DNA, so that these sequences are transmitted in a Mendelian fashion to future offspring. In many instances, the injected gene is also transcribed by the mouse. This provides an excellent way of studying what sequences are necessary to direct proper developmental and tissue-specific expression of a given gene. The process is diagrammed in Figure 5.22. Figure 5.23 shows a picture of a mouse that was derived from such an experiment, in which the injected gene was a growth hormone gene engineered in such a way as to produce large quantities of the hormone. The resulting increase in size of the mouse relative to its normal littermate is apparent.

Finally, gene transfer can be accomplished by use of a retrovirus (Fig. 5.24). Retroviruses are RNA viruses that encode a reverse transcriptase so that they are transcribed into DNA upon entering a host cell. The virus contains specific sequences that promote its integration into the host genome. Retroviruses can be engineered in such a way to delete their usual genes and replace them with DNA sequences coding for a gene one wishes to transfer into cells. The advantage of this technique is the very high efficiency, which can approach 100%, with which such vectors can enter cells. In fact, retroviruses have many properties that make them ideal candidates for gene therapy, as is discussed in Chapter 12.

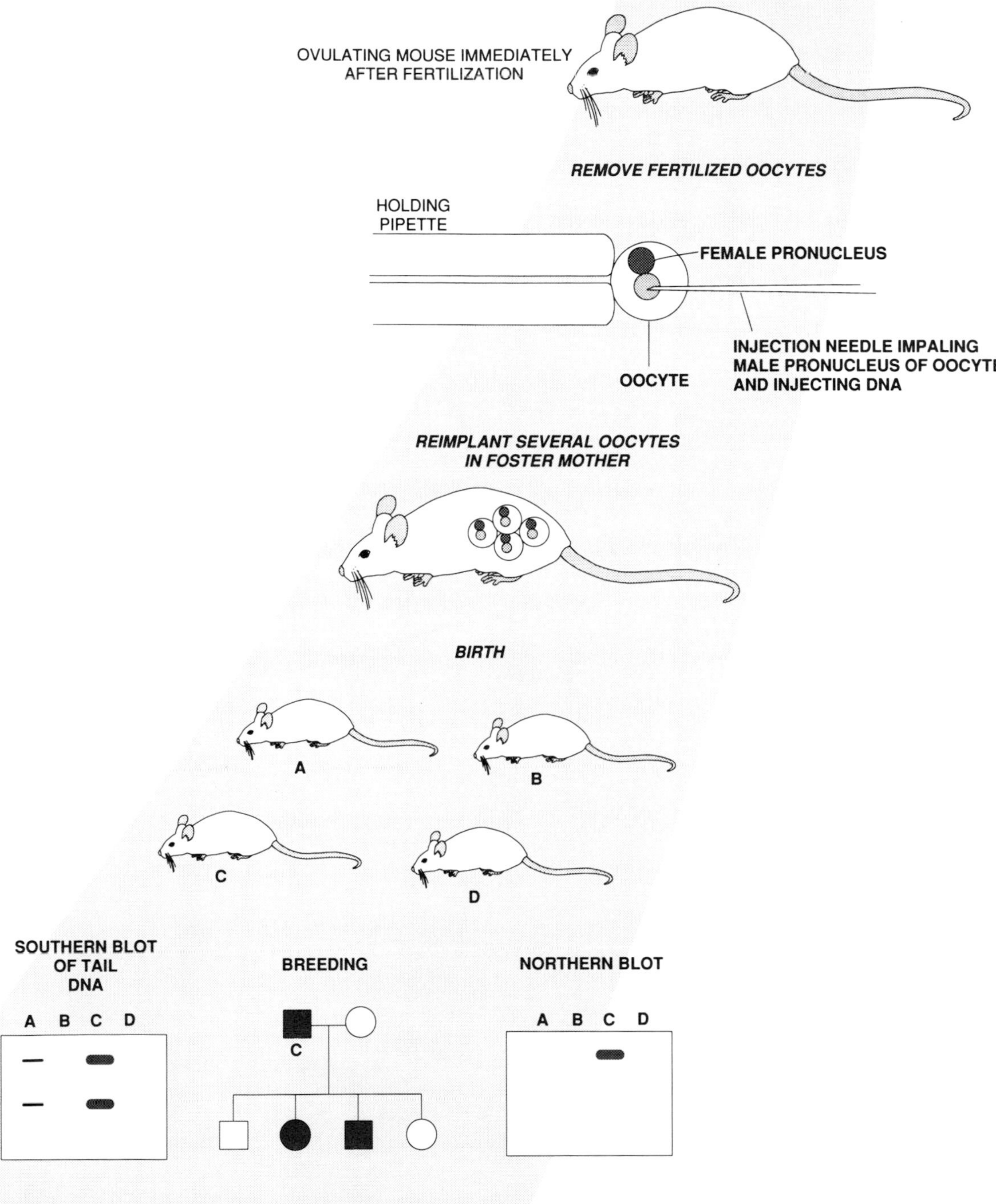

Figure 5.22. Generation of transgenic mice. With the aid of a microscope, oocytes are obtained surgically just after fertilization, before the male and female pronuclei have fused. Under direct vision, the cloned DNA to be transferred to the mouse genome is injected into the male pronucleus; the pronuclei then fuse, and in a proportion of eggs the injected DNA will be covalently integrated into a random site in the mouse genome. The oocytes are then reimplanted surgically into a foster mother whose uterus has been primed suitably by hormonal treatment. After delivery, the animals can be checked for the presence of the injected DNA by a Southern blot of a small amount of DNA, most conveniently prepared from a tail tip. Transcription of this sequence can be assessed by Northern blotting. In this example, animals *A* and *C* have incorporated the injected DNA, whereas *B* and *D* are negative. *C* has more DNA copies than *A* (commonly 1–200 copies occur) and also expresses the gene, whereas *A* does not. The transgene ordinarily is transmitted to offspring in Mendelian dominant fashion.

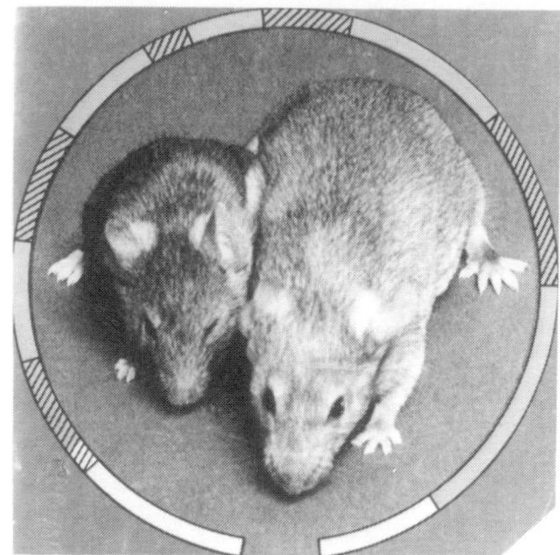

Figure 5.23. Mouse and supermouse. The smaller mouse on the *left* is a normal (nontransgenic) animal, whereas the larger mouse is transgenic for a rat growth hormone gene, which was constructed in such a way that growth hormone is overproduced. The transgenic mouse has attained a weight two to three times normal as a result of this intervention. (From Palmiter RD, Norstedt G, Gelinas RE, Hammer RE, Brinster RL: Metallothionein-human GH fusion genes stimulate growth of mice. Science 222:809–814, 1983.)

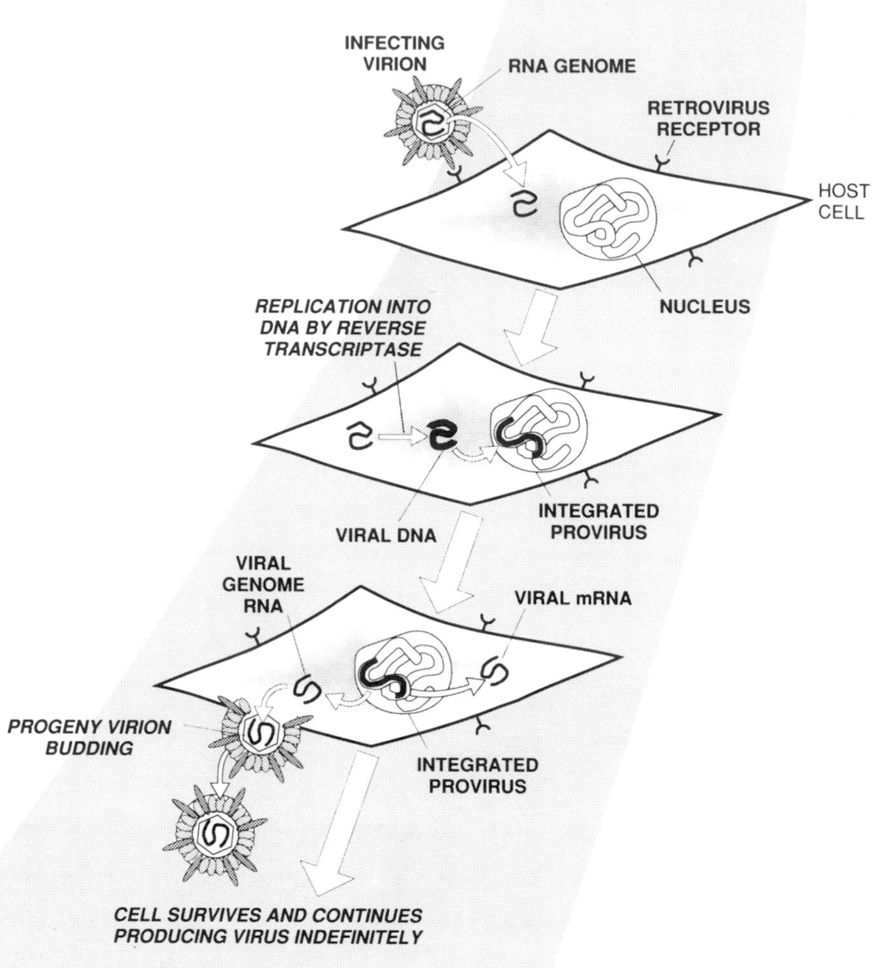

Figure 5.24. Overview of the life cycle of a retrovirus. The infecting virion, which carries its own reverse transcriptase, enters the cell and has its RNA genome copied to DNA. Special sequences in the viral DNA genome promote its incorporation into the host genome, where it can direct the synthesis of multiple copies of itself. The efficiency of this process makes retroviruses an attractive system for attempting gene therapy (see Chapter 12).

ANATOMY OF A HUMAN GENE

With a few notable exceptions, all of the cells of the human body contain the complete genome. Yet, in any given tissue only a relatively small proportion of these genes are being expressed. Therefore, the control of gene expression is fundamental to understanding virtually all aspects of human biology.

In general, it is the mature protein product of a gene that carries out its controlling influence. The level of this mature protein can be altered by (*a*) the rate of transcription of the gene into RNA; (*b*) the processing of this RNA; (*c*) the transport of the mRNA from nucleus to cytoplasm; (*d*) the rate of translation of the mRNA into protein on cellular ribosomes; (*e*) the rate of degradation of the mRNA; (*f*) posttranslational modifications of the protein; and (*g*) the rate of degradation of the protein. All of these control mechanisms have been implicated in specific instances. The most economical method of control, however, and one which is widespread in eukaryotes is to control the protein production at its earliest level, namely that of transcription of the gene. Fig-

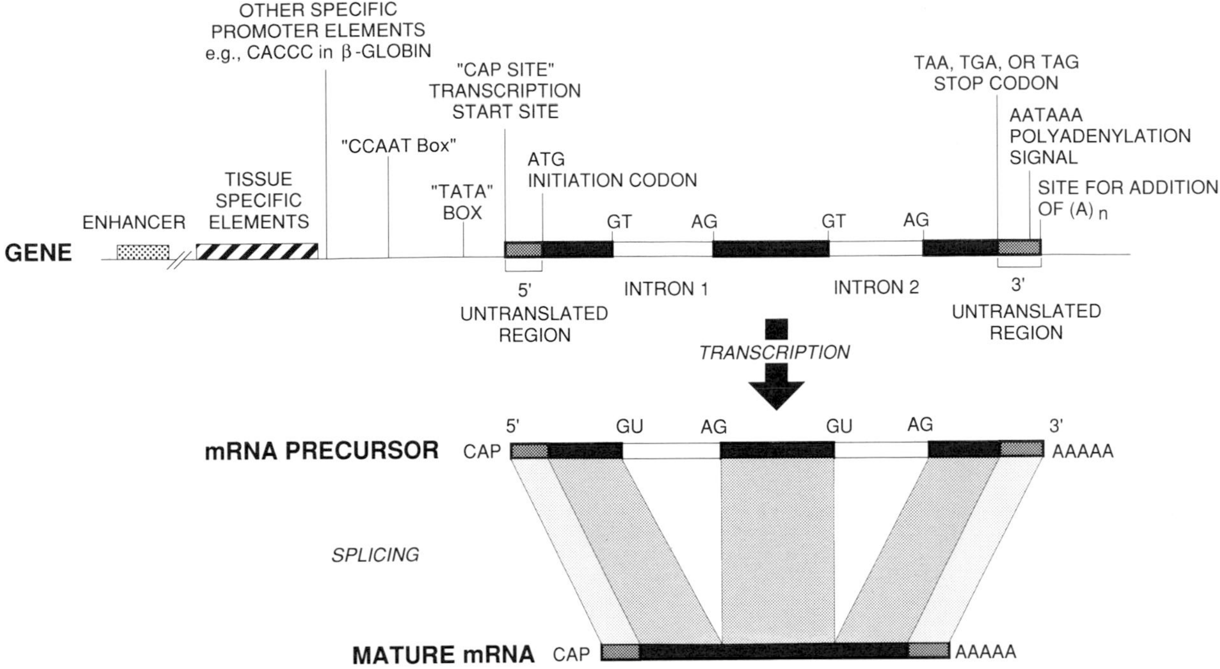

Figure 5.25. Structure and expression of an idealized gene, including various promoter elements, an enhancer, and the transcribed region of the gene. In the example shown, the gene has two introns, each beginning with GT and ending with AG; these are spliced out to generate the mature mRNA. As described in the text, not only promoter elements but also enhancers can be tissue specific.

ure 5.25 shows a schematic of the control elements of an idealized human gene. The important sequence elements have been identified by a variety of methods, including mutational analysis, evolutionary comparison, and functional assays using gene transfer into cultured cells or transgenic mice.

The Promoter

The promoter is somewhat loosely defined as the sequence elements located 5′ to the gene; these elements fix the site of transcription initiation and control mRNA quantity and sometimes tissue specificity. While in some situations the promoter elements may extend for several kilobases, in many instances the important promoter elements seem to be located in the region 300–400 bp 5′ to the gene.

Most but not all human genes contain a conserved "TATA box" sequence, which is located 25–30 bp 5′ to the start of transcription, and seems to be involved in the precise localization of the start. Further upstream, there is often a "CCAAT box" sequence located 75–80 bp 5′ to the start site, although this is less commonly present than the TATA box. In those genes with a CCAAT box, its presence seems to be required for quantitatively efficient transcription, at least in gene transfer experiments. Notably, some "housekeeping" genes, which encode enzymes that are present in virtually all cells, are usually lacking both of these boxes and contain promoters that are highly enriched in C and G nucleotides.

The tissue of expression of many genes is tightly regulated, and such regulation must be mediated by sequences in the vicinity of the gene that interact with tissue-specific factors. Such sequences would not be expected to be the same, therefore, between genes expressed in dif-

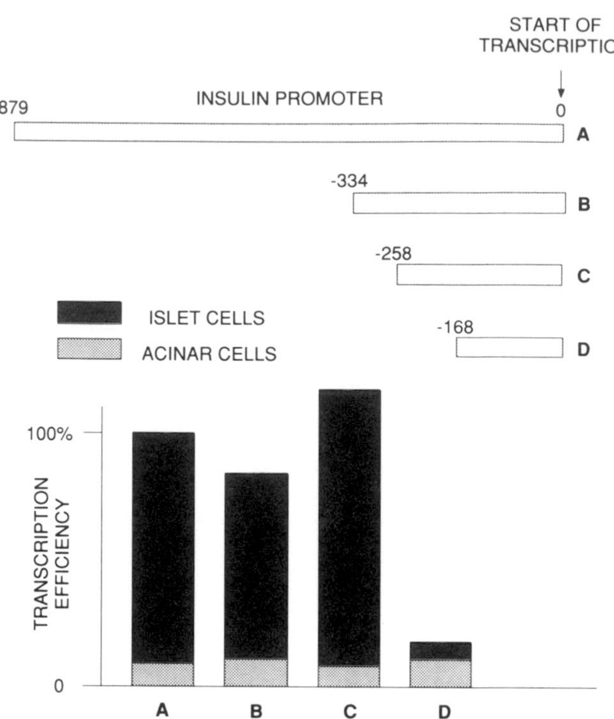

Figure 5.26. The insulin promoter. Sequences in the region 5′ to the start of transcription are responsible for the fact that the insulin gene is efficiently expressed in pancreatic islet cells, which normally produce insulin, but not in acinar cells, which do not. By deleting successively greater amounts of DNA from the 5′ end, the efficient transcription in islet cells is lost when a sequence located in the −168 to −258 region is removed, suggesting that an important promoter element lies in this region.

ferent tissues, and thus their identification by simple sequence comparison has been difficult. The most successful approaches to this important issue have involved deletion or mutation of portions of the gene, followed by gene transfer into cultured cells or transgenic mice. In the insulin gene, for example, elements located 168–258 bp 5′ to the initiation site have been identified, which are capable of conferring pancreatic islet cell specificity (see Fig. 5.26).

Promoter elements also serve to fix the start site of transcription to a particular location, although some degree of heterogeneity of starts in a 10–20-bp region is often seen, especially with genes lacking a TATA box. A particular modified nucleotide, 7-methylguanosine, called a "cap," is added to the 5′ end of the growing mRNA chain. Thus, the site of initiation of transcription is also often called the "cap site."

Splicing

As noted previously, most eukaryotic genes have their coding regions interrupted by introns, which must be removed, in a process called splicing, in order to generate a mature mRNA that can be trans-

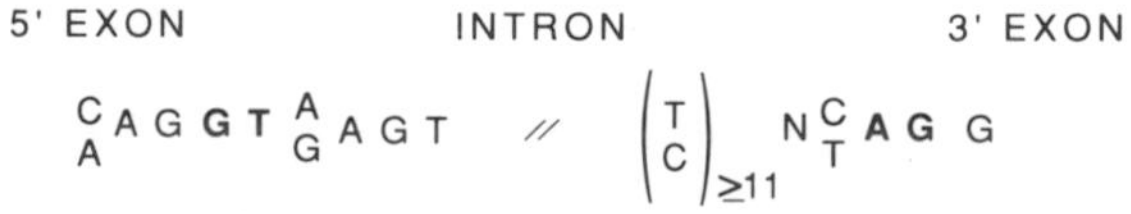

5′ EXON INTRON 3′ EXON

$^{C}_{A}$AG**GT**$^{A}_{G}$AGT // $\left(^{T}_{C}\right)_{\geq 11}$ N$^{C}_{T}$**AG** G

Figure 5.27. Consensus sequences found at 5′ and 3′ splice sites. The GT at the beginning of the intron and the AG at the end are invariant, whereas some deviation from the rest of the consensus sequence is usually seen. The position marked *N* can be any nucleotide (A, C, G, or T).

lated into a functional protein. While the function of introns remains unclear, the mechanism of splicing is beginning to be understood. At the beginning and end of an intron, certain nucleotide sequences are found (Fig. 5.25). The intron always begins with a GT (the splice donor) and ends with an AG (the splice acceptor), and other adjacent bases tend to follow a certain sequence (referred to as a consensus (Fig. 5.27)). However, these consensus sequences, while necessary, are not entirely sufficient for recognition by the splicing apparatus; one can find consensus splice donor or acceptor sequences in transcribed genes which are not used. Interestingly, inactivation of the normal splice signal by mutation occasionally activates one of these "cryptic" splice signals.

The mechanism by which a particular splice donor "finds" the correct acceptor remains unclear. A 5′ to 3′ scanning model would be one possibility, but is not consistent with the pattern of splicing seen in the presence of certain splice acceptor mutations. A random search mechanism, however, is not tenable, given the fact that some genes such as collagen (Chapter 7) contain up to 50 separate introns and yet always connect the correct donor to the correct acceptor.

Polyadenylation

Messenger RNAs that code for protein are characterized by the addition of a string of about 200 adenosine residues at their 3′ end (polyadenylation), which seems to be involved in their transport out of the nucleus. A hexanucleotide signal AAUAAA in the 3′-untranslated region is a consistent feature of such mRNAs, although other sequences in the vicinity also may play a role in correct polyadenylation. The A residues are added at a point 18–20 bp downstream from this AAUAAA signal.

Enhancers

Enhancers are DNA sequences defined by the following properties: (*a*) they increase transcription from a nearby gene; (*b*) they operate over considerable distances and are relatively unaffected by altering this distance; and (*c*) they are effective even if inverted. The first enhancers characterized were those of certain DNA viruses such as SV40, which bears a 72-bp twice-repeated sequence meeting these criteria, capable of increasing transcription from a large number of genes in almost any tissue tested. More recently, tissue-specific enhancers have been discovered. Perhaps the best example of the latter is the enhancer located in the immunoglobulin gene, which has been shown to be functional in B cells (which synthesize immunoglobulin) but not in other tissue types.

DNA REARRANGEMENTS

In general, DNA remains in the form present in the germline throughout all of the somatic cells of the human organism. Notable exceptions occur, however, in the cells of the immune system. The immunoglobulin molecule consists of two light chains and two heavy chains, and the highly variable (*V*) regions permit these antibodies to bind to a wide repertoire of antigens. Each B cell, however, makes just one kind of antibody. DNA rearrangement of the heavy and light chains of the immunoglobulin molecule is responsible for this "commitment" and is shown for the heavy chain gene in Figure 5.28. In the unexpressed germline configuration, a large number of variable (*V*) regions are fol-

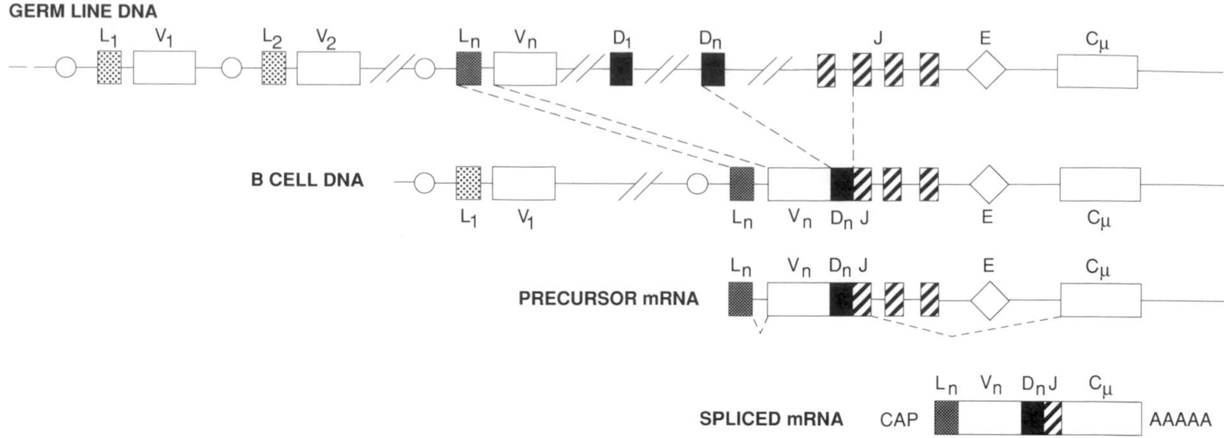

Figure 5.28. Organization and rearrangement of the immunoglobulin heavy chain locus. On the *top line* is depicted the germ line configuration. *Stippled blocks* marked by L_1, L_2, etc. represent leader sequence exons and are each preceded by a promoter *(circle)* and followed by a variable region coding exon (V_1, V_2, etc.). The numerous *V* region exons are followed by a smaller number of diversity regions *(D, dark blocks),* which are in turn followed by junction regions *(J, crosshatched).* Within the intron between the last *J* region and the constant region coding block (*C*) is located a tissue-specific enhancer (*E*) sequence. At the time of B-cell commitment, a rearrangement occurs at the DNA level to generate the structure shown in the *second line,* where a specific L_n-V_n region has attached to a particular D_n region, deleting the intervening DNA, and this has joined to a particular *J* region, also by deletion. Note that this rearrangement brings the promoter for the L_n-V_n region into relative proximity to the enhancer sequence, which may at least partially account for its transcriptional activation. Transcription starts at the beginning of the leader exon and proceeds through the entire rearranged gene; the precursor mRNA is then processed by splicing and polyadenylation to generate the mature mRNA, which is transported to the cytoplasm and translated to generate a heavy chain. The large number of possible outcomes of heavy chain and light chain gene rearrangement allows for an enormous potential repertoire of antibodies.

lowed by several diversity (*D*) regions, six joining (*J*) regions, and then several constant regions, which determine which type of immunoglobulin chain (IgM, IgG, IgA, etc.) is going to be produced. At the time of commitment of a B cell, an irreversible DNA rearrangement takes place that brings one of the V regions, one of the D regions, and one of the J regions into contiguity. The intervening segments of DNA are deleted. Note that this is occurring at the *DNA* level. This rearrangement juxtaposes the necessary transcription signals to allow the onset of RNA production from a locus that has successfully rearranged. In particular, the promoter for the specific V region that has been involved in the rearrangement is brought in close enough proximity to the enhancer (*E*) in Figure 5.28 to activate its transcription. A similar process occurs for the light chain gene. The resulting combinatorial diversity of protein production allows for an enormous range of antigen recognition sites. A similar somatic DNA rearrangement takes place in certain T cells of the immune system to allow the production of antigen-specific T-cell receptors.

CONCLUSION

We have reviewed the gross and detailed structure of genes and gene families and the powerful methods of recombinant DNA technology that have made possible such a remarkable understanding of human molecular biology. Armed with this background about normal structure and function, we are now ready to move forward into an analysis of the molecular basis of human disease, which will occupy us for the next two chapters.

SUGGESTED READINGS

Botstein D, White RL, Skolnick M, Davis RW: Construction of a genetic linkage map in man using restriction fragment length polymorphisms. Am J Hum Genet 32:314–331, 1980.

Caskey CT: Disease diagnosis by recombinant DNA methods. Science 236:1223–1229, 1987.

Mitchell PJ, Tjian R: Transcriptional regulation in mammalian cells by sequence-specific DNA binding proteins. Science 245:371–378, 1989.

Nakamura Y, et al.: Variable number of tandem repeat (VNTR) markers for human gene mapping. Science 235:1616–1622, 1987.

Orkin SH: Molecular genetics and inherited human disease. In: Scriver CR, Beaudet AL, Sly WS, Valle D, eds. *The Metabolic Basis of Inherited Disease.* 6th Ed. New York, McGraw-Hill, 1989, pp. 165–175.

Palmiter R, Brinster RL: Germline transformation of mice. Annu Rev Genet 20:465–499, 1986.

Watson JD, Tooze J, Kurtz DT: *Recombinant DNA. A Short Course.* Scientific American Books, New York, WH Freeman, 1983.

Watson JD, Hopkins NH, Roberts JW, Steitz JA, Weiner AM: *Molecular Biology of the Gene.* 4th Ed. Menlo Park, CA, Benjamin/Cummings, 1986.

5/ Study Questions

1/ A gene for an enzyme is made up of three exons. Shown below is the sequence of the DNA of the sense strand for the first two exons (*capital letters*) as well as some of the sequence (*lower case letters*) around these exons.

. . . accggcagtagATATCAGACCATGCTAATCGCTCCCCGACAGgtaagttgca . . .

atgaacgcaatatccttcctctcgacagGGGTAGTTT . . .

a. How many bases are in the first exon? How many amino acids in the enzyme are encoded by this exon? Write them down. (Hint: Where does translation of this exon start?)
b. Where will the 7-methylguanosine cap be placed in the mRNA made from this gene?
c. What is the effect on expression of this gene if base number 14 in the first exon were changed from C to T?
d. Where is the stop codon?
e. What is the effect on expression of changing base number 26 in the first exon from C to T?
f. Write a "D" and arrow pointing to the splice donor site(s) and an "A" and arrow pointing to the splice acceptor site(s).

2/ You have identified an enzymatic activity in cell extracts that catalyzes the conversion of metabolite A to product B. Outline three different strategies you could use to isolate a cDNA representing the mRNA that encodes all or part of the protein for this enzyme.

3/ Shown below is a Southern blot of human DNA cut with three different restriction enzymes. Each *lane* is labeled B, E, or H representing DNA digested with *Bam* HI, *Eco* RI, and *Hin* dIII, respectively, alone or with two of the enzymes in a double digestion. The probe is a 2.3-kb *Hin* dIII fragment of human genomic DNA. Draw the two possible maps of the restriction endonuclease sites in and around the probe sequence.

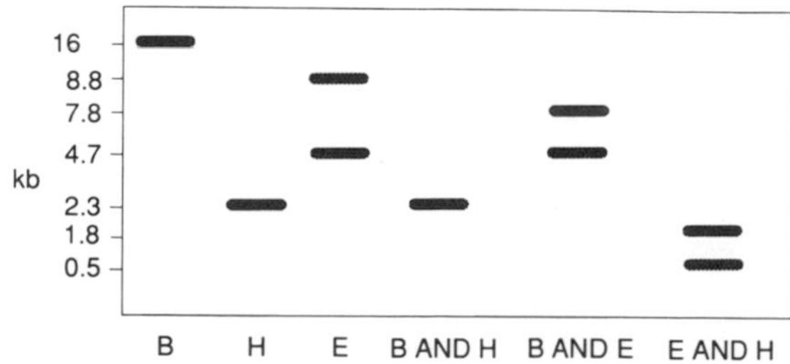

6

Molecular Genetics of Human Disease: Hemoglobinopathies

"Making a discovery is such a wonderful thing. It's like falling in love and getting to the top of the mountain all in one."

—Nobel Laureate Max Perutz, who met Cupid on the top of the mountain called the Structure of Hemoglobin

The preceding chapter had as its goal the introduction of the basic anatomy of a human gene and the various techniques of molecular biology and recombinant DNA that are used to analyze such genes. The current chapter seeks to bring these issues into even sharper focus by showing how, in one well-studied system, namely the human hemoglobin genes, these principles have a direct bearing on the occurrence of genetic disease. In fact, as pointed out in Chapter 1, many of the central facts in our understanding of the anatomy of genes and their developmental and tissue-specific control have been arrived at using the hemoglobin genes as a model system. Therefore, it is quite correct to say that the pathway between basic genetics and clinical medicine is indeed two-way for this system.

THE HEMOGLOBIN PROTEIN

Red blood cells, which are produced in the bone marrow of adults, are nonnucleated, having lost their nuclei just prior to release from the marrow. Young red blood cells, called reticulocytes, still contain some messenger RNA, but this disappears after a few days. For the rest of their approximately 120-day life span, red blood cells circulate in the system as membrane-surrounded flexible bags of protein, approximately 70% of which is hemoglobin. Hemoglobin is a tetramer consisting of two α chains and two β chains, which spontaneously assemble by hydrogen bonding to form a stable structure (Fig. 6.1). Each globin

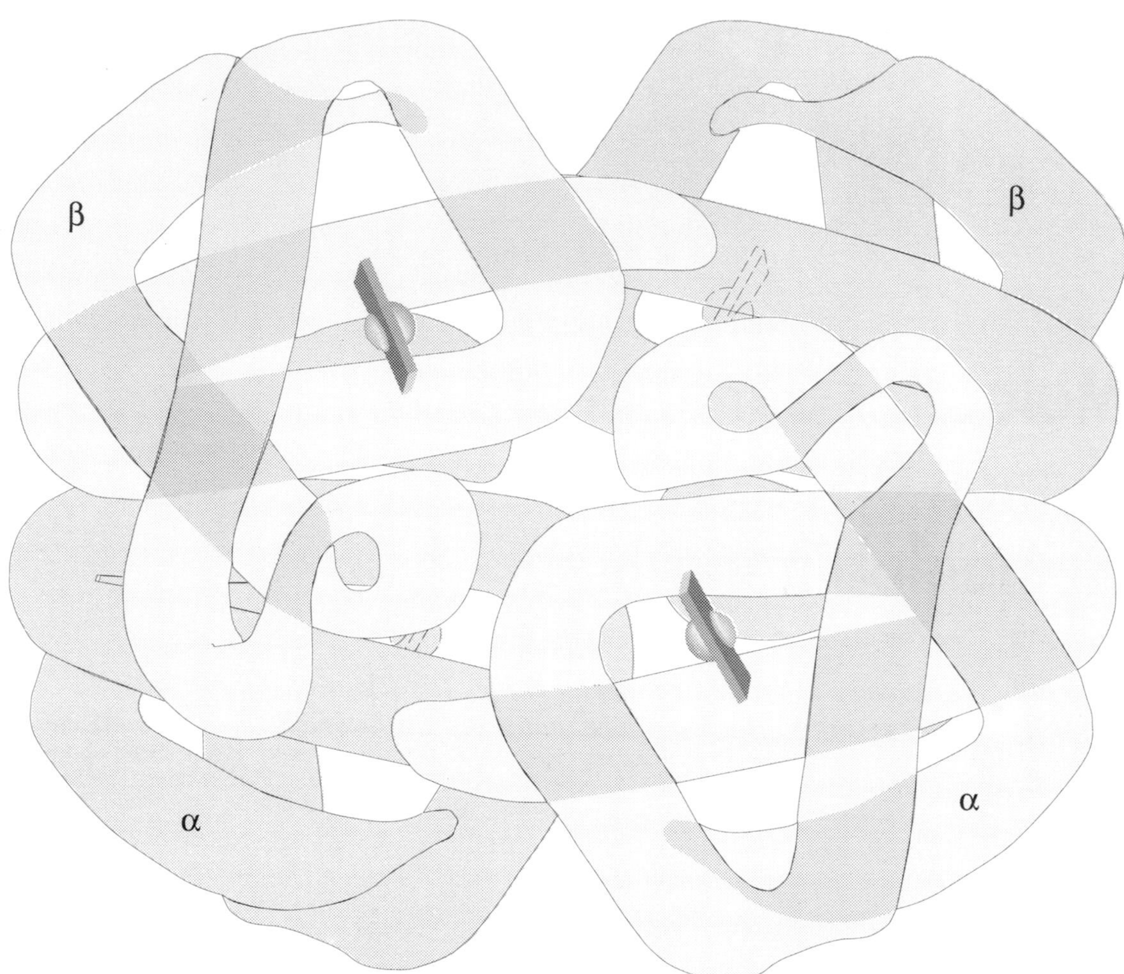

Figure 6.1. Diagram of the hemoglobin tetramer. The two α and two β chains, each of which binds a molecule of heme (the planar structure in the center of each subunit), are shown. (From Dickerson RE, Geis I: *Hemoglobin: Structure, Function, Evolution, and Pathology.* Menlo Park, CA, Benjamin/Cummings, 1983. © Irving Geis.)

chain also contains a heme molecule, the product of a complex enzymatic pathway involving multiple steps and resulting in a tetracyclic organic compound. In concert with iron, the heme molecule binds molecular oxygen.

There are several reasons why the hemoglobin system is so well-studied. One is that red blood cells provide such a convenient source of material because they are removable and renewable. No extensive protein purification of hemoglobin is necessary because the protein is present in such high concentrations already. This same natural enrichment has been of considerable use in studying the molecular genetics of hemoglobin; reticulocytes have α- and β-globin mRNA as their major polyadenylated RNA constituents, so that, as pointed out in Chapter 5, it is possible to clone the α- and β-globin cDNAs in a relatively straightforward fashion. Finally, hemoglobin is particularly well-studied because of the large number of genetic disorders that involve this system, including sickle cell anemia, the first "molecular disease," which will be discussed in detail below.

THE HEMOGLOBIN GENES

A scale drawing of the α- and β-globin gene regions of humans is shown in Figure 5.2. Both the α and β genes actually are part of gene clusters, with the β-globin cluster on chromosome 11 and the α-globin cluster on chromosome 16. These clusters contain, in addition to the major adult genes, α and β, other expressed sequences, which are used at different points in development. In both clusters, the genes are arranged so that their 5′ to 3′ direction of transcription is the same for all genes, and the genes used earliest in development are at the 5′ end of the cluster, and those used last, at the 3′ end. As noted in Chapter 5, both clusters contain pseudogenes, remnants of once functioning genes, which have undergone mutations rendering them no longer capable of producing a protein. In both clusters, the majority of the DNA is located in intergenic regions of unknown and possible dispensable function.

Figure 6.2 shows the pattern of expression of the functional genes in both of these clusters, plotted as a function of developmental age. In the first few weeks of life, hemoglobin synthesis occurs in the yolk sac. The major hemoglobin at that time is a tetramer of two ζ chains (encoded within the α cluster), and two ϵ chains transcribed from the β cluster. Very soon, however, production of these two globin chains rapidly diminishes and the α-globin cluster begins to transcribe α as its major product. There are actually two α genes, $\alpha 2$ and $\alpha 1$, but these are identical in their coding regions and therefore produce a single protein. The α genes then stay on for the remainder of the life of the individual.

The β-globin cluster, however, contains an additional set of genes, the fetal hemoglobin genes. This consists of a pair of genes, ${}^{G}\gamma$ and ${}^{A}\gamma$, which differ in their coding region by only one amino acid, which is glycine for ${}^{G}\gamma$ and alanine for ${}^{A}\gamma$ at position 136. As shown in Figure 6.2, the γ genes turn on as the embryonic genes are turning off, and during fetal life the major products from the β-globin cluster are ${}^{G}\gamma$ and ${}^{A}\gamma$. Beginning somewhat before birth and continuing for several months after birth, there is a smooth and carefully regulated switch from γ production to β production, so that at all times the sum of the two is kept

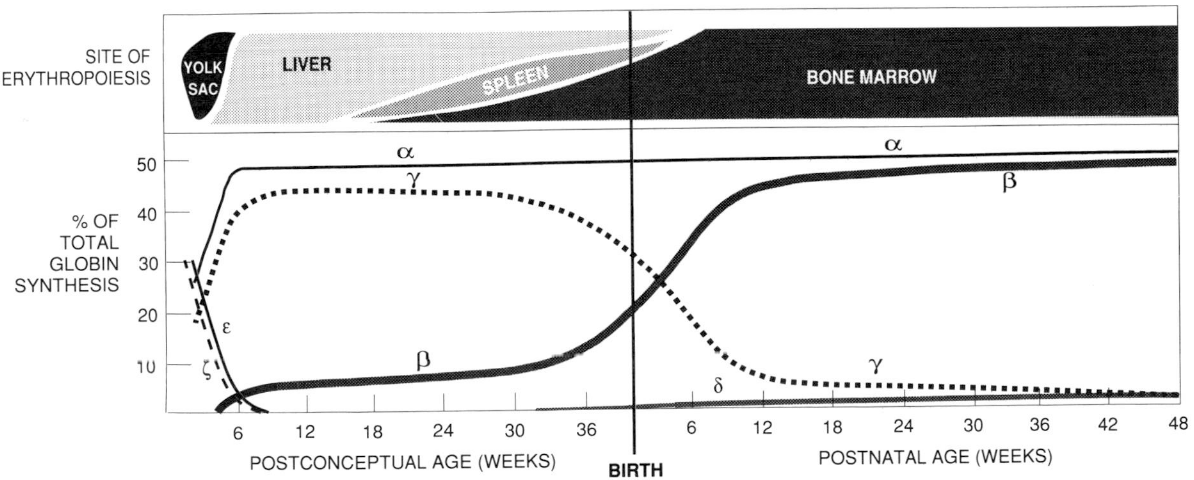

Figure 6.2. Developmental pattern of expression of human hemoglobin. The time course of production of the various globin chains is shown. At the *top* of the figure is diagrammed the primary site of hematopoiesis during these various stages. (From Weatherall DJ, Clegg JB: *The Thalassemia Syndromes.* 3rd Ed. Oxford, Blackwell Scientific Publications, 1981.)

approximately constant. This development switch cannot be attributed to the change in environment that occurs at birth because the switch is already underway by that time. It also cannot be attributed to a change in the site of hemoglobin production, although red cell production does switch at about the same time from the fetal liver to the bone marrow (Fig. 6.2). If one looks in the bone marrow at the time of birth, however, both γ and β are being produced at that site; thus, the switch occurs on a cell-by-cell basis.

Figure 6.3 shows the possible hemoglobin tetramers during this developmental pattern. All of these have been identified and have been given somewhat anachronistic names prior to an understanding of their molecular basis. In embryonic life, the major hemoglobin is hemoglobin Gower I. Hemoglobin Gower II and hemoglobin Portland are seen transiently during the time when the embryonic genes are turning off and the fetal genes are turning on. During fetal life the major hemoglobin is hemoglobin F, which includes both $\alpha_2{}^G\gamma_2$ and $\alpha_2{}^A\gamma_2$. In adult life, the major globin is hemoglobin A, which is a tetramer of two α and two β chains. There is also a minor adult globin called hemoglobin A_2, which is a tetramer consisting of two α chains and two δ chains. The δ gene has developmental timing similar to β, but it has acquired a number of abnormalities in its promoter, particularly in the CCAAT box region, which render it relatively inefficient. At least partly for this reason, the amount of δ mRNA is considerably lower than that of β mRNA. The net result is that a normal adult individual has approximately 97.5% hemoglobin A, about 2% hemoglobin A_2, and about 0.5% hemoglobin F.

The expression of the γ genes in a fetal developmental program is a relatively recent evolutionary event, having appeared only in primates. It is speculated that this additional hemoglobin had advantages because of the longer gestation time in these species, which requires a more efficient means of insuring adequate oxygen delivery to the growing fetus over an extended period of time. Fetal hemoglobin has a somewhat higher oxygen affinity than adult hemoglobin and thus is capable of extracting oxygen more efficiently across the placenta from the maternal circulation.

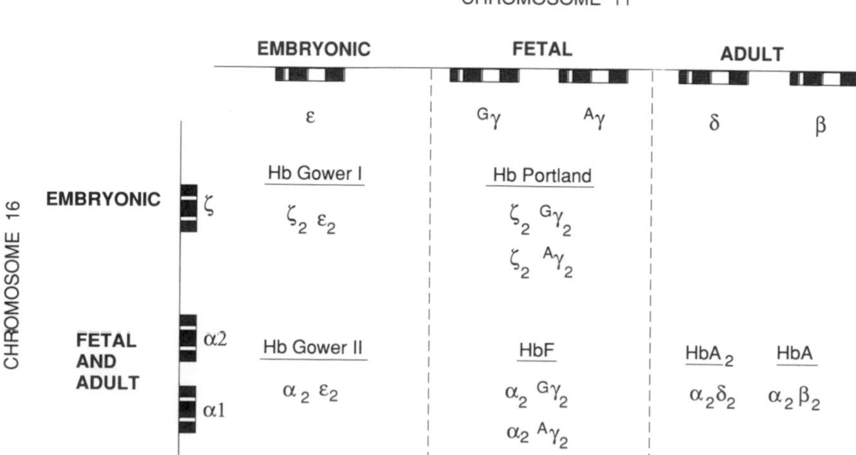

Figure 6.3. A matrix diagram showing the possible tetrameric products of the α-globin cluster on chromosome 16 and the β-globin cluster on chromosome 11, together with their historical names.

NORMAL ANATOMY AND EXPRESSION OF THE β-GLOBIN GENE

The general features of eukaryotic genes described in Chapter 5 are well-exemplified by the human β-globin gene, which is diagrammed in Figure 6.4. The promoter region of the β-globin gene contains a TATA box, but in this instance the sequence is actually just ATA. There is also a CCAAT box, and somewhat further upstream a sequence, CACCC, which is repeated once and is present in many other globin genes. Human β globin is exquisitely tissue-specific, being expressed in significant levels only in red blood cells and their precursors. While the DNA sequences responsible for this tissue specificity have not been entirely defined, there is evidence for an enhancer sequence located on the 3′ side of the gene, which may also have its function most strongly expressed in red blood cell precursors. There is also evidence that other sequences at considerable distances from β play a significant role in tissue specificity.

The β-globin gene consists of three exons and two introns, with the second intron considerably larger than the first. As shown in Figure 6.4, there are short 5′ and 3′ untranslated regions, and capping, polyadenylation, and splicing all proceed in the usual fashion. The resultant mRNA is then transported to the cytoplasm and its complete sequence is shown in Figure 6.5. Note the presence of the 7-methyl guanosine at the cap site, followed by a short stretch of untranslated RNA. The first AUG codon is surrounded by a box and denotes the start of translation of this RNA. This initial methionine is subsequently cleaved off of the polypeptide, so that the first amino acid of the mature protein is valine, which is coded for by GUG. There are a total of 146 amino acids in the mature polypeptide, and translation is terminated upon encountering

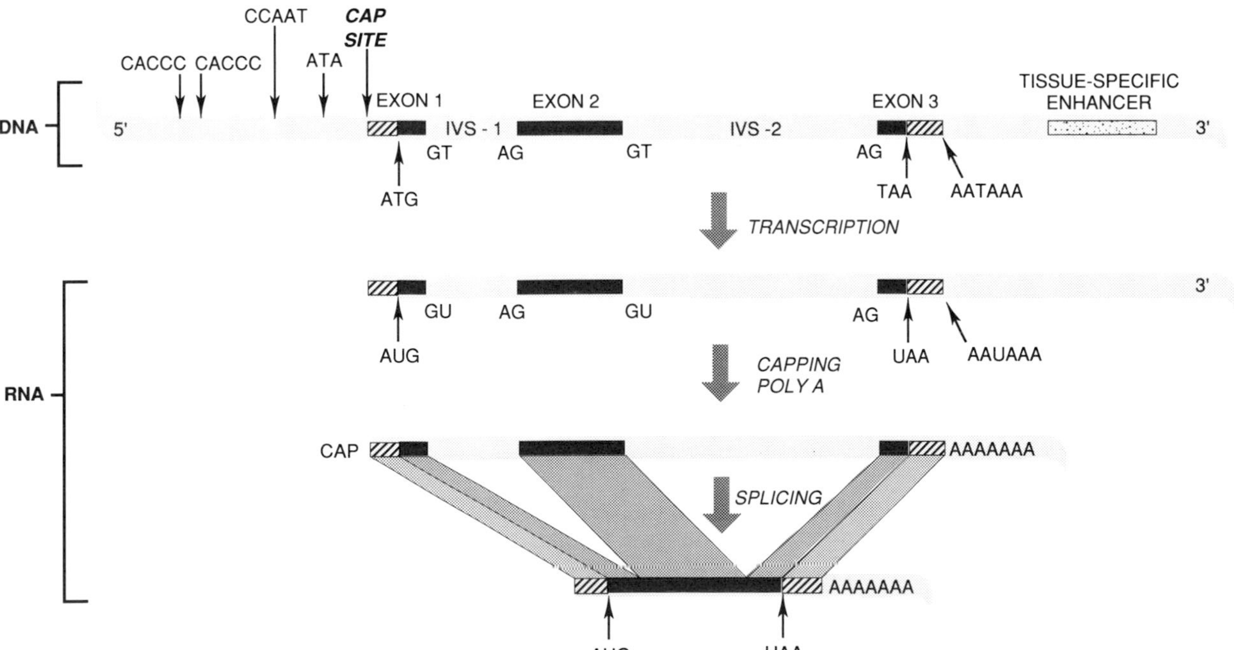

Figure 6.4. A schematic of the human β-globin gene. Shown at the *top* is a diagram of the genomic DNA, with important elements in the promoter and 3′-flanking region indicated. The introns and their junctions with exons are also noted, as is the polyadenylation (AATAAA) site. The transcription of this gene into RNA is depicted, as is the processing of that RNA into a mature cytoplasmic message.

											–15					–10		
									m7GpppAC	AUU	UGC	UUC	UGA	CAC	AAC	UGU	GUU	CAC
		–5					0					5					10	
UAG	CAA	CCU	CAA	ACA	GAC	ACC	AUG	GUG	CAC	CUG	ACU	CCU	GAG	GAG	AAG	UCU	GCC	GUU
			15					20					25					30
ACU	GCC	CUG	UGG	GGC	AAG	GUG	AAC	GUG	GAU	GAA	GUU	GGU	GGU	GAG	GCC	CUG	GGC	AGG
				35					40					45				
CUG	CUG	GUG	GUC	UAC	CCU	UGG	ACC	CAG	AGG	UUC	UUU	GAG	UCC	UUU	GGG	GAU	CUG	UCC
50					55					60					65			
ACU	CCU	GAU	GCU	GUU	AUG	GGC	AAC	CCU	AAG	GUG	AAG	GCU	CAU	GGC	AAG	AAA	GUG	CUC
	70					75					80					85		
GGU	GCC	UUU	AGU	GAU	GGC	CUG	GCU	CAC	CUG	GAC	AAC	CUC	AAG	GGC	ACC	UUU	GCC	ACA
		90					95					100					105	
CUG	AGU	GAG	CUG	CAC	UGU	GAC	AAG	CUG	CAC	GUG	GAU	CCU	GAG	AAC	UUC	AGG	CUC	CUG
			110					115					120					125
GGC	AAC	GUG	CUG	GUC	UGU	GUG	CUG	GCC	CAU	CAC	UUU	GGC	AAA	GAA	UUC	ACC	CCA	CCA
				130					135					140				
GUG	CAG	GCU	GCC	UAU	CAG	AAA	GUG	GUG	GCU	GGU	GUG	GCU	AAU	GCC	CUG	GCC	CAC	AAG
145					150					155					160			
UAU	CAC	UAA	GCU	CGC	UUU	CUU	GCU	GUC	CAA	UUU	CUA	UUA	AAG	GUU	CCU	UUG	UUC	CCU
	165					170					175					180		
AAG	UCC	AAC	UAC	UAA	ACU	GGG	GGA	UAU	UAU	GAA	GGG	CCU	UGA	GCA	UCU	GGA	UUC	UGC
CUA	AUA	AAA	AAC	AUU	UAU	UUU	CAU	UGC	POLY A									

Figure 6.5. The nucleotide sequence of human β-globin messenger RNA. The AUG initiation codon is *boxed*, marked with an *arrow*, and numbered as *0*. The termination codon UAA (codon 147) is also marked. The polyadenylation signal near the 3′ end of the message is also *boxed* and is followed 19 nucleotides later by a string of A residues.

the UAA stop codon. The remainder of the 3′ portion of the RNA represents untranslated sequence. The AAUAAA sequence, which is used in the nucleus as a signal for polyadenylation, is boxed, and a string of adenosine residues is attached 19 nucleotides to the 3′ side of this.

We are now ready to take a look at the wide variety of mutations that have been described in the globin genes. These mutations can be divided into those causing qualitative abnormalities (often called hemoglobinopathies) and those causing quantitative abnormalities (the thalassemias).

MUTATIONS CAUSING QUALITATIVE ABNORMALITIES IN GLOBIN: THE HEMOGLOBINOPATHIES

Missense Mutations

As described in Chapter 2, a missense mutation results from a nucleotide change that alters the amino acid encoded by a particular 3-base codon. Because of the intense scrutiny to which the α- and β-globin genes have been subjected, a very large number of missense mutations have been described. Many of these do not cause any phenotypic abnormalities. Figure 6.6 is a schematic drawing showing how numerous the described mutations are, with each marked amino acid identifying a position in which a mutation has been identified. As can be seen, more than half of the amino acids in both the α- and the β-globin genes have had missense mutations identified. Correlation of the phenotypes of these mutations with functional abnormalities seen in some of the

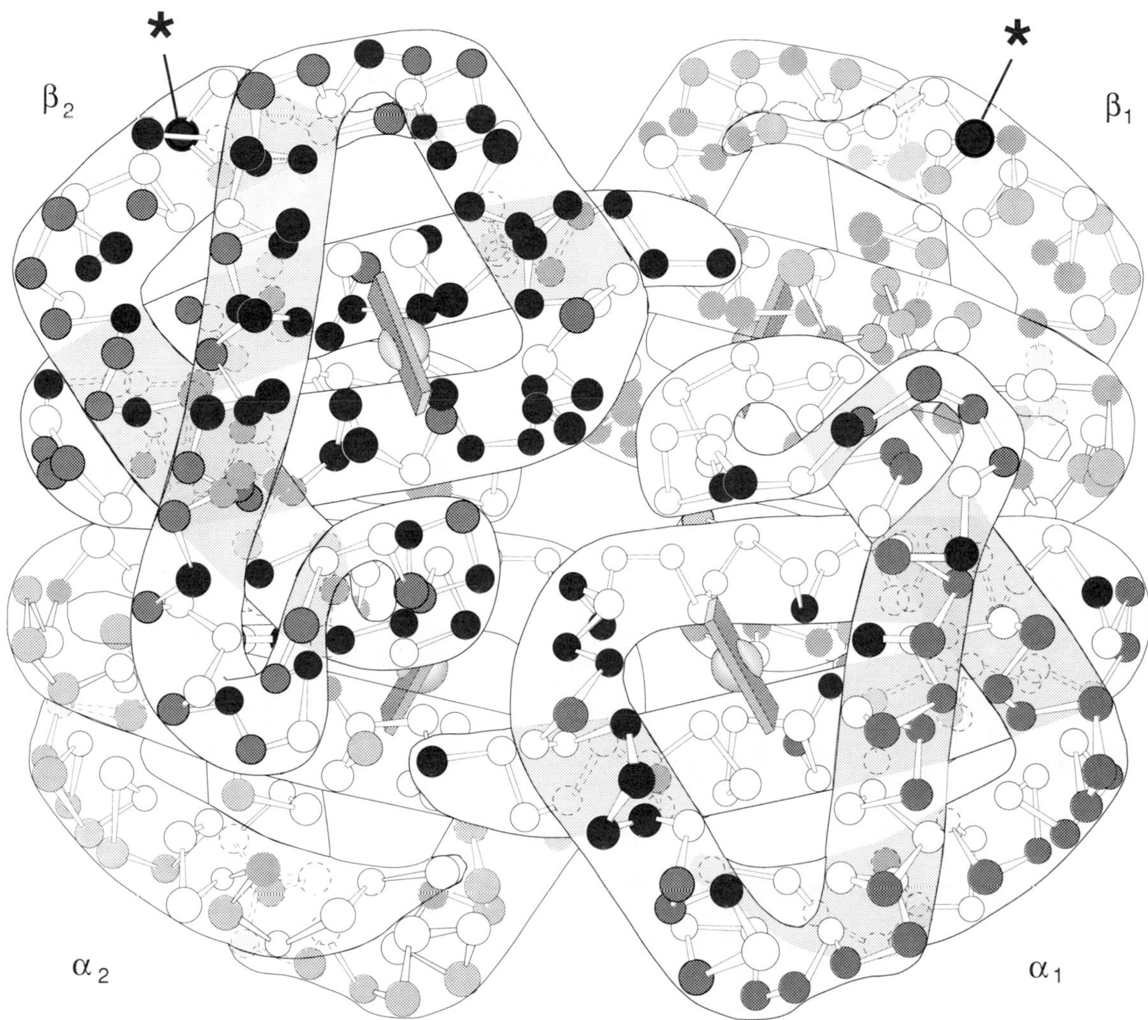

Figure 6.6. Schematic drawing of the hemoglobin molecule, indicating the positions in α and β at which missense mutations have been described. The very large number of abnormal hemoglobins detected thus far is immediately apparent. *Shaded circles* indicate positions where altered amino acids have been observed, and mutations leading to abnormal hemoglobin function are indicated in *dark red* in the two closest subunits, α_1 and β_2. The β6 location of the sickle mutation is indicated with an *asterisk*. (From Dickerson RE, Geis I: *Hemoglobin: Structure, Function, Evolution, and Pathology*. Menlo Park, CA, Benjamin/Cummings, 1983. © Irving Geis.)

mutations has led to a much better understanding of the functional domains of the hemoglobin tetramer, which are responsible for its properties. The general strategy of correlating the effect of mutations at specific locations in a molecule with the functional properties of that molecule is a powerful one with far-reaching implications.

The most common missense mutation in the β-globin gene leads to sickle cell anemia in the homozygote. The incidence of this disease in the black population is approximately 1 in 500 births, and the disease causes significant morbidity and mortality. The disorder is recessive, but carriers are easily detected. Using the Hardy-Weinberg law, described in Chapter 4, one can predict that, if the incidence of the disease (q^2) is 1 in 500, the carrier frequency (2pq) is approximately 8%, and carrier screening confirms this result. Given that homozygous sickle cell anemia causes severe disease with shortening of life and decrease in reproductive potential, it may seem remarkable that this gene has

DNA

	codon 5	6	7
β^A	. . . CCT	GAG	GAG . . .
β^S	. . . CCT	GTG	GAG . . .
β^C	. . . CCT	AAG	GAG . . .

PROTEIN

	5	6	7
β^A	. . . Pro	Glu	Glu . . .
β^S	. . . Pro	Val	Glu . . .
β^C	. . . Pro	Lys	Glu . . .

Figure 6.7. The DNA and protein abnormalities in codon 6, which lead to sickle hemoglobin (β^S) and hemoglobin C (β^C).

reached such a high frequency in the black population. As described in Chapter 4, however, there appears to be a clear-cut explanation for this occurrence. Specifically, heterozygotes for sickle cell anemia are moderately protected from the most severe and lethal consequences of infection with the malarial parasite, which apparently has led to selection for this gene over the long term. Thus, even though the homozygotes (1 in 500) are selected against, the moderate selection for heterozygotes (1 in 12) has allowed the gene to reach its high frequency in areas of the world where malaria has been endemic.

The molecular abnormality in sickle cell anemia was first postulated by Linus Pauling and represents the first true example of a molecular disease. Using careful analysis of the hemoglobin protein, Vernon Ingram subsequently demonstrated that the sickle cell β-globin gene differed by a single amino acid at position 6. The normal residue at this position is glutamic acid, whereas in sickle cell anemia valine is present instead. Subsequently, cloning and sequencing the respective genes has revealed the expected change in the DNA sequence, namely that the sequence for codon 6 is changed from GAG in the normal gene to GTG in sickle cell disease. Interestingly, another relatively common β-globin chain missense mutation, called hemoglobin C, also results from an alteration at codon 6, changing GAG to AAG and resulting in a lysine at this position (Fig. 6.7).

It is remarkable indeed that a single nucleotide change of the 3 billion nucleotides in the haploid human genome results in the wide array of severe clinical problems experienced by individuals with sickle cell anemia. The basis of these problems is diagrammed in Figure 6.8. The underlying problem is that the valine for glutamic acid replacement results in hemoglobin tetramers that, when deoxygenated, can aggregate into arrays rather than remaining soluble. As shown in Figure 6.8, these arrays can become nearly crystalline in their structure. Thus, every time a red cell carrying sickle hemoglobin travels through the circulation and becomes deoxygenated, the hemoglobin within it aggregates. This in turn deforms the red cell, makes it relatively inflexible, and renders it unable to traverse the fine capillary beds, which have diameters smaller than the red cell itself. After repeated cycles of deoxygenation and reoxygenation, some cells become irreversibly sickled. The result of all this is plugging of the circulation, particularly in areas of low oxygen tension. Bones are particularly affected, leading to the frequent and severe bone pain experienced in a sickle cell "crisis." Over the long term, this recurrent plugging of the circulation leads to significant damage to internal organs, especially the heart, lungs, and kidneys. Cerebrovascular accidents are another serious complication. Because of the destruction of red cells containing hemoglobin crystals, sickle cell patients are chronically anemic, and that contributes to the cardiac stress.

The diagnosis of sickle cell anemia usually can be readily made by examination of the blood smear (Fig. 6.8) in the presence of a typical clinical syndrome. Carriers can be diagnosed by exposing their red blood cells to very low oxygen tension, under which circumstances even blood from a heterozygote can be made to sickle. It is important to note, however, that heterozygotes (often referred to as having sickle trait) are not symptomatic, with the possible exception of very low oxygen tension environments such as high altitude unpressurized flight.

To be certain of the diagnosis, however, hemoglobin electrophoresis is usually carried out. As shown in Figure 6.9, hemoglobins that differ in charge can be separated by their migration in an electric field.

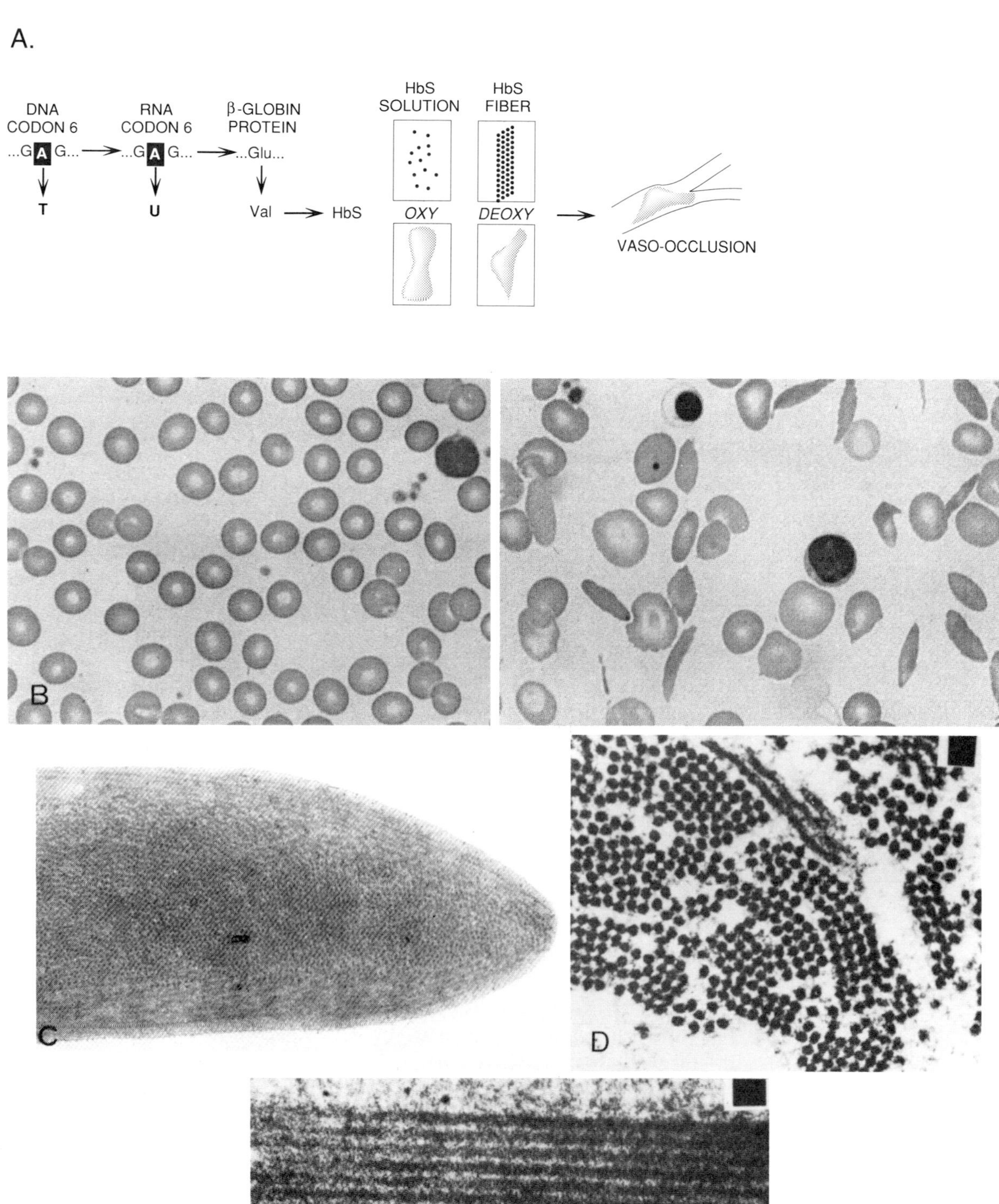

Figure 6.8. Molecular pathogenesis of sickle cell anemia. A, Deoxygenated sickle hemoglobin crystallizes within the red cells leading to rigidity and inability to traverse small capillaries. **B,** The sickled cells are visible in a blood smear on the *right*, with a normal blood smear on the *left* for comparison. **C,** Electron micrographs of deoxygenated sickle cells reveal fibers of hemoglobin, seen at higher magnification in both transverse (**D**) and longitudinal (**E**) orientation. (From Bunn HF, Forget BG: *Hemoglobin: Molecular, Genetic, and Clinical Aspects.* Philadelphia, WB Saunders, 1986.)

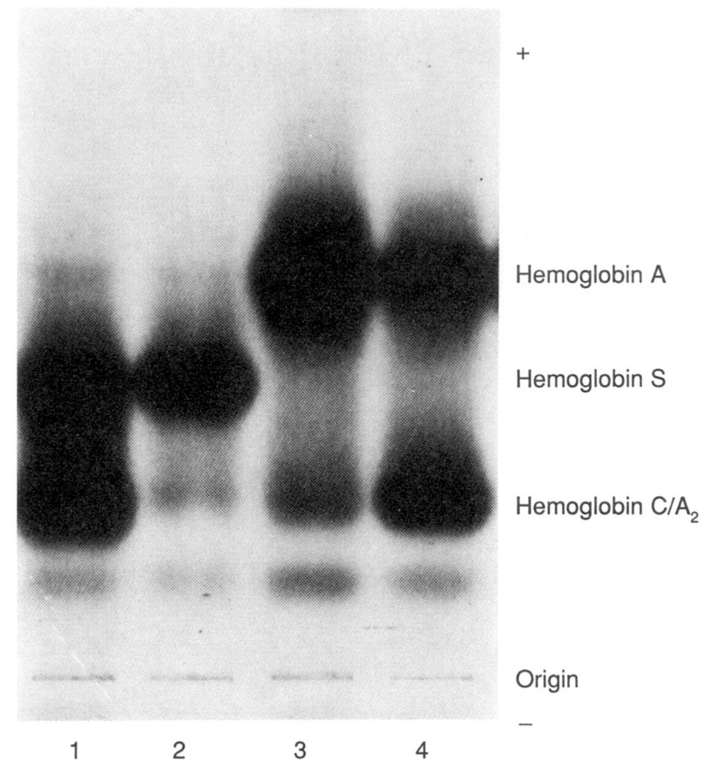

Figure 6.9. Hemoglobin electrophoresis. Hemoglobin samples are loaded at the position marked *origin* and then placed under an electric field; the distance travelled reflects total charge of the molecule. This allows separation of hemoglobins A, S, C, and A_2 (C and A_2 travel very close together). A normal individual (*AA, lane 3*) has primarily hemoglobin A with a small amount of hemoglobin A_2. A sickle homozygote (*SS, lane 2*) has only hemoglobin S and A_2. Hemoglobin samples from AC (*lane 4*) and SC (*lane 1*) individuals are also shown. (From Weatherall DJ, Clegg JB: *The Thalassemia Syndromes.* 3rd Ed. Oxford, Blackwell Scientific Publications, 1981.)

Because the sickle mutation alters a negatively charged amino acid (glutamic acid) to a neutral one (valine), the result is a significant alteration in the migration of the protein on a gel in an electric field. Such gels can also detect the small amount of hemoglobin F and hemoglobin A_2 in the blood; these appear in a different position than hemoglobin A. Hemoglobin C, which, as noted above, represents a two-charge difference from hemoglobin A because of the mutation of a negatively charged amino acid to a positively charged amino acid (lysine) at codon 6, results in a band on the gel that migrates even more slowly than hemoglobin S toward the positive electrode and travels very close to the position of hemoglobin A_2. Many of the other missense mutations shown in Figure 6.6 were initially detected by the presence of an abnormal band in hemoglobin electrophoresis.

When red blood cells are available, electrophoresis of the hemoglobin itself may be the most direct way to diagnose these abnormalities. However, in some situations such as prenatal diagnosis, it is risky or impossible to obtain a pure blood sample from the individual to be tested. Since the DNA encoding the β-globin gene is represented in all cells of the organism, it is possible to diagnose the presence of the sickle mutation by directly analyzing the DNA from any available source of cells. As will be described in a later chapter, such cells can be obtained by amniocentesis or chorionic villus biopsy far more easily than one could obtain a blood sample.

One method by which one can diagnose the presence of the sickle mutation in a DNA sample is diagrammed in Figure 6.10. As shown, the enzyme *Mst*II recognizes the sequence CCTNAGG, where N is any nucleotide. Thus, the sequence of codons 5 and 6 and the first base of codon 7 normally constitute a restriction site for this enzyme. The sickle mutation, however, abolishes this *Mst*II site because the mutation of A to T makes this region no longer a match for the restriction enzyme. This is a somewhat fortuitous occurrence. Restriction enzyme recogni-

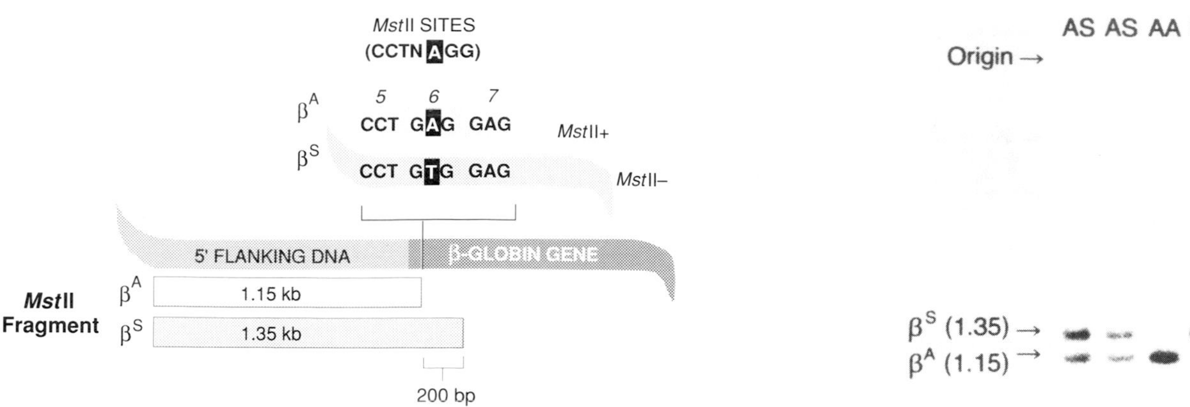

Figure 6.10. Diagnosis of the sickle mutation using Southern blotting analysis. The abolition of the normal *Mst*II site in codons 5, 6, and 7 by the sickle mutation is shown. On the *right* is the result of a Southern blot of DNA from individuals who are homozygous A, homozygous S, or AS heterozygotes. The probe is a genomic fragment from 5′ flanking DNA. (From Bunn HF, Forget BG: *Hemoglobin: Molecular, Genetic, and Clinical Aspects.* Philadelphia, WB Saunders, 1986.)

tion sites do not comprise an infinite set; most single base changes causing disease in humans do not alter a restriction site and cannot be detected by this direct approach. Since the sickle mutation does destroy a restriction site, heterozygotes and homozygotes can be identified by cutting their DNA with *Mst*II and analyzing the results with a Southern blot, as shown in Figure 6.10. The normal β-globin allele, which contains the *Mst*II site at codon 6, leads to a 1.15-kilobase (kb) band when probed with a sequence from the 5′-flanking region of the gene. This fragment is 1.35 kb, however, in the sickle allele because the site at codon 6 is lost, and the next adjacent site is located 200 base pairs (bp) further to the 3′ side (within the β-globin gene). Homozygous normal individuals, heterozygotes, and homozygous affected individuals can then be distinguished using this approach.

Sickle cell anemia is one of the few genetic diseases where this direct approach to DNA diagnosis can be applied. This is possible because 1) the mutation is known at the DNA level; 2) all individuals with the disease have the same mutation, i.e., there is no allelic heterogeneity; and 3) fortuitously, a restriction enzyme recognizes the mutation itself. Many other methods can also be applied. An example using the polymerase chain reaction (PCR) and allele-specific oligonucleotides (ASOs) was given in Figure 5.18.

Frameshift Mutations

As described in Chapter 2, frameshift mutations occur when there is an insertion or deletion of a small number of nucleotides that are not a multiple of three. When the RNA from such a mutant gene is translated, the amino acid sequence beyond the point of the frameshift is completely garbled. There are several possible effects of this. If the frameshift occurs near the 5′ end of the coding region, the protein may bear little resemblance to its normal counterpart or may be rapidly degraded and impossible to identify. The net result of this is a virtual absence of a recognizable protein product, which falls in the thalassemia category we will consider shortly. However, if the frameshift mutation is near the end of the protein, the result can be a qualitative abnormality where the carboxy-terminal end of the polypeptide has acquired an entirely new stretch of amino acids. An example of this, shown in Figure

6.11, is hemoglobin Cranston. (Abnormal hemoglobins are often named by the geographic location where the patient in whom the abnormality was first described resided.) Here a 2-nucleotide insertion has occurred between codons 144 and 145 of the β-globin gene, almost at the end of the coding region. The result of this is that the normal termination codon 6 nucleotides further along is shifted out of frame and is therefore not read as stop. Thus, translation proceeds obliviously into the normally 3′-untranslated region, and a protein consisting of 157 amino acids is produced before the next fortuitous termination codon is encountered.

A similar situation occurs in hemoglobin Constant Spring, which is an analogous mutation of an α-globin gene. In this situation the normal termination codon, UAA, is mutated to CAA, which codes for glutamine instead of stop. Therefore, this is not truly a frameshift but can be thought of as the opposite of a nonsense mutation. The result is that translation continues to read into the normally 3′-untranslated region of the α-globin RNA, continuing for an additional 31 amino acids until encountering an in-frame stop at codon 173 (Fig. 6.11). Thus, the resulting α-globin chain is entirely normal for the first 141 amino acids but contains this unusual carboxy-terminal tail. As it turns out, this renders the α-globin protein somewhat unstable, so that the result is a combined qualitative and quantitative abnormality in α-globin production.

Another interesting and important source of mutation is a phenomenon called unequal crossing over. As described in Chapter 2, homologous chromosomes line up based on their similar sequence over the entire length of a chromosome during meiosis I; at this time crossing over between homologous chromosomes occurs. If a stretch of duplicated nucleotide sequence exists, it is possible for the lining up process

A.

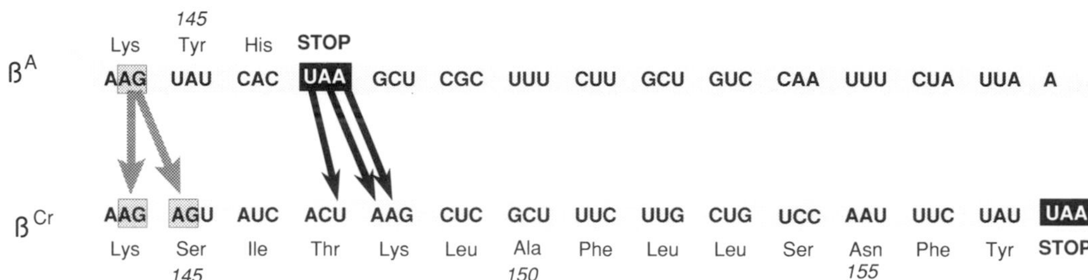

B.

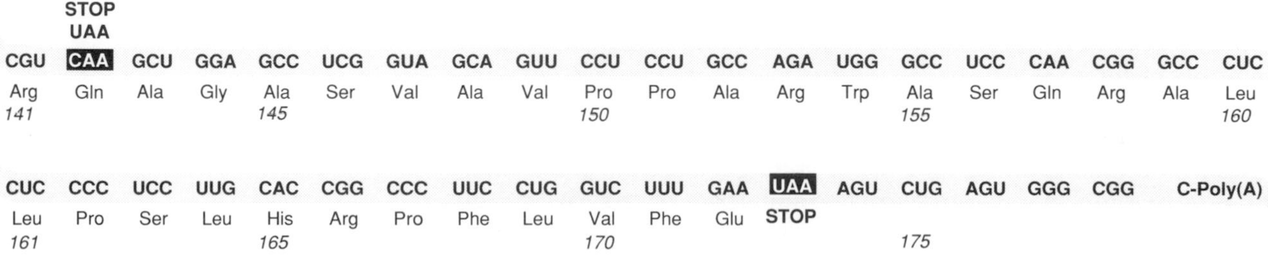

Figure 6.11. **A**, A frameshift mutation near the end of the β-globin gene, leading to hemoglobin Cranston (β^{Cr}). **B**, Mutation of the normal α-globin termination codon 142 to result in hemoglobin Constant Spring, containing an extra 31 amino acids at the carboxy terminus.

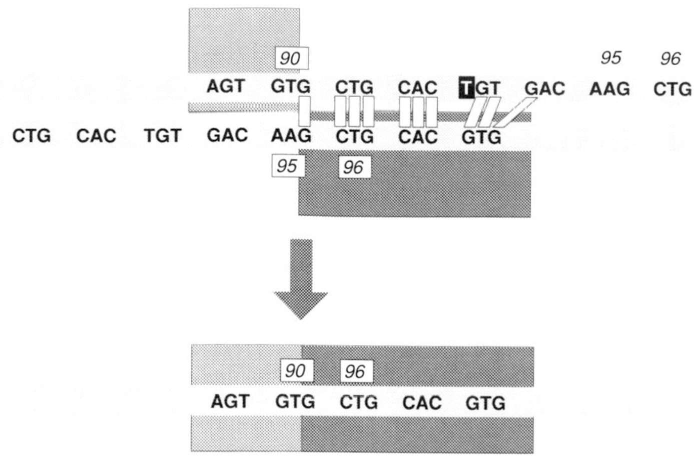

Figure 6.12. Generation of hemoglobin Gun Hill by unequal crossing over between homologous regions during meiosis.

to occur improperly. Should a crossover occur between chromosomes that are misaligned, the net result will be a deletion or duplication. An example is shown in Figure 6.12. A nearly perfect duplication of the sequence GCTGCACGTG is found in codons 91–94 and in codons 96–98 of the β-globin gene. If the first copy of this sequence lines up with the second (rather than with itself), and a crossover occurs within this region, the result is the deletion or duplication of amino acids 91–95. This deletion has in fact been observed and is denoted as hemoglobin Gun Hill. This deletion of 15 nucleotides keeps the reading frame intact, so that the amino acids from 96 on are still correct in the translated protein.

A much larger deletion can occur if the δ- and β-globin genes, which are approximately 90% homologous to each other, happen to line up improperly during meiosis and participate in a crossover. This event is diagrammed in Figure 6.13. The chromosome resulting from a crossover (indicated by the *gray line*) would thus be a hybrid adult globin gene consisting of the 5′ end of the δ gene and the 3′ end of the β gene. Several such variants have been observed, depending upon the precise localization of the point of crossover; all are called Lepore hemoglobins. Since, as noted above, the promoter of the δ-globin gene has sustained a number of mutations, which render it relatively inefficient, the Lepore hemoglobin is produced at reduced amounts. Thus, this is another example of a combined quantitative and qualitative abnormality.

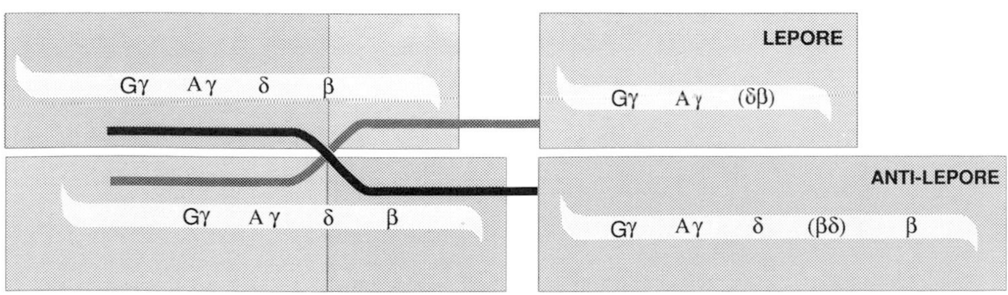

Figure 6.13. Unequal crossing over between the δ and β genes to generate hemoglobins Lepore (a hybrid $\delta\beta$ gene) and anti-Lepore (a hybrid $\beta\delta$ gene).

Note that this sort of unequal crossover has an alternative outcome. As shown by the *red line* in Figure 6.13, the result will be a chromosome with intact δ and β genes, with a hybrid β-δ gene inserted between them. In this situation the hybrid gene has the 5′ sequences of β and the 3′ sequences of δ. This is known as an "anti-Lepore" hemoglobin. Individuals with this chromosome will make relatively normal amounts of δ and β, but in addition will produce the novel anti-Lepore hemoglobin. The level of production of anti-Lepore is lower than that of β, probably because the anti-Lepore gene is lacking the 3′ β enhancer sequence shown in Figure 6.4.

GLOBIN CHAIN IMBALANCE: THE THALASSEMIAS

Until this point we have been considering primarily qualitative abnormalities of δ- and β-globin chains that are due to alterations in the coding region of these genes. The thalassemias, on the other hand, are hereditary abnormalities of hemoglobin production in which the primary difficulty is a *quantitative* deficiency of either β-globin, leading to β-thalassemia, or α-globin, leading to α-thalassemia. Thalassemia derives from the Greek word thalassa, which means "sea." This name was applied because of the relatively high frequency of these disorders in individuals living around the Mediterranean Sea. In fact, the thalassemias are common not only in the Mediterranean area but also in parts of Africa and Southeast Asia. As in sickle cell anemia, the distribution of the thalassemias coincides with the frequency of malaria, and the high frequency of thalassemia alleles in these areas is felt to be a reflection of the advantage that a heterozygote for one of these conditions has when infected with the malarial parasite.

The pathogenesis of the thalassemias is diagrammed in Figure 6.14. In the normal situation, equal amounts of α- and β-globin chains are produced, so that they are able to combine stoichiometrically to generate appropriate hemoglobin tetramers. As a result, red blood cells in a normal adult are loaded with a high concentration of hemoglobin and have a mean cell volume of about 100 μm^3. α-Thalassemia is characterized by a relative deficiency of α-globin chains but normal production of β-globin chains. If some α chains are still being made, a small amount of normal tetramers will form, but there will be a large excess of β chains. Under these circumstances, β is capable of forming homotetramers (β_4). This hemoglobin, which is called hemoglobin H (HbH), can be visualized as inclusion bodies within the red cells of individuals with

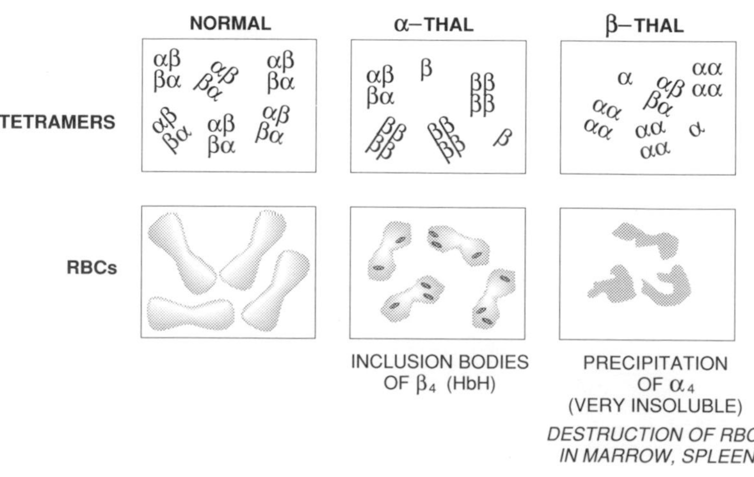

Figure 6.14. Schematic diagram of the pathogenesis of the thalassemias. *RBCs*, red blood cells.

α-thalassemia. HbH has markedly reduced ability to function as an oxygen carrier. The result of this β chain excess and α chain deficiency is that the red cells are reduced in size (50–80 μm^3, depending on the severity of the disease), and in number, resulting in anemia.

In β-thalassemia, it is the β-globin chains that are deficient. Under these circumstances, α-globin is in excess and is also capable of forming homotetramers. These tetramers, however, are *very* insoluble and precipitate within red blood cells, leading to their premature destruction in the bone marrow and marked trapping in the spleen. Again, red cells from individuals with β-thalassemia are reduced in size (50–80 μm^3), as well as in number.

α-Thalassemia

The genetics of α-thalassemia were initially puzzling, as individuals with this disorder seemed to have a wide range of α-globin production, extending from none at all (leading to stillbirth) to very near normal levels. Much of this confusion was clarified by the realization that each chromosome 16 carries two functioning α-globin genes, leading to a total of four genes in the normal situation. The α-thalassemias generally involve inactivation of anywhere from one to all four of these genes, and therefore the wide range of severity has a reasonable explanation. The possible outcomes of inactivating α-globin genes are diagrammed in Figure 6.15. If three of the four genes are functioning, the clinical abnormalities are extremely subtle and such individuals are completely asymptomatic. This is denoted as the "silent carrier" state; it is also anachronistically called α-thalassemia 2. A somewhat more transparent designation for this genotype is $\alpha\alpha/\alpha-$ or $\alpha-/\alpha\alpha$ (Fig. 6.15). If two of the four α-globin genes have been inactivated, this is denoted as "α-thalassemia trait" or α-thalassemia 1. There are two possible ways in which this could occur; in one situation, commonly seen as the cause of α-thalassemia 1 in Southeast Asia, both α-globin genes on one chro-

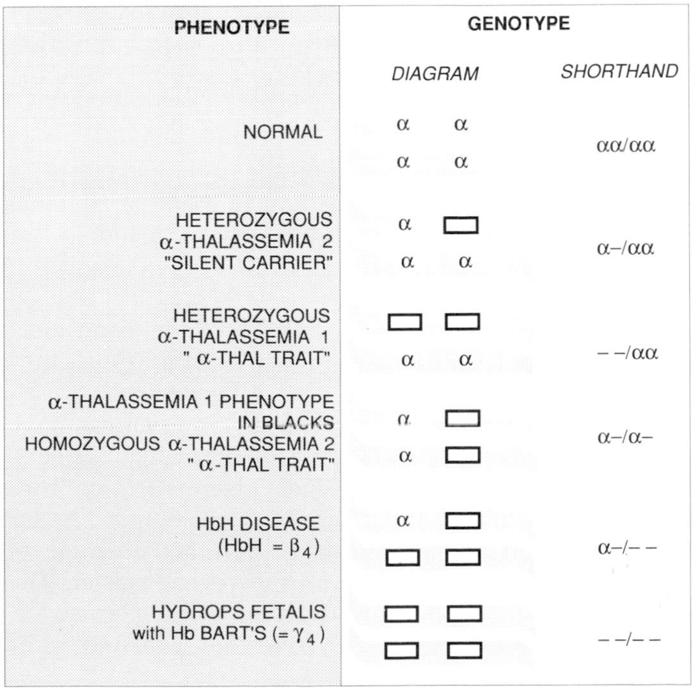

PHENOTYPE	GENOTYPE	
	DIAGRAM	SHORTHAND
NORMAL	α α α α	αα/αα
HETEROZYGOUS α-THALASSEMIA 2 "SILENT CARRIER"	α □ α α	α−/αα
HETEROZYGOUS α-THALASSEMIA 1 " α-THAL TRAIT"	□ □ α α	− −/αα
α-THALASSEMIA 1 PHENOTYPE IN BLACKS HOMOZYGOUS α-THALASSEMIA 2 " α-THAL TRAIT"	α □ α □	α−/α−
HbH DISEASE (HbH = β_4)	α □ □ □	α−/− −
HYDROPS FETALIS with Hb BART'S (= γ_4)	□ □ □ □	− −/− −

Figure 6.15. Gradation and severity of α-thalassemia, ranging from the normal situation where all four genes are functioning to the lethal hydrops fetalis, where no α-globin production occurs.

mosome are defective, whereas both α-globin genes on the other chromosome are normal ($\alpha\alpha/--$). Blacks with α-thalassemia 1, however, usually have the alternative arrangement where one α-globin gene on each chromosome is functioning normally ($\alpha-/\alpha-$). Therefore, these individuals are homozygous for an α-thalassemia 2 chromosome. The α-thalassemia 1 phenotype is also relatively benign; the mean cell volume is reduced, but these individuals are relatively asymptomatic.

A more severe situation arises if only one of the four α genes is functioning. This could arise, for example, if one parent ($\alpha-/\alpha\alpha$) carried an α-thalassemia 2 chromosome and the other parent carried the Southeast Asian variety of α-thalassemia 1 ($\alpha\alpha/--$). If both parents passed along their thalassemia chromosomes to a child, then the child ($\alpha-/--$) would be fairly markedly deficient in α-globin production. The net result of this would be a 4 to 1 predominance of β-globin chains leading to quite detectable levels of β_4 tetramers. In fact, the presence of significant amounts of β_4 has led to the designation of this situation as hemoglobin H disease. These individuals have moderate to marked anemia, which is present at birth. Their mean cell volume is quite low (about 50). This is not, however, a lethal condition.

The most severe situation, in which there are no functioning α-globin genes ($--/--$), leads to stillbirth or early neonatal death. In this situation, the predominant fetal hemoglobin is a tetramer of γ chains known as hemoglobin Bart's. This hemoglobin has virtually no oxygen-carrying capacity, so that the fetal tissues are deprived of oxygen, except for the small amount that is dissolved in the blood. In addition, there is a profound anemia. Heart failure results because of the efforts of an unoxygenated heart to pump the small amount of dissolved oxygen in the blood to oxygen-starved tissues. As the heart fails, marked edema (hydrops fetalis) occurs, and this condition is generally incompatible with life. This genotype can only arise when each parent carries a $--/$ chromosome. Most commonly, this results from both parents having the Southeast Asian variety of α-thalassemia 1 ($\alpha\alpha/--$), although occasionally one parent carries hemoglobin H disease ($\alpha-/--$). Hydrops fetalis is most commonly seen in individuals of Southeast Asian origin and is relatively rare in the black population because most α-thalassemia alleles in the black population are of the $\alpha-/$ type.

The causes of α-thalassemia are diverse at the molecular level. The most common abnormality, leading to loss of one α-globin gene on a chromosome, is unequal crossing over. As shown in Figure 6.16, there is a high degree of homology of the nucleotide sequence including and surrounding the $\alpha 2$ and $\alpha 1$ globin genes. The X and Y blocks shown in the figure represent regions that are greater than 90% identical to each other, and the Z block is greater than 99% identical. This is an ideal setup, therefore, for unequal crossing over. If the two homologous chromosomes align incorrectly, with the Z block of the $\alpha 1$ gene lined up with the Z block of the other $\alpha 2$ gene, a crossover in this interval can have two outcomes. In one situation, as shown at the top of the figure, a deletion occurs with the 5′ end of the resulting single α gene deriving from $\alpha 2$, and the 3′ end deriving from $\alpha 1$. In fact, most α-thalassemia 2 alleles have arisen by this mechanism. Alternatively, the other outcome of such an event leads to a chromosome with a triple α gene cluster. The exact anatomy of the chromosome depends upon the point of crossover, which can occur in the X and Y blocks as well as the Z. In support of

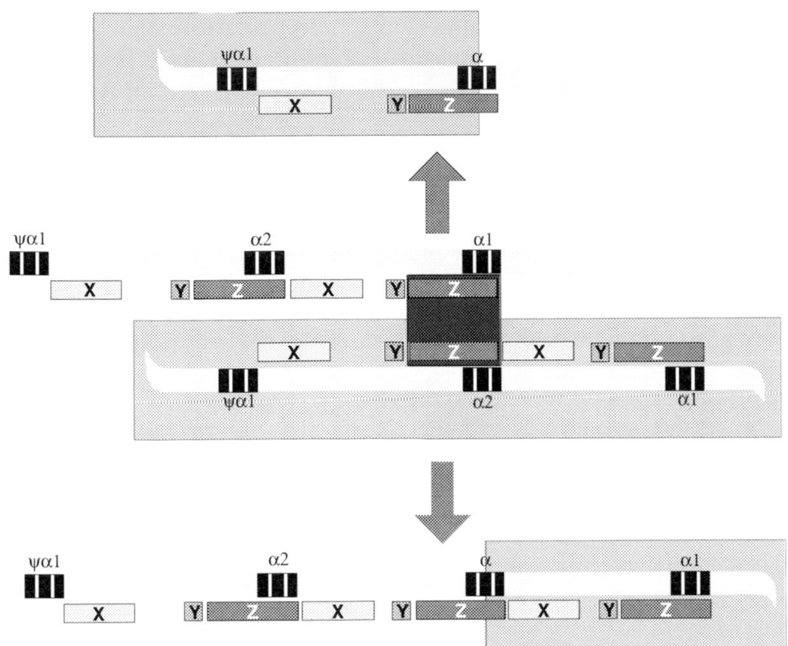

Figure 6.16. Misalignment of the α-globin cluster during meiosis leading to α-thalassemia. In the *middle* of the figure are shown two chromosomes that have lined up incorrectly so that α1 from one chromosome is matched with α2 from the homologous chromosome. If a crossover occurs in the Z box region, the outcome can be either a chromosome with only a single α gene (shown above), or a chromosome with three α genes (shown below).

this hypothesis, the triple α-globin gene chromosome is also seen at reasonably high frequency in most populations.

This mechanism, however, cannot explain the loss of *both* α-globin genes on one chromosome (— —/). Such chromosomes also are usually found to harbor deletions; in this instance the deletions are large, remove both α-globin genes, and cannot be easily explained by unequal crossing over. Finally, in a few situations, loss of function of an α-globin gene has been shown to arise from more subtle mutations such as nonsense or frameshift abnormalities; but in contrast to β-thalassemia (see below), these mutations are in the minority.

β-Thalassemia

In β-thalassemia it is the β-globin chains that are deficient. Since there is only one β-globin gene per chromosome 11, the potential for unequal crossing over is much reduced. When this does occur between δ and β, it results in hemoglobin Lepore as noted above; because the homology between δ and β is considerably less than the two α-globin genes, this is a relatively rare event. Loss or decreased function of the β-globin gene, therefore, is in general found to be due to other mechanisms.

The genetics of β-thalassemia are complicated by the large number of mutations that can result in decreased or absent function of a β-globin gene. The disease is inherited in an autosomal recessive fashion. Carriers are detectable, however, by the fact that their red cells have reduced volume, and they have characteristic mild increases in hemoglobin A_2 and hemoglobin F by hemoglobin electrophoresis. As in α-thalassemia, the genetic analysis is somewhat complicated by the large number of possible mutations and by the historical terminology that developed before the molecular basis of β-thalassemia was understood.

Figure 6.17 shows the possible phenotypes arising from mutations at the β-globin locus and the genotypes that can underlie them. Beginning at the most severe, β-thalassemia major represents the homozygous

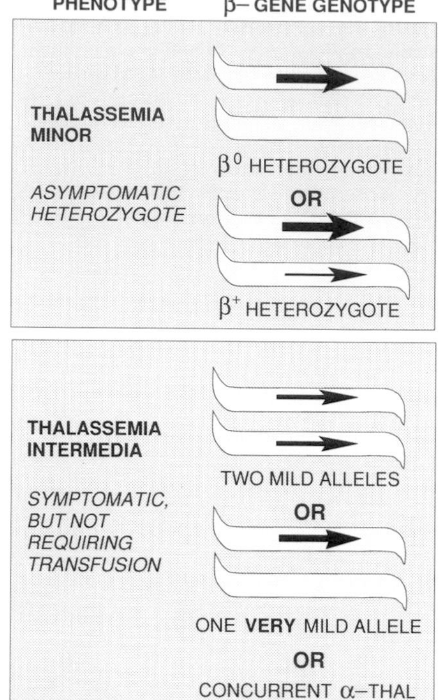

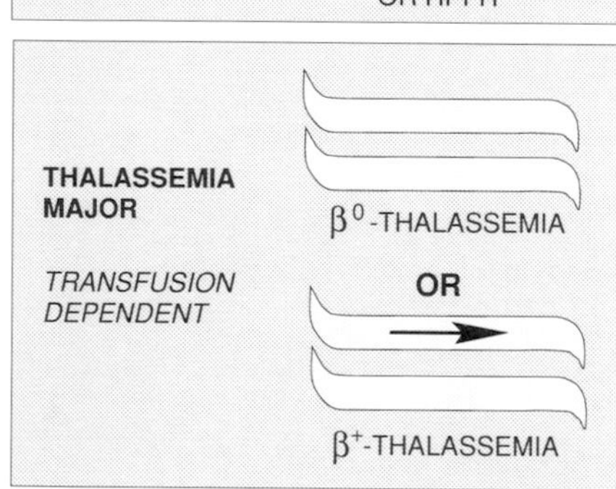

Figure 6.17. Possible genotypes that can give rise to phenotypes of β-thalassemia minor, β-thalassemia major, or β-thalassemia intermedia. The thickness of the *arrow* indicates the level of transcription from each β-globin gene. Note that concurrent α-thalassemia can lead to less severity of disease because of an improvement in balance of chain synthesis (Fig. 6.14). Hereditary persistence of fetal hemoglobin (*HPFH*) is also beneficial in β-thalassemia because the increased γ chains can partially make up for the deficiency in β.

state in which both β-globin genes contain mutations that prevent them from producing normal amounts of β-globin protein. If both β genes are completely nonfunctional, there will be no hemoglobin A whatsoever; this is denoted as β^0-thalassemia. If one or both of the mutations still allows the production of small amounts of β-globin, then this is denoted as β^+-thalassemia. Individuals with β-thalassemia major are transfusion-dependent and experience a variety of major medical problems, which will be described below.

Heterozygotes for β-thalassemia are said to have "thalassemia minor" and are asymptomatic. In general, they carry one normal β-globin gene and one which has a mutation that reduces or destroys its function. It is usually impossible to tell by looking at the level of β-globin in such an individual whether the thalassemia allele carried is a β^+ or a β^0 mutation because the normal chromosome is producing the vast majority of β-globin in both situations.

A somewhat confusing term is the designation "thalassemia intermedia," which has been used clinically to designate individuals who are significantly anemic and symptomatic but do not require transfusion. Such individuals have abnormalities in both of their β-globin genes, but one or both of these mutations is relatively mild so that a significant amount of β-globin production still occurs. An alternative mechanism for thalassemia intermedia is for an individual to be homozygous for β^+-thalassemia and for α-thalassemia. As can be appreciated from Figure 6.14, if *both* α- and β-globin production are reduced, the phenotype will be milder because of a lack of the destructive α_4 precipitates within red cells.

While α-thalassemias are primarily due to deletions, β-thalassemia is usually due to more subtle mutations. Intense work over the past decade has demonstrated a dizzying array of mutational events that can give rise to this phenotype. There are now more than 60 different mutations causing β-thalassemia, so this disorder is a prime example of allelic heterogeneity. Because of this wide diversity of mutations, most individuals with β-thalassemia major are in fact compound heterozygotes, having inherited a different mutation from each parent.

A diagram of some of the β-thalassemia mutations is shown in Figure 6.18. The mutations in the β-globin gene are scattered throughout the length of the gene, including the 5′-flanking region where the promoter lies. One of the points to carry away from this analysis is that almost every feature of the gene has been a target for thalassemia mutations. Thus, this is an example of "Murphy's Law of the Genome"—anything that can go wrong, will.

It is not important to absorb all of the details of this array of mutational events, but it is useful to consider some of the categories in a bit more detail. One interesting category consists of individuals with point mutations in the promoter of the gene, as shown in Figure 6.19. Four different mutational events that have occurred in the ATA box are shown, as well as three mutations in the CACCC sequence, which was previously described as being a consistent feature of β-globin genes. Individuals with any one of these mutations do make β-globin mRNA from the mutated gene, but at approximately 10% of the normal amount. This represents the ultimate proof that these sequences are crucial for efficient transcription of the β-globin gene. Thus far, no mutations in the CCAAT box have been identified.

Chain terminator mutations, in which translation is stopped prematurely, can result from nonsense mutations or frameshift mutations.

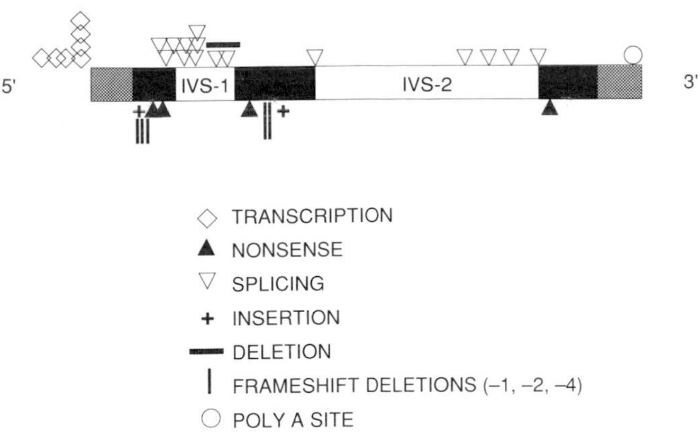

Figure 6.18. **Schematic diagram of some of the mutations that have been shown to cause β-thalassemia.** (From Stamatoyannopoulos G, Nienhuis AW, Leder P, Majerus PW: *The Molecular Basis of Blood Disease.* Philadelphia, WB Saunders, 1987.)

In most of these situations in Figure 6.18, the abnormality occurs early enough in the coding region that the resulting protein is missing one-half or more of its structure and is totally nonfunctional. This contrasts with hemoglobin Cranston and hemoglobin Constant Spring described above, where the abnormality occurs very near the end of the protein, and therefore function is still maintained. Chain terminator mutations early in the coding region usually lead to a product that is very unstable and is rapidly degraded within the cell. Thus, homozygotes for these mutations have β^0-thalassemia.

An interesting array of abnormalities occurs in the splicing signals, and these mutations have added considerably to our understanding of the normal splicing process. Some of these splicing abnormalities are relatively easy to understand, as they alter the invariant GT sequence at the beginning of an intron or the AG at the end. Since these sequences are absolutely required for normal splicing, it is not surprising that these lead to β^0-thalassemia. Somewhat more subtle, however, are mutations that do not occur in the invariant nucleotides but affect the consensus region of the donor or the acceptor. In Figure 6.20, for example, mutations in the donor sequence of the first intron are shown. Those that alter the first nucleotide, abolishing the normal GT sequence, lead to

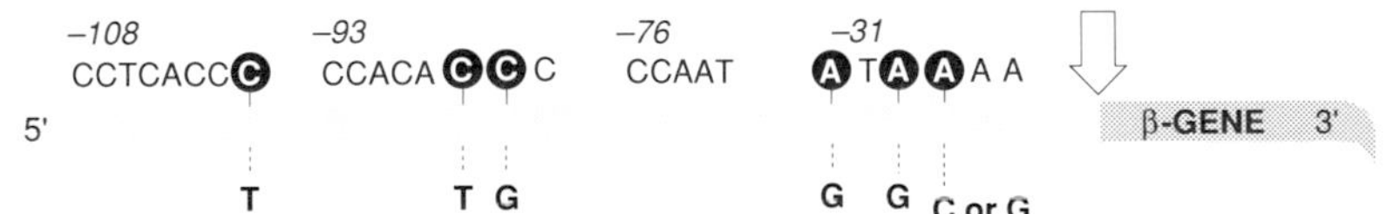

Figure 6.19. **Mutations in the β-globin promoter that have been found to give rise to β^+-thalassemia.**

	EXON 1	INTRON 1	PHENOTYPE
NORMAL	GCCAG	GT TGGTAT. . .	NORMAL
IVS - pos. 1	GCCAG	A TTGGTAT. . .	β^0
IVS - pos. 1	GCCAG	T TTGGTAT. . .	β^0
IVS - pos. 5	GCCAG	GTTG T TAT. . .	β^+
IVS - pos. 5	GCCAG	GTTG C TAT. . .	β^+
IVS - pos. 6	GCCAG	GTTGG C AT. . .	β^+
CONSENSUS DONOR	C/A AG	GT A/G AGT	

Figure 6.20. **Five mutations that have been described in the beginning of the first intron of the β-globin gene.**

β^0-thalassemia, but mutations at positions 5 and 6 within the intron lead to reduced ability of this RNA to splice correctly but still result in detectable amounts of normal β-globin. Thus, these mutations in the homozygous state lead to β^+-thalassemia.

A particularly instructive mutation, and the most common cause of β^+-thalassemia in the Mediterranean region, is a mutation within intron 1 that does not actually affect the sequence of the normal donor or acceptor site. This mutation, shown in Figure 6.21, is a simple point mutation of a G to an A at position 110 of intron 1 and occurs 21 nucleotides upstream of the normal splice acceptor site. The result of this mutation is the creation of an AG sequence, which previously did not exist at that location. This AG sequence is preceded by a long run of pyrimidines, and although the sequence is not an ideal fit for the consensus acceptor sequence, it functions extremely well. As shown in Figure 6.21, when this mutation is present, 90% of the splicing events use the new AG as the acceptor site, and only 10% splice into the correct site. The abnormally spliced RNA contains an additional 19 nucleotides in the mature RNA, which normally would have been removed during splicing. Because this is not a multiple of 3, the result is a frameshift mutation in all subsequent coding regions. Therefore, the abnormally spliced RNA does not give rise to useful protein, and only the 10% of the RNA that is normally spliced is useful. The phenotype is thus β^+-thalassemia in a homozygote.

An even more bizarre mutation is represented by hemoglobin E. This represents a puzzling combination of a qualitative and quantitative abnormality. As shown in Figure 6.22, hemoglobin E arises from a point mutation in codon 26 where the normal GAG codon is mutated to an AAG, resulting in a change from glutamic acid to lysine. One would

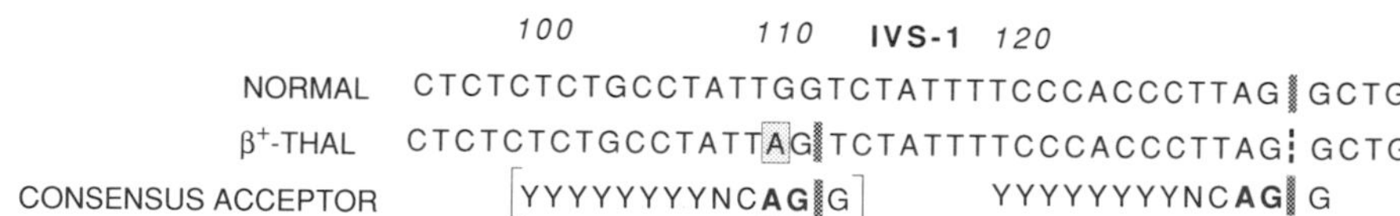

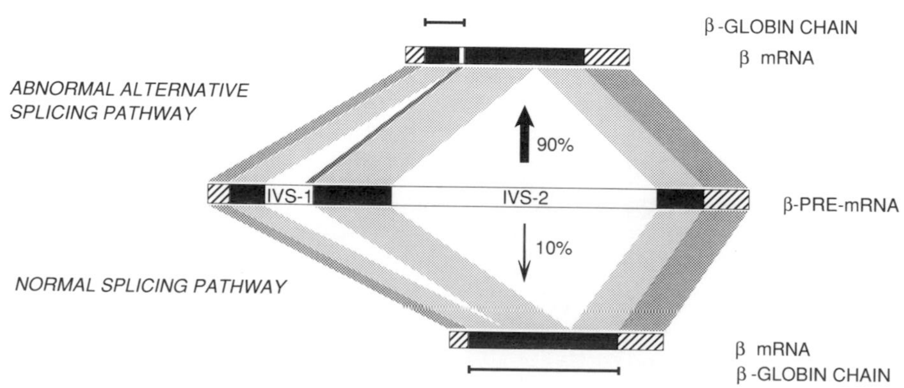

Figure 6.21. β^+-Thalassemia caused by a G to A mutation at position 110 of the first intron. This leads to creation of an abnormal splice acceptor site, as the new sequence contains an AG. As shown in the lower part of the diagram, this abnormal splicing pathway is used about 90% of the time. Only 10% of the message is spliced properly and can give rise to normal β-globin chains. Y = C or T; N = any nucleotide. The invariant AG in the consensus acceptor is *underlined*. *Vertical lines* indicate location of splice.

MECHANISM

NORMAL β GLOBIN	Gly	Gly	Glu	Ala
NORMAL GENE	GGT	G**GT**	**G**AG	GCC
CODON NUMBER	24	25	26	27
β^E GENE	GGT	G**GT**	**A**AG	GCC
β^E GLOBIN	Gly	Gly	Lys	Ala
"CONSENSUS" DONOR SIGNAL	C/A A	G**GT**	A/G AG	T

CONSEQUENCE

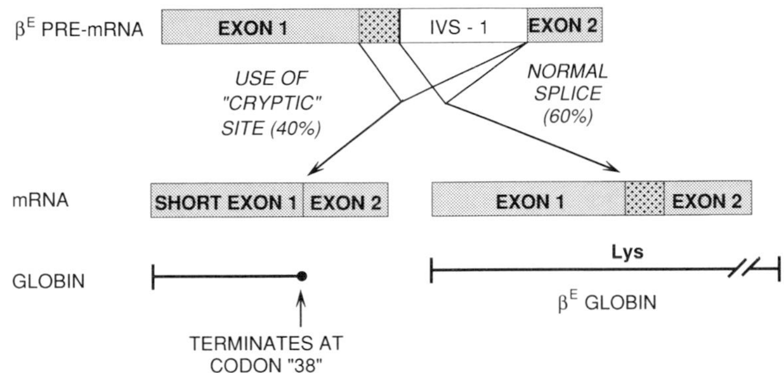

Figure 6.22. The mutation in hemoglobin E, which gives rise to both a quantitative abnormality, due to activation of a cryptic splice donor site, and a qualitative abnormality, because the properly spliced message will contain a lysine instead of glutamic acid at codon 26. The A in codon 26 is apparently enough to activate this otherwise cryptic splice donor site, which is then used in 40% of the splicing events.

predict that this would lead to a hemoglobin with abnormal electrophoretic mobility; this is, in fact, observed. However, individuals with this mutation produce only about 60% of the normal amount of β-globin from this mutant allele, and the reduction cannot be explained on the basis of protein stability. The reason for this additional quantitative reduction in protein production became clear when the pattern of splicing of the mutant gene was investigated. As shown in Figure 6.22, the sequence of codons 24–27 is actually a rather good fit for the consensus donor signal for splicing. In the normal situation, of course, this potential donor signal is not used at all. The nucleotide immediately following the GT in an ideal intron donor can be either A or G, but A is preferred, occurring about twice as often as G in this position. Apparently, the β^E mutation, which converts a G in this position to an A, activates this "cryptic" splice site so that it begins to function in a rather efficient way. The result of this event is that about 40% of the splices remove the sequence from codon 25 to the end of exon 1, or a total of 16 nucleotides. Again, because this is not a multiple of 3, the abnormally spliced message is out of frame in exon 2, resulting in termination at an out-of-frame stop codon. Thus, the 40% abnormally spliced RNA does not give rise to any detectable β-globin protein. The normally spliced RNA contains the β^E mutation. Thus, the result of this is a combined quantitative and qualitative abnormality from a single mutation.

A final interesting mutation shown in Figure 6.18 is a point mutation in the signal for polyadenylation, where the AATAAA is converted to an AACAAA. While transcription occurs normally, the cleavage and addition of A residues, which is required for normal processing and transport to the cytoplasm, is impaired, with the net outcome being a β^+-thalassemia phenotype.

CLINICAL ASPECTS OF β-THALASSEMIA MAJOR

Thalassemia major, also called Cooley's anemia after Dr. Thomas Cooley who first described this disorder, is usually not apparent at birth because the switch of fetal to adult hemoglobin is still incomplete and the deficiency of β-globin chains is not yet of consequence. However, during the first year of life, as fetal globin production progressively drops, symptoms of severe anemia become apparent. Because of this anemia, the bone marrow, within which the majority of red blood cells are destroyed before ever being released into the circulation, makes a massive effort at blood production. The cortex of the bones becomes thinned, which can lead to pathologic fractures as well as distortion of the bones of the face and the skull. The liver and spleen are also markedly enlarged and act as additional sites of red blood cell production (Fig. 6.23). If not treated, death usually occurs in the first decade of life due to severe anemia, debilitation, and infection.

These symptoms can be effectively alleviated by blood transfusion, since this supplies normal red blood cells and suppresses the overactive bone marrow. However, in the long run, transfusion is a two-edged sword. The reason for this relates to the mechanism of iron metabolism. Normally the total amount of iron in the body is regulated completely at the level of absorption. No efficient mechanism exists for increasing iron excretion when body stores accumulate. In the process of transfusion, total body levels of iron rise continuously, and with no means of excretion, the iron deposits in the heart, liver, pancreas, and other organs. This leads to a gradual failure of these organs, particularly the heart, and an inexorable downhill course. In Figure 6.24 is shown a survival curve for individuals with thalassemia major treated with transfusion. While survival is relatively normal in the first decade of life, the effects of iron overload become apparent after this, leading to death in the teens and twenties.

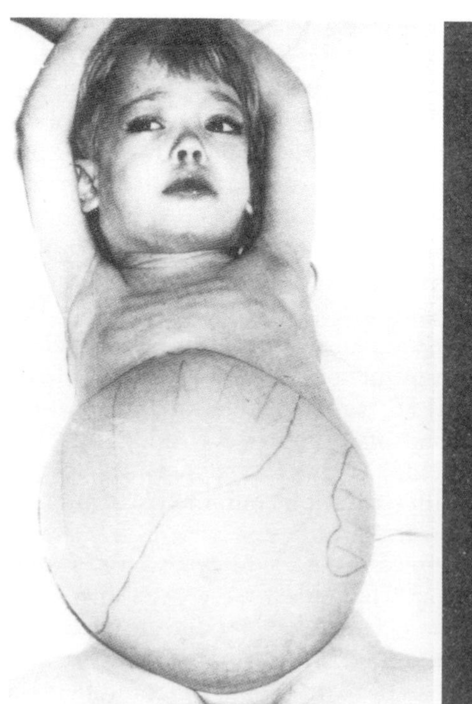

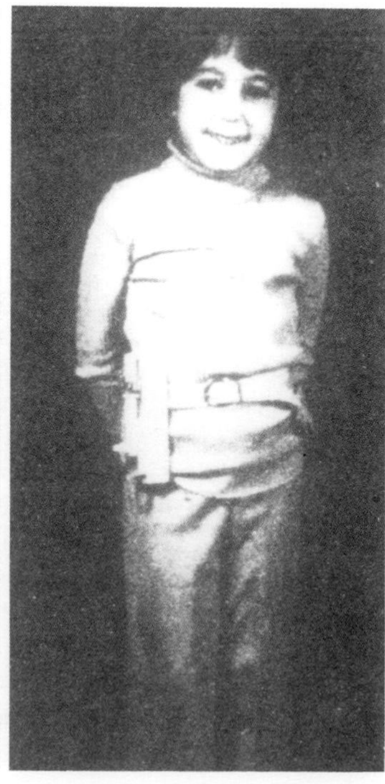

Figure 6.23. The clinical picture of thalassemia major. The individual on the *left* is 18 months old and has received no treatment. She shows marked enlargement of the liver and spleen (the borders of which have been marked on her abdomen), which are attempting to increase blood production. The individual on the *right* has been treated with a transfusion program and has a normal appearance. She is wearing an infusion pump that subcutaneously administers desferrioxamine, in order to handle the iron overload, which is an otherwise eventually fatal complication of transfusion therapy. (From Weatherall DJ, Clegg JB: *The Thalassemia Syndromes.* 3rd Ed. Oxford, Blackwell Scientific Publications, 1981.)

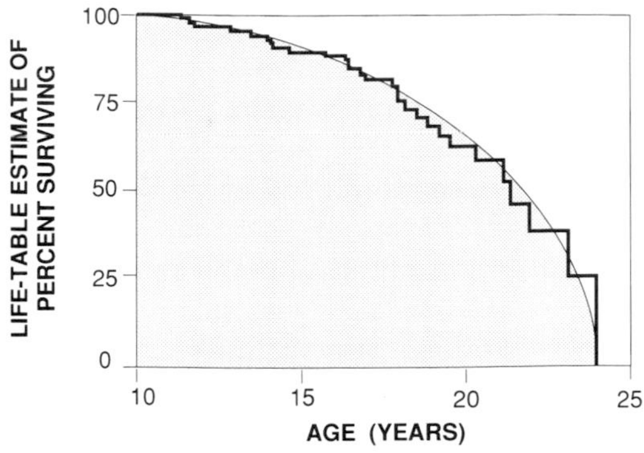

Figure 6.24. Survival curve for individuals with thalassemia major treated with transfusion but without iron chelation therapy. Survival has been improved over this curve by the introduction of agents that stimulate iron excretion, although it is not yet clear whether these will lead to a completely normal life span. (From Weatherall DJ, Clegg JB: *The Thalassemia Syndromes*. 3rd Ed. Oxford, Blackwell Scientific Publications, 1981.)

Some hope has been provided for this situation by the availability of drugs that chelate iron and lead to its excretion in the urine. The most commonly used drug, desferrioxamine, appears to be capable of chelating enough iron to keep up with chronic transfusions, but only if given continuously and subcutaneously through an infusion pump (Fig. 6.23). This is an inconvenient and painful method of administration, and an effective iron chelator that could be given orally is badly needed.

Future prospects for treatment of thalassemia major include bone marrow transplantation, which has been tried in a few patients and is curative if the marrow transplant is successfully carried out. However, the current high morbidity and mortality of bone marrow transplantation has limited the application of this approach to a small number of patients. Other approaches, which are still experimental and will be described in Chapter 12, include gene therapy, in which a normal β-globin gene is transferred into the bone marrow of an individual with β-thalassemia major, or methods of turning back on the fetal hemoglobin genes to compensate for the defective adult genes.

HEREDITARY PERSISTENCE OF FETAL HEMOGLOBIN

A final group of mutations to be considered in this chapter is that in which the developmental timing of globin production is altered. Individuals with hereditary persistence of fetal hemoglobin (HPFH) continue to produce increased amounts of hemoglobin F (greater than 1% of total) as adults, in the absence of other causes. In some instances these individuals may even produce 100% fetal hemoglobin. Somewhat surprisingly, this is a benign condition, and such individuals are usually unaware of the hemoglobin abnormality. One might expect that fetal hemoglobin, with its somewhat increased oxygen affinity, might lead to symptoms if its production continued throughout adult life, but these are sufficiently subtle that they do not cause overt clinical disease.

The significance of HPFH is two-fold. In the first place, mutations in developmental timing may provide clues to the general control of gene expression, which would advance our understanding in this area. Secondly, an ability to understand the control of fetal globin gene expression might allow manipulation of this situation in individuals with sickle cell anemia or β-thalassemia, in which turning the fetal globin genes back on would probably be curative.

The molecular basis of HPFH turns out to be heterogeneous (Fig. 6.25). Many such individuals have large deletions of the δ- and β-globin extending a considerable distance to the 3′ side. The fetal globin genes are not deleted, however, and by a poorly understood mechanism continue to be transcribed at high levels throughout life, rather than turning off at about the time of birth. Not all large deletions that remove the δ- and β-globin genes have this phenotype, however. Figure 6.25*A* also shows three mutations of the same type in which the fetal genes do turn off in their usual fashion. Since the δ and β genes are missing on the affected chromosome, the phenotype is therefore $\delta\beta$-thalassemia. The reason why some deletions lead to HPFH and others to thalassemia is still not understood.

Other individuals with HPFH do not have major deletions in the β-globin cluster. In general, these individuals overproduce either $^{G}\gamma$ or $^{A}\gamma$, but not both, and also continue to make substantial amounts of β-globin from their affected chromosome. Cloning and sequencing studies have demonstrated that these individuals carry point mutations in the promoter region of the overexpressed fetal globin gene, and the point mutations so far identified are shown in Figure 6.25*B*. As can be seen, these are scattered over a region 5′ to the start of transcription of the gene and presumably identify sequences involved in the normal switching mechanism. One of these mutations, located 117 bp 5′ to the start of transcription, is immediately adjacent to one of the duplicated CCAAT boxes, but most of the other mutations fall in regions of the promoter not previously suspected to be important for control. One hypothesis for the mechanism of these mutations would be that they fall in a binding site for a repressor that is normally involved in shutting off

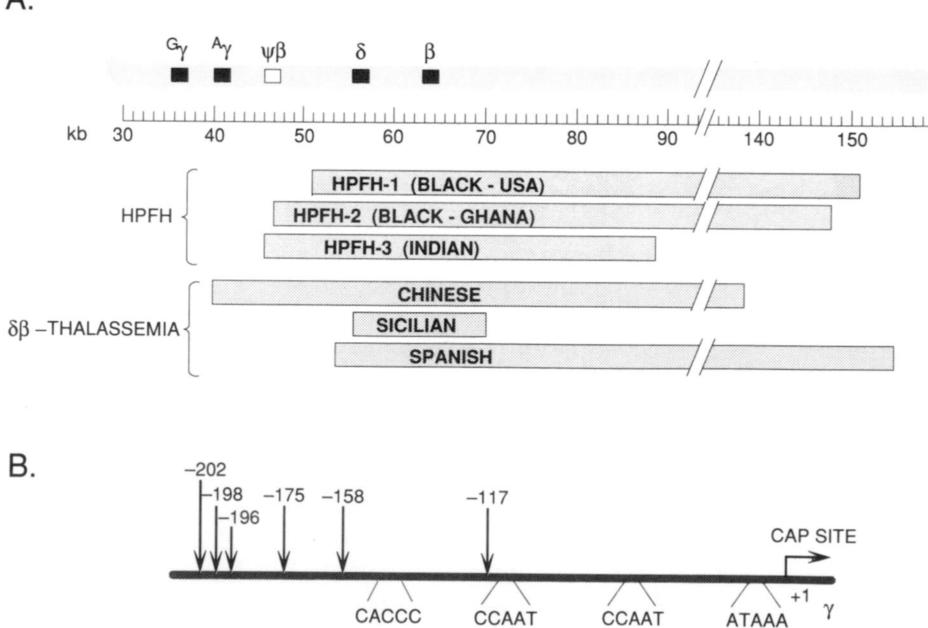

Figure 6.25. Molecular mechanisms leading to HPFH. In **A** are shown three HPFH deletions that remove large segments of DNA at the 3′ end of the β-globin cluster including the adult genes. Not all such deletions lead to HPFH, however, as shown by the three $\delta\beta$-thalassemia mutations also diagrammed. In **B** are shown the location of mutations (numbered relative to the cap site) in the promoter of either the $^{G}\gamma$ or the $^{A}\gamma$ fetal globin genes that have been found in individuals with HPFH (marked with *arrows* above the *line*). These positions presumably mark the location of important control sequences, but most do not involve the usual promoter elements (CACCC, CCAAT, or TATA).

fetal globin production but which cannot bind as well in the presence of a mutation. This hypothesis is under active study. What is learned from an analysis of HPFH mutations may well turn out to have clinical use in the attempt to develop effective treatments for sickle cell anemia and β-thalassemia.

CONCLUSION

In this chapter we have considered a wide variety of mutational events occurring in the human hemoglobin genes. Currently this system is the best studied of any set of loci in humans, and the rich array of mutational events is likely to foreshadow the findings with many other genes as our understanding of molecular genetics increases. For the student of genetics, the exact details of these mutations are not particularly critical; what is important, however, are the principles that emerge and the profound implications that an understanding of the mechanism of these mutations has for normal gene function. Truly, as Bateson advised some 70 years ago, "Treasure your exceptions."

SUGGESTED READINGS

General

Bunn HF, Forget BG: *Hemoglobin: Molecular, Genetic, and Clinical Aspects.* Philadelphia, WB Saunders, 1986. A superb and thoroughly referenced work on human hemoglobin, from protein structure and function through molecular biology.

Collins FS, Weissman SM: The molecular biology of human hemoglobin. Prog Nucleic Acid Res Mol Biol *31*:315–458, 1984. In-depth review of hemoglobin molecular biology.

Dickerson RE, Geis I: *Hemoglobin: Structure, Function, Evolution, and Pathology.* Menlo Park, CA, Benjamin/Cummings, 1983. A beautifully illustrated short volume on the structure of the hemoglobin protein.

Orkin SH, Kazazian HH: The mutation and polymorphism of the human β-globin gene and its surrounding DNA. Annu Rev Genet *18*:131–171, 1984. Review of mutations leading to β-thalassemia, by the authors who described the majority of these.

Stamatoyannopoulos G, Nienhuis AW, Leder P, Majerus PW: *The Molecular Basis of Blood Disease.* Philadelphia, WB Saunders, 1987. Also a superb reference text. Chapters on hemoglobin molecular biology and hemoglobin switching are particularly relevant.

Weatherall DJ, Clegg JB: *The Thalassemia Syndromes.* 3rd Ed. Oxford, Blackwell Scientific Publications, 1981. Encyclopedic work on the clinical and laboratory aspects of thalassemia. Most of the information in the book predates the explosion of information made possible by recombinant DNA, however.

Classic References

Ingram VM: A specific chemical difference between the globins of normal human and sickle cell anemia hemoglobin. Nature 178:792, 1956.

Pauling L, Itano H, Singer SJ, et al.: Sickle cell anemia: A molecular disease. Science 110:543, 1949.

6/ Study Questions

1/ Which of the following strategies would *not* be beneficial to a patient with β-thalassemia major?

A. Transfusion and iron chelation therapy
B. Increasing α-globin production
C. Increasing β-globin production
D. Increasing fetal hemoglobin production
E. Decreasing α-globin production

2/ A polymerase chain reaction (PCR, Chapter 5) test has been developed to detect sickle cell anemia. The sickle mutation alters codon 6 of the β-globin gene from GAG to GTG, eliminating an *Mst*II site that is normally present there. The primers used for the PCR are shown below:

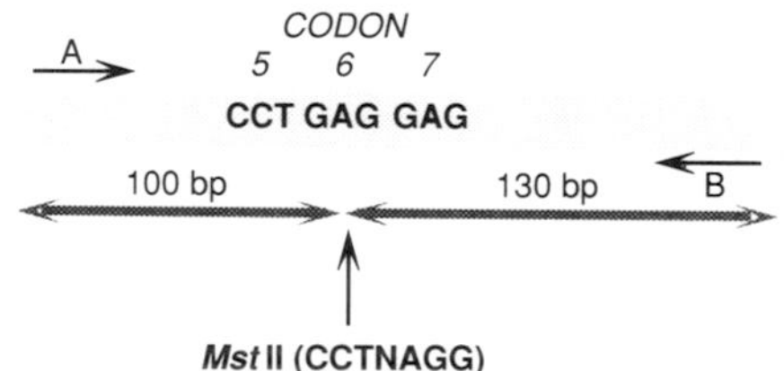

What are the expected sizes of PCR products for AA (homozygous normal), AS (heterozygous "sickle trait"), and SS (homozygous affected) individuals after *Mst*II digestion?

What would be the expected result for an individual homozygous for hemoglobin C (codon 6 AAG) and for an individual homozygous for codon 6 frameshift β-thalassemia (one base deletion of codon 6)?

3/ You are investigating a patient with thalassemia major. On taking a family history, you are surprised to find that, although the mother is from Greece where thalassemia is common, the father and all of his known ancestors are from Russia.

(a) What are some possible explanations?
(b) You perform paternity testing on the father and find that it is very likely (>99%) that he is, in fact, the biological father of the child. However, his blood shows absolutely no evidence that he has thal trait (thal minor). How could this be explained?
(c) What is the chance that this couple's next child will have thal major? Thal minor?

(d) Intrigued by this situation, you decide to clone the β-genes from this patient. You obtain two clones. By sequencing, one has a nonsense mutation at codon 30, a common defect in Mediterranean populations. This mutation creates a restriction site for the enzyme *Mae*I, which recognizes the sequence CTAG:

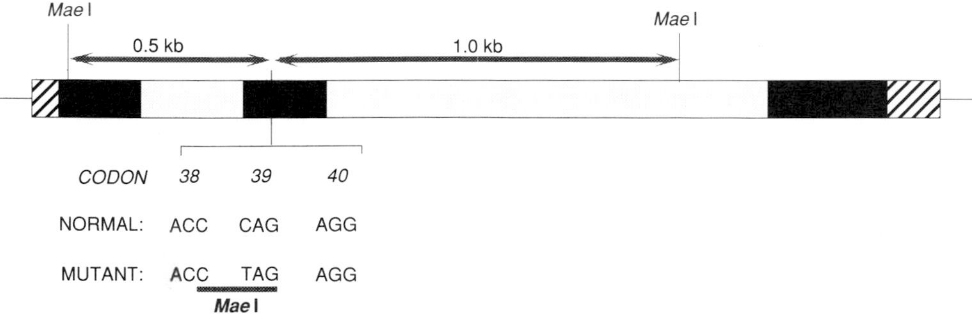

Using Southern blotting, how can you determine whether this is the mutant gene inherited from the mother? Be specific about how you set up the test. Assume you have available DNA on the mother, the father, the affected child, and any cloned DNA fragments you want from the β gene. How would you do the test using PCR?

(e) The other clone does not have this same mutation. Suspecting it may harbor a heretofore undescribed mutation, and with visions of fame in your head, you sequence the clone. The entire β gene is normal except for one nucleotide change at the end of the second intron:

```
                    intron 2              exon 3
Normal—CCTCTTATCTTCCTCCCACAG|CTCCTGGG . . .
Mutant—CCTCTTATCTTCCTCCCAC[T]G|CTCCTGGG . . .
```

How would this cause thalassemia?

Would you expect this to be a β^0-thal or β^+-thal allele?

4/ You are counseling a Greek couple because both parties have been found to be carriers of β-thalassemia in a population survey. They have one son who tests normal (not a carrier). They wish to know whether a current pregnancy is affected. You obtain fetal DNA by amniocentesis. Using a probe 10-kb 5′ to the β gene, which detects a *Hin*cII RFLP, you obtain the following blot:

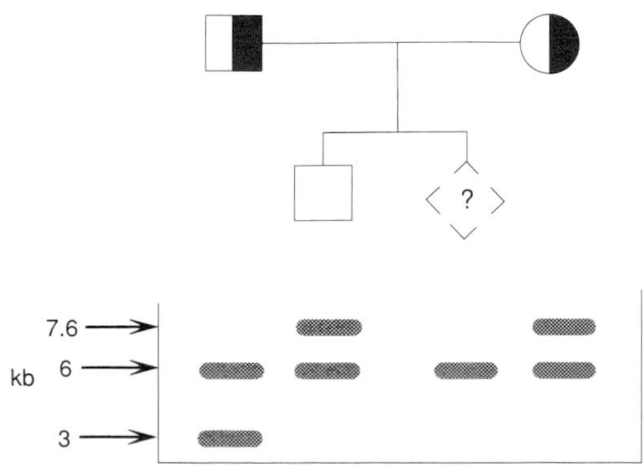

Is the fetus affected?

7

Biochemical and Molecular Genetics of Human Disease

"It is an old experience that through her errors, Nature often grants us unexpected insights into her secrets which are otherwise a closed domain."

—A. Loewy and C. Neuberg (From Über Cystiurie. Hoppe-Seyler's Physiol Chem 43:338–354, 1904)

"Whatever it is you're studying, you're better off if you have a mutant."

—Anonymous

In the previous chapter, the detailed dissection of the molecular pathology of the human hemoglobin molecule illustrated the rich diversity of mutational mechanisms that cause human genetic disease and introduced the principles of the molecular genetics of human disease. In this chapter, we will consider several other genetic diseases that are also well understood at a biochemical and molecular level. The examples chosen are not intended to be exhaustive; rather the specific diseases have been chosen because they illustrate specific principles of medical genetics. Sir Archibald Garrod's pioneering studies on alkaptonuria established the field of biochemical genetics and introduced the concept of the "inborn errors of metabolism." His insights into the principles of biochemical genetics, based on careful studies of human patients, are a paradigm of clinical investigation. The fortuitous observation of drug-induced anemia and the elucidation of glucose-6-phosphate dehydrogenase deficiency defined the field of pharmacogenetics. α_1-Antitrypsin deficiency illustrates how a single mutation in a nonenzymatic protein, a protease inhibitor, can predispose to a common serious disease, emphysema, by interacting with an all-too-common environmental toxin, cigarette smoke. The brilliant investigations of familial hypercholesterolemia illustrate beautifully the dynamic interface between basic genetics and clinical medicine, clarifying on one hand the normal cellular process of receptor-mediated endocytosis and, on the other hand, a major cause of coronary artery disease. Studies on urea cycle defects illustrate the impact of rapid advances in biochemical and molecular genetics on the diagnosis and therapy of previously lethal genetic diseases. Finally, molecular analysis of collagen disorders is increasing our understanding of "protein suicide" and the mechanisms by which dominantly inherited disorders of structural proteins cause disease.

INBORN ERRORS OF METABOLISM

In 1908, Archibald Garrod delivered the prestigious Croonian lectures to the Royal College of Physicians of London on the topic of "The Inborn Errors of Metabolism." He presented the results of his studies on four rare disorders in humans: alkaptonuria, pentosuria, cystinuria, and albinism. Alkaptonuria is characterized by black urine and degenerative arthritis of the spine and large joints. The urine is actually colorless when passed, but quickly turns black when exposed to air, secondary to the oxidation of the large amounts of homogentisic acid present in it. The deposition of endogenous homogentisic acid autooxidation products in cartilage and collagenous tissues accounts for the blue or black pigmented palate, black deposits in the sclerae of the eyes, and the degenerative changes in the large joints and in the intervertebral discs of the spine (Fig. 7.1). The ochre color of these cartilaginous deposits, when viewed under the light microscope, gave rise to the term ochronosis to describe this form of arthritis.

Garrod found that when homogentisic acid was fed to alkaptonuric subjects, it was excreted quantitatively in the urine; none was

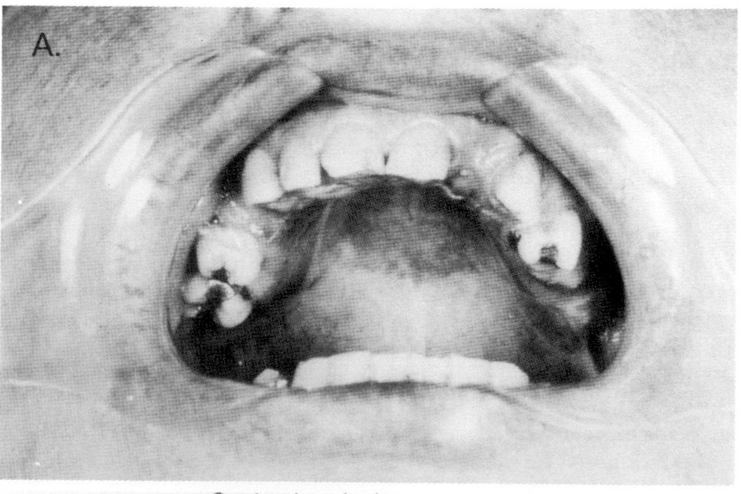

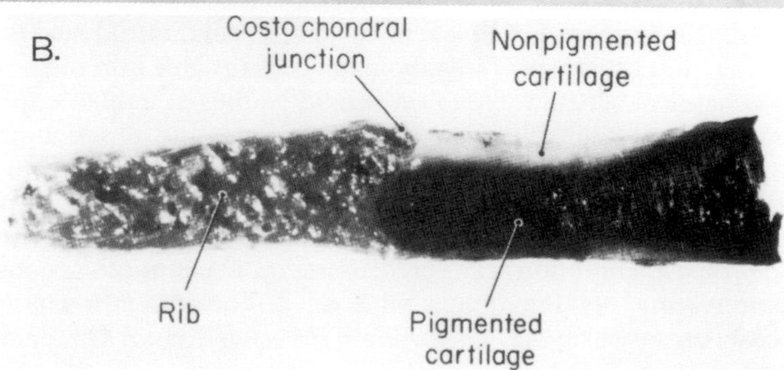

Figure 7.1. **A**, Pigmentation of the hard palate in a patient with alkaptonuria. **B**, Deeply pigmented costal cartilage in a patient with alkaptonuria. (Reproduced by permission from McKusick, VA: *Heritable Disorders of Connective Tissue.* 4th Ed. St. Louis, 1972, The C. V. Mosby Co.)

excreted by normal subjects. Furthermore, the amount of endogenous homogentisic acid excreted by alkaptonuric patients was increased by feeding them a high-protein diet and specifically by feeding the amino acids phénylalanine and tyrosine. Normal individuals fed these amino acids did not excrete any measurable homogentisic acid. Garrod interpreted these observations to indicate that homogentisic acid was a normal metabolic product of phenylalanine and tyrosine metabolism and that it was immediately converted to another metabolite and did not accumulate; however, in individuals with alkaptonuria, its further metabolism was blocked, and it accumulated and was excreted in the urine in large amounts. His hypothesis was proven 50 years later by the demonstration that the livers of alkaptonuric patients had no detectable homogentisic acid oxidase, the enzyme responsible for the further metabolism of homogentisic acid (Fig. 7.2). Garrod generalized from his studies on alkaptonuria that individual steps in metabolism were the work of unique enzymes. He wrote in 1908:

> The conception of metabolism in block is giving place to that of metabolism in compartments. The view is daily gaining ground that each successive step in the building up and breaking down . . . of individual fractions of proteins and of individual sugars is the work of special enzymes set apart for each particular purpose.

Garrod was also struck by the familial distribution of alkaptonuria. He noted that the abnormality is:

> . . . apt to occur in several brothers and sisters whose parents do not exhibit the anomaly and direct transmission from parent to child is very rare.

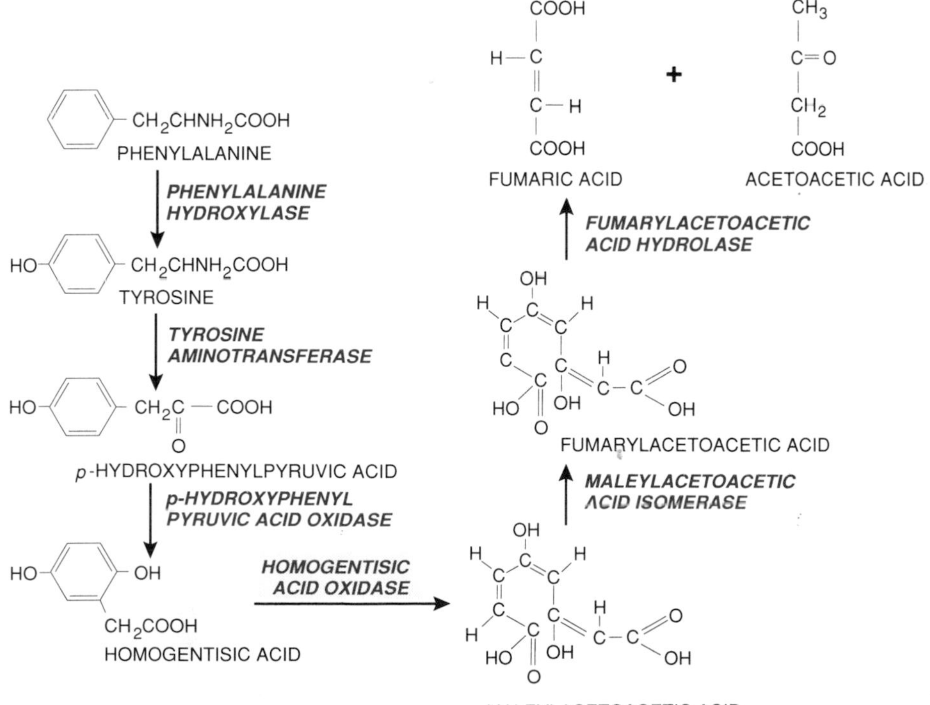

Figure 7.2. Enzymatic steps in the catabolism of phenylalanine and tyrosine to acetoacetic acid.

In 8 of 17 families with alkaptonuria, the parents were first cousins. Garrod consulted his friend, the distinguished English biologist William Bateson (who coined the term "genetics"). Bateson interpreted this familial pattern in light of the newly rediscovered laws of Mendel, pointing out that the mating of first cousins gives exactly the conditions most likely to enable a rare, recessive character to show itself. Alkaptonuria was thus the first autosomal recessive human disease recognized. The implication of this insight was that the normal allele was in some way necessary for the production of a specific enzyme in the unaffected individual. This was the first clue that genes may exert their effects by coding for enzymes. Garrod's work presaged the concept of one gene-one enzyme, which was established in the 1940s and 1950s by the pioneering work of George Beadle and Edward Tatum. Beadle and Tatum, studying the mold *Neurospora,* used UV light and x-rays to create nutritional, or auxotrophic, mutants, which lacked the ability to catalyze specific metabolic steps. They showed that individual metabolic steps in *Neurospora* were controlled by individual enzymes and that single mutations altered single functions. Beadle and Tatum had done their work in ignorance of Garrod's observations; however, Beadle paid tribute to Garrod in his Nobel Prize acceptance speech in 1958:

> . . . we had rediscovered what Garrod had seen so clearly so many years before. By now we knew of his work and were aware that we had added little if anything new in principle.

Finally, Garrod recognized the concept of biochemical and genetic individuality:

> The existence of chemical individuality follows of necessity from that of chemical specificity. Even those idiosyncrasies with regard to drugs and articles of food which are summed up in the proverbial saying that what is one man's meat is another man's poison presumably have a chemical (and genetic) basis.

Thus, Garrod laid the groundwork for the study of pharmacogenetics, discussed below, as well as the conceptual framework for the genetic basis of susceptibility to disease caused in part by exogenous agents.

Garrod's views were well ahead of his time. Despite his dominant position in English medicine (he succeeded Sir William Osler as the Regius Professor of Medicine at Oxford), his work on the inborn errors of metabolism had little immediate impact on clinical medicine. Garrod predicted that many more inborn errors would be found, suggesting that there was an "almost countless variety of such sports." In fact, few additional inborn errors of metabolism were discovered for many years, most likely because serious inborn errors caused death early in infancy and went unrecognized at a time when infectious diseases were a major cause of infant mortality.

The explosion in knowledge about inborn errors of metabolism had to wait until the introduction of antibiotics, which dramatically reduced the frequency of death in infancy from infectious causes, and the improvement in nutrition and control of such disorders as infant diarrhea. In addition, certain technical advances were also very important. These included the development of paper chromatography to separate amino acids and other metabolites from each other in urine and blood, the development of human cell culture techniques, which allowed investigators to study tissue from patients without requiring constant access to the patients, and subsequently the development of molecular techniques, which allowed a much more sophisticated approach to human biochemical disorders.

PHARMACOGENETICS

During World War II, when United States soldiers were given the drug primaquine for antimalarial prophylaxis, approximately 10% of black servicemen developed an acute but self-limited anemia secondary to the intravascular breakdown of red blood cells (hemolysis). A smaller number of white soldiers, usually of Mediterranean origin, developed a similar but often more severe hemolytic anemia. The basis for the drug-induced hemolytic anemia was found to be a genetically determined deficiency of the enzyme glucose-6-phosphate dehydrogenase (G6PD), which catalyzes the first step in the hexose monophosphate shunt pathway. One function of this minor pathway of glucose metabolism is the generation of NADPH, which in turn is necessary to maintain reduced sulfhydryl groups to protect cellular proteins against oxidative damage (Fig. 7.3).

Approximately 10% of black men were found to have a G6PD that was altered in electrophoretic mobility and had only 15% of normal enzymatic activity. These men were clinically entirely normal unless they were exposed to certain drugs such as primaquine or the antibiotic Furadantin, or to certain infections such as viral hepatitis or bacterial pneumonias. Under these circumstances, they developed an acute hemolytic anemia. Young red blood cells from affected individuals were found to be more resistant to oxidant damage and to have higher levels of G6PD activity than did older red blood cells. It was subsequently found that the abnormal G6PD, designated A$^-$, had decreased stability in vivo with a reduction in half-life from 62 to 13 days. Although the same defect was found in other cell types, the clinical phenotype was limited to anemia. This is because mature red blood cells lack a nucleus and ribosomes and thus are unable to synthesize new proteins to replace those that are degraded. Thus, an oxidant stress would selectively hemolyze old red cells with diminished G6PD activity. In an otherwise healthy individual, the bone marrow is able to respond to this stress with increased production of red blood cells. These young red blood cells, because of their normal levels of G6PD, would be resistant to the oxidant stress. Therefore, as long as the bone marrow was able to increase red cell production, the hemolytic anemia was self-limited even in the continued presence of the offending drug.

Recent studies have defined the molecular defect in G6PD A$^-$ (Table 7.1). An A → G change at nucleotide 376 in exon 5 results in a substitution of aspartic acid for asparagine at amino acid position 126. This same mutation is found in G6PD A, an electrophoretic variant with normal enzymatic activity, which is also common in the black population. The substitution of the acidic amino acid aspartic acid for the basic amino acid asparagine presumably accounts for the more rapid electrophoretic mobility of the A and A$^-$ variants relative to the B, or wild-type, G6PD. A second mutation in G6PD A$^-$, a G → A change in nucleotide 202 in exon 4, results in a substitution of methionine for valine at amino acid 68 and presumably accounts for the decreased stability of the variant.

In the Mediterranean variant of G6PD, the activity of the enzyme is considerably lower (3–4% of normal activity) and there is a greater risk of hemolytic anemia. A C → T transition at nucleotide 563 in exon

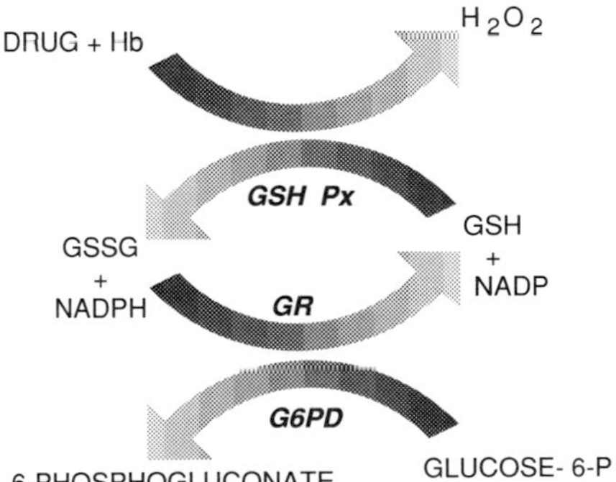

Figure 7.3. Role of G6PD in the generation of NADPH used to protect the red blood cell against oxidative damage. NADPH is necessary for the glutathione reductase (GR)-catalyzed reduction of oxidized glutathione (GSSG) to reduced glutathione (GSH). The latter is oxidized by glutathione peroxidase (GSH Px) in the presence of peroxides.

Table 7.1. Mutations in G6PD Variants[a]

Variant	Enzyme Activity in Red Blood Cells (% of Normal)	Clinical Expression	Exon Number	Base Position	Base Change	Codon Change	Amino Acid Position	Amino Acid Substitution
B (wild-type)	100	None						
A	100	None	V	376	A → G	AAT → GAT	126	Asn → Asp
A^-	15	Acute hemolytic anemia	V	376	A → G	AAT → GAT	126	Asn → Asp
			IV	202	G → A	GTG → ATG	68	Val → Met
Mediterranean	4	Acute hemolytic anemia	VI	563	C → T	TCC → TTC	188	Ser → Phe

[a]From Vulliamy TJ, D'Urso M, Battistuzzi G, Estrada M, Foulkes NS, Martini G, Calabro V, Poggi V, Giordano R, Town M, Luzzatto L, Persico MG: Diverse point mutations in the human glucose-6-phosphate dehydrogenase gene cause enzyme deficiency and mild or severe hemolytic anemia. Proc Natl Acad Sci USA 85:5171–5175, 1988.

6 results in the substitution of phenylalanine for serine at amino acid 188 (Table 7.1) and presumably accounts for the decreased catalytic activity and stability of this variant enzyme. In some Mediterranean G6PD-deficient individuals, especially children, ingestion of fava beans (the common broad bean in the Mediterranean region) causes a dramatically severe acute hemolytic crisis (favism), often requiring blood transfusion. As early as the 5th century BC, the Greek historian Herodotus had described an unusual response of some Greeks to the ingestion of fava beans. Thus, G6PD deficiency is a striking confirmation of Garrod's prediction that idiosyncratic reactions to drugs and articles of food could be the result of inborn errors of metabolism.

Family studies indicated that G6PD was encoded by a gene, designated Gd, on the X chromosome, and the gene was subsequently mapped to the end of the long arm of the X chromosome, very close to the hemophilia A locus. More than 300 allelic mutations have been described, many of which occur at polymorphic frequencies. G6PD variants have provided interesting models for studying structure-function relationships in a human enzyme. There are a variety of different defects affecting this molecule, ranging from alterations in the K_m for the substrate glucose 6-phosphate, to alterations in the K_i for NADPH, to differences in synthetic rates and stability. Some variants cause no disease at all (for example, the electrophoretic variant G6PD A), whereas others cause severe chronic hemolytic anemia even in the absence of offending drugs or infections. Most mutant alleles are named after the geographic area in which they were first described and cover the alphabet from Aachen in West Germany to Zhitomir in the Ukraine.

G6PD deficiency is common, affecting approximately 400 million people worldwide. It is found in high frequency in African, Mediterranean, and Asiatic populations in which malaria has been endemic, leading to the suggestion that resistance to malaria may account for this balanced polymorphism. Although there appears to be no benefit to the G6PD-deficient hemizygote, women heterozygous for the mutant G6PD A^- have been found to have lower parasite counts and are relatively resistant to malaria infection.

G6PD deficiency is a paradigm of pharmacogenetics, the study of the genetic basis for differences in response to drugs. Several other polymorphisms have been described that specifically affect drug metabolizing enzymes and may account for differences in therapeutic efficiency of drugs as well as for idiosyncratic reactions to drugs among different individuals. Genetic differences in drug metabolizing enzymes among different races may account for observed racial differences in therapeutic efficiency of drugs (for example, differences in β-blocker effects between Orientals and Caucasians) and for the greater susceptibility of Orientals to alcohol-induced facial flushing and palpitations. Garrod's concept of chemical individuality also suggested that there might be genetic differences in response to exogenous pathogenic agents that might account for differences in susceptibility to disease. α_1-Antitrypsin deficiency provides an excellent example of just such a situation.

α_1-ANTITRYPSIN DEFICIENCY

The serine proteases are a group of closely related proteolytic enzymes, with serine in their active site, which play a key role in coagulation and fibrinolysis and in kinin and complement activation. The activities of these enzymes are controlled at least in part by specific inhibitors known collectively as serine protease inhibitors, or serpins. The serine protease inhibitor found in highest concentration in plasma is α_1-antitrypsin, a 52-kDa glycoprotein, which accounts for 90% of the total α_1-globulin in plasma. Despite its name, the major function of α_1-antitrypsin is to inhibit the activity of elastase generated by neutrophils in the lung. The major phenotype of α_1-antitrypsin deficiency is destruction of pulmonary alveoli resulting in chronic obstructive pulmonary disease or emphysema.

The gene for α_1-antitrypsin is highly polymorphic, with more than 70 different alleles described in the European population. The different forms of α_1-antitrypsin, frequently designated as Pi for proteinase inhibitor, are commonly distinguished by differences in electrophoretic mobility. The most common allele in the European population is Pi^M, with an allele frequency of 0.95; 90% of white Europeans have the MM genotype. Two mutant alleles, S and Z, account for most of the disease associated with α_1-antitrypsin deficiency. The frequency of the important Pi genotypes and the activity associated with each is indicated in Table 7.2. Pi^{ZZ} is associated with 10–15% of normal activity and is found in approximately 1 in 2500 whites of Northern European descent. This mutant accounts for most of the illness associated with α_1-antitrypsin deficiency. Homozygous Pi^{SS} reduces α_1-antitrypsin activity by only 50–60% and does not cause disease. However, heterozygous Pi^{SZ} individuals have 30–35% of normal activity and may develop emphysema. In addition, a dozen rare alleles have been described that cause severe deficiency or absence ("null alleles") of detectable α_1-antitrypsin.

Individuals with α_1-antitrypsin deficiency have at least a 20-fold increased risk of developing emphysema; 80–90% of deficient individuals eventually develop this condition. Activated neutrophils elaborate elastase that, if unchecked by the proteinase inhibitor, can cause

Table 7.2. Clinically Important Pi Genotypes

	Pi Genotype				
	MM	MZ	SS	SZ	ZZ
Frequency	0.90	0.038	0.001	0.0012 (1/800)	0.0004 (1/2500)
Activity (% control)	100	60	50–60	30–35	10–15

destruction of lung tissue. Furthermore, they release oxygen radicals and chlorinated oxidants that can oxidize the methionine at the active site of α_1-antitrypsin. Such oxidation decreases the rate of association of the inhibitor with neutrophil elastase 2000-fold, markedly reducing its ability to inhibit elastase activity. The unopposed elastase activity is thought to cause destruction of the lung.

Clinical and epidemiologic studies indicate that α_1-antitrypsin deficiency causes much more severe disease in cigarette smokers than in nonsmokers. The basis for this is probably the effect of smoking on the elaboration of oxygen radicals by neutrophils and macrophages. There is a 2½-fold increase in superoxide anion and an 8-fold increase in peroxides formed by alveolar macrophages in the lungs of smokers. These levels of oxygen radicals, in vitro, decrease the ability of normal α_1-antitrypsin to inhibit neutrophil elastase activity by 60%. Thus, the interaction of an environmental agent, cigarette smoke, with a genetic predisposition, deficiency of α_1-antitrypsin, results in severe lung disease. Nonsmokers with α_1-antitrypsin deficiency also develop emphysema, but they tend to do so later in life than smokers, and while life expectancy is decreased relative to unaffected individuals, it is not nearly so severely decreased as it is in deficient subjects who are cigarette smokers (Fig. 7.4).

Individuals with Pi^{ZZ} also develop liver disease, thought to be the result of accumulation of the abnormal protein secondary to failure of the hepatocyte to secrete it. Approximately 10–15% of affected patients develop a neonatal cholestatic hepatitis and approximately 20% of those children develop juvenile cirrhosis. Approximately 20% of adults with α_1-antitrypsin deficiency also develop cirrhosis of the liver and with it an increased risk of primary carcinoma of the liver.

The gene for α_1-antitrypsin has been cloned and mapped to the long arm of chromosome 14. The Pi^S variant results from a GAA to GTA mutation in exon 3 causing the substitution of valine for glutamic acid at position 264. This results in the production of an inhibitor with decreased stability. The Pi^Z variant results from a mutation in exon 5

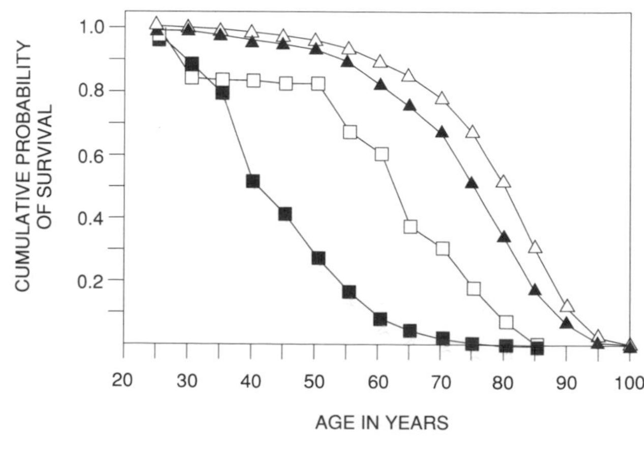

Figure 7.4. Cumulative probability of survival, given that 20 years of age is reached, in smoking and nonsmoking Pi^{ZZ} individuals compared with all Swedish individuals. (From Larsson C: Natural history and life expectancy in severe α_1-antitrypsin deficiency, Pi Z. Acta Med Scand 204:345–351, 1987.)

changing GAG, encoding glutamic acid at position 342, to AAG, encoding lysine. This change has been shown to cause decreased processing and secretion of the abnormal α_1-antitrypsin in the liver, a major source of its biosynthesis, as well as in mononuclear macrophages. In addition, the altered protein appears to be less effective as an inhibitor of neutrophil elastase than is the normal form.

Although the α_1-antitrypsin gene is highly polymorphic, only two mutations, Z and S, cause the great majority of disease associated with a deficiency of this protease inhibitor. Therefore, it is feasible to offer prenatal DNA diagnosis for this condition using allele-specific oligonucleotide probes, a technique discussed in Chapter 5. The relevant regions of DNA can be amplified using the polymerase chain reaction (Chapter 5) and probed with allele-specific oligonucleotides specific for the normal or mutant sequence (Fig. 7.5). In addition, restriction frag-

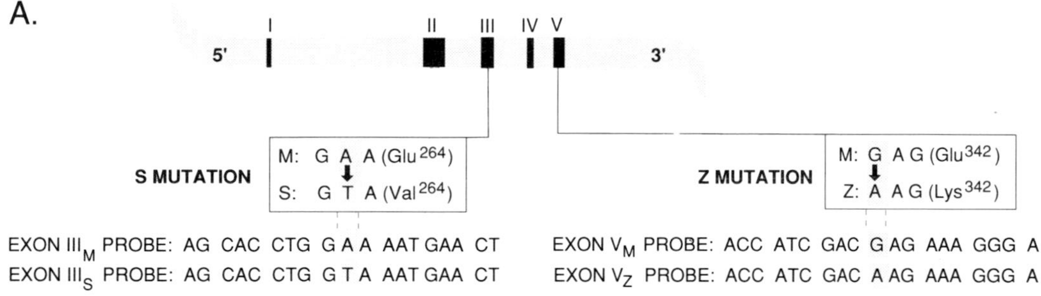

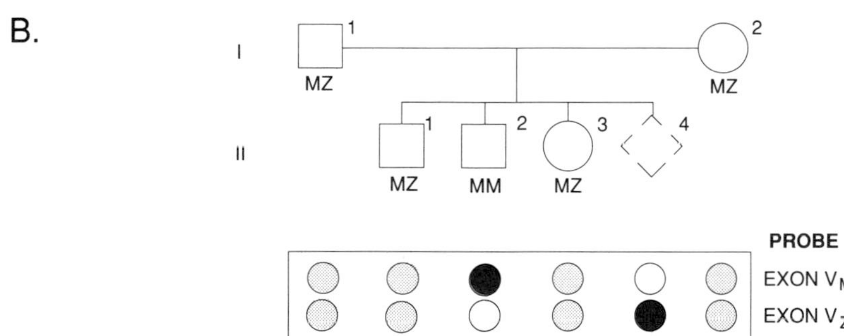

Figure 7.5. The strategy to recognize the S and Z mutations in the α_1-antitrypsin gene using synthetic allele-specific oligonucleotide probes. A, The structure of the α_1-antitrypsin gene is shown with its five exons (*solid boxes* labeled I-V). The *boxes* below the gene structure indicate the mutations encoding the S and Z forms of α_1-antitrypsin. The pairs of 19-mer oligonucleotide probes used to detect these two mutations are shown at the *bottom* of the figure. (Modified with permission from Nukiwa T, Brantly M, Garver R, Paul L, Courtney M, LeCrocq J-P, Crystal RG: Evaluation of "at-risk" α_1-antitrypsin genotype SZ with synthetic oligonucleotide gene probes. J Clin Invest 77:528–537, 1986.© permission of the American Society for Clinical Investigation. **B**, Prenatal diagnosis of a fetus with Pi ZZ α_1-antitrypsin deficiency using synthetic allele-specific oligonucleotide probes. Genomic DNA was obtained from the individuals shown in the pedigree, including the fetus at risk, and amplified using the polymerase chain reaction. Amplified DNA was applied to nylon filter membranes as "dot blots" and hybridized with labeled oligonucleotide probes specific for the Z and M sequences. Radioactivity was detected by autoradiography. Pi typing in the parents and siblings of the fetus at risk was carried out by standard electrophoretic techniques. DNA from I-1 and I-2 and II-1 and II-3 hybridized with both probes confirming heterozygosity for Pi MZ; DNA from II-2 hybridizes only with the M-specific probe. DNA from the fetus hybridized only with the Z-specific probe, indicating homozygosity for the mutant allele.

ment length polymorphisms have been identified using genomic probes. Highly accurate prenatal diagnosis can be accomplished using a combination of allele-specific oligonucleotide probes and RFLPs.

Therapy of α_1-antitrypsin deficiency has been attempted by replacement of human inhibitor purified from plasma. Studies in a series of patients with already established pulmonary disease have indicated that weekly injections of purified inhibitor can restore α_1-antitrypsin levels in blood and alveolar fluid to levels that ought to be protective against neutrophil elastase activity. Obviously, patients with α_1-antitrypsin deficiency, even more than unaffected individuals, must be strongly encouraged not to smoke cigarettes. Future prospects for replacement therapy include the delivery of inhibitor directly to the lungs by aerosol and the use of low molecular weight inhibitors of neutrophil elastase such as eglin C, an inhibitor isolated from the medicinal leech.

Gene therapy is also being explored (see Chapter 12). Mouse fibroblasts have been transfected with human α_1-antitrypsin cDNA and found to synthesize the inhibitor both in vitro and after implantation of the cells into the peritoneal cavity of nude mice. As noted earlier, the wild-type or normal α_1-antitrypsin has methionine at its active site and is susceptible to oxidative damage. Therefore, investigators have used site-directed mutagenesis to substitute valine for methionine in the active site and expressed this protein in bacteria. These studies have shown that α_1-antitrypsin containing valine in its active site appears to be fully active in vitro and to be resistant to damage by oxygen radicals generated by stimulated neutrophils. Thus, it is possible that molecular manipulations may allow the development of an even better α_1-antitrypsin molecule for replacement therapy. Unfortunately, replacement either with purified inhibitors or by somatic cell gene therapy will not prevent the liver disease associated with the ZZ genotype unless endogenous mutant gene expression can be turned off.

α_1-Antitrypsin deficiency is a very common autosomal recessive disorder in the white population. Although many individuals with this condition appear to be asymptomatic until late in life when they develop pulmonary emphysema or cirrhosis of the liver, they are at high risk if exposed to a specific environmental agent, cigarette smoke. Thus, α_1-antitrypsin is a paradigm of an "ecogenetic" disorder, resulting from the interaction of an unfortunately common environmental factor with a specific genetic predisposition to disease. Biochemical and molecular investigations have determined the nature of the two common mutations that cause disease associated with α_1-antitrypsin deficiency, have provided techniques for highly accurate prenatal diagnosis of this disease, and have offered possible ways to manipulate the α_1-antitrypsin gene to produce a more effective inhibitor that is less sensitive to oxidative damage.

FAMILIAL HYPERCHOLESTEROLEMIA

Familial hypercholesterolemia is an autosomal dominant disease affecting 1 in 500 individuals and is found in approximately 5% of myocardial infarction patients under the age of 60. The disease is characterized by elevated serum cholesterol (300–600 mg/dl, normal less than 230) and a low density lipoprotein (LDL) cholesterol of greater than 200 mg/dl. Approximately 50% of affected adults manifest deposits of cholesterol (xanthomas) in extensor tendons, typically an irregular thickening of the Achilles tendons, and xanthelasmata, yellowish fatty deposits of the eyelids. Most significantly, patients with familial hypercholesterolemia have early onset of atherosclerotic cardiovascular disease. The medical and family history of W. H. presented in Chapter 3 (Fig. 3.3) is typical for this condition. It is important to emphasize that, given the autosomal dominant inheritance, diagnosis of an affected individual immediately identifies a population at high risk of hypercholesterolemia and premature atherosclerotic heart disease. All first degree relatives have a 50% chance of being affected and should be tested for this condition. Hypercholesterolemia is present in childhood so that the condition can be detected early and dietary and drug intervention begun before atherosclerotic heart disease develops. Because the disease is relatively common, mating between heterozygotes occasionally occurs (1/500 × 1/500 = 1/250,000) and homozygous affected offspring occur with a frequency of approximately 1 in 1 million. Homozygous affected individuals have very high blood cholesterol levels (600–1,200 mg/dl), frequently suffer heart attacks in childhood, and often die from coronary artery disease in the second or third decade of life. Familial hypercholesterolemia is important not only because it is common and treatable, but because the elegant investigations of Michael Brown and Joseph Goldstein, for which they were awarded the Nobel Prize in 1985, beautifully illustrate the dynamic interface between medicine and genetics.

The Cellular Defect in Familial Hypercholesterolemia

Brown and Goldstein astutely selected cultured skin fibroblasts from homozygous affected individuals as their model system. They demonstrated that fibroblasts from such patients had high levels of β-hydroxy-β-methylglutaryl-CoA reductase (HMG-CoA reductase), the rate-limiting enzyme in cholesterol biosynthesis, that were not normally repressed by incubation in the presence of LDL. The defect, however, was not in the regulation of HMG-CoA reductase per se, and thus not in cholesterol biosynthesis, but rather in the delivery of the regulatory signal, cholesterol. Using radioiodinated LDL, they demonstrated specific, saturable binding of LDL to the surface of normal cells. Electron microscopic studies indicated that the LDL receptor was not distributed randomly on the cell surface but rather was located in specialized structures called coated pits that contain a specific protein, clathrin. Binding of LDL particles to LDL receptors in coated pits resulted in their subsequent internalization and in the degradation of the apoprotein to amino acids and the cholesterol esters in the LDL particle to free cholesterol. Free intracellular cholesterol triggered three important regulatory events: a marked decrease in the synthesis of HMG-CoA reductase, resulting in decreased endogenous synthesis of cholesterol; increased activity of acyl-CoA cholesteryl transferase, resulting in increased cholesterol esterification and storage; and importantly, decreased synthesis of LDL receptors, resulting in a decrease in cellular uptake of exogenous cholesterol (Fig. 7.6).

Fibroblasts from patients homozygous for familial hypercholesterolemia failed to bind and internalize LDL and thus to repress HMG-CoA reductase. Therefore, the defect in familial hypercholesterolemia appeared to be a deficiency of functional LDL receptors. Patients with the more common partial deficiency of LDL receptors, i.e., those het-

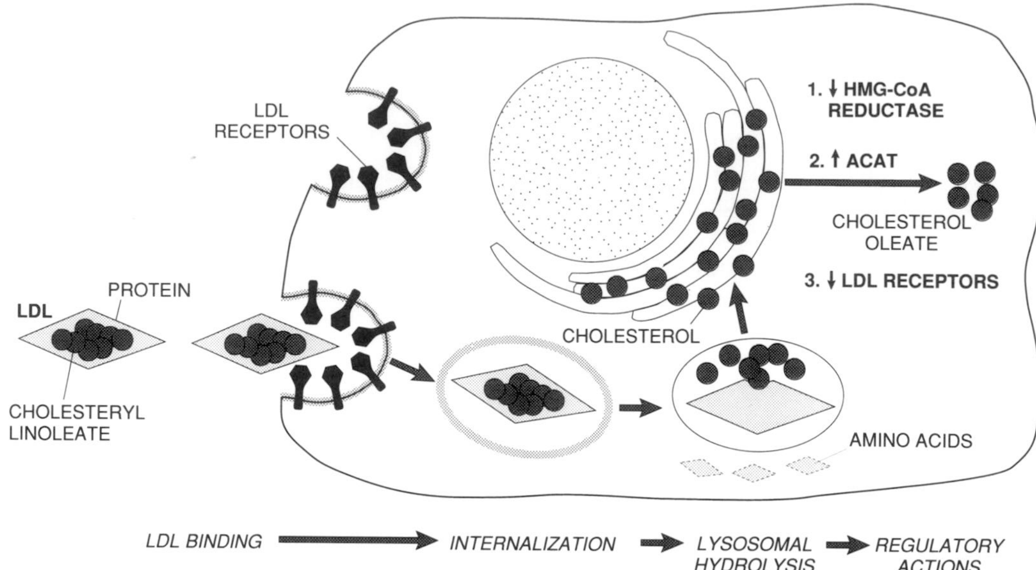

Figure 7.6. Sequential steps in the LDL receptor pathway in cultured mammalian cells. *HMG-CoA reductase* denotes β-hydroxy-β-methylglutaryl coenzyme A reductase; *ACAT* denotes acyl-CoA:cholesterol acyltransferase; *vertical arrows* indicate the directions of regulatory effects. (From Brown MS, Goldstein JL: Receptor-mediated endocytosis: Insights from the lipoprotein receptor system. Proc Natl Acad Sci USA 76:3330–3337, 1979.)

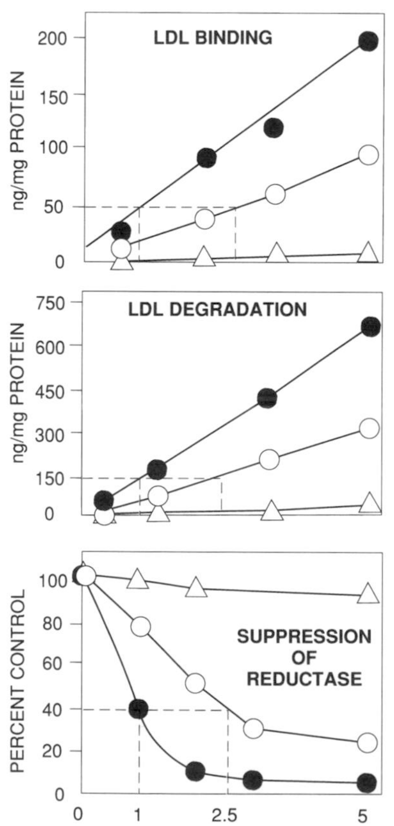

Figure 7.7. LDL binding, LDL degradation, and suppression of HMG-CoA reductase in cultured skin fibroblasts from a normal individual *(closed circles)*, a heterozygote for FH *(open circles)*, and a homozygote with FH *(open triangles)*. (From Goldstein JL, Brown MS: Familial hypercholesterolemia, genetic regulatory defect in cholesterol metabolism. Am J Med 58:147–150, 1975.)

erozygous for familial hypercholesterolemia who have one normal allele encoding a normal LDL receptor, show an intermediate defect. Cultured fibroblasts from heterozygotes show normal regulation of HMG-CoA reductase by LDL but only at higher concentrations of ambient LDL than are necessary in normal fibroblasts (Fig. 7.7). Thus, normal regulation occurs at the expense of an increased LDL cholesterol level. These studies, in addition to defining the molecular defect in familial hypercholesterolemia, also elucidated a very important normal cellular process, namely, receptor-mediated endocytosis, a process by which cells specifically bind and internalize a variety of important ligands including hormones, such as insulin, and nutritional signals, such as the iron-binding protein transferrin.

The LDL Receptor

Purification of the LDL receptor and cloning of its cDNA and gene indicated that the receptor is synthesized on the endoplasmic reticulum, glycosylated during its passage through the Golgi complex, and is inserted into the membrane as an integral membrane protein of approximately 160-kDa apparent molecular mass. The domain structure of the LDL receptor was defined by analysis of its amino acid sequence as well as study of specific mutations (Fig. 7.8). The N-terminal end of the molecule contains the ligand binding domain that has a strongly negative charge and is composed of seven repeated units of 40 amino acids, each containing 6 cysteines. This domain is followed by a domain that resembles the precursor to epidermal growth factor (EGF). A short stretch containing O-linked sugars is followed by a membrane-spanning region and a 50-amino acid cytoplasmic tail at the carboxyl end of the molecule. The latter two domains appear to be important in anchoring the receptor and properly locating it in coated pits in the cell membrane.

The LDL receptor gene is 45 kb in length, has 18 exons, and has been mapped to chromosome 19. The gene encodes a 5.3-kb mRNA.

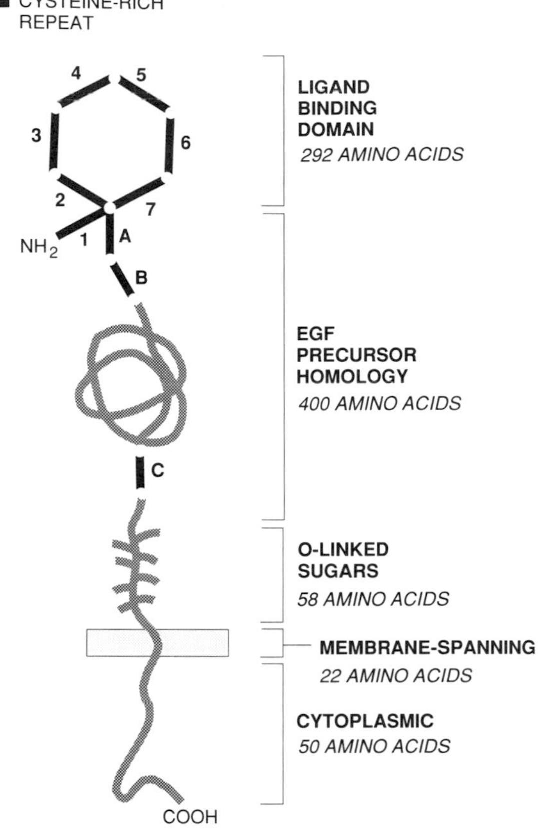

Figure 7.8. Domain structure of the human LDL receptor. Cysteine-rich repeat units are indicated by *red bars* numbered *1–7* and *A–C*. Repeats 2–7 are believed to constitute the major binding site for LDL. (From Esser V, Limbird LE, Brown MS, Goldstein JL, Russell DW: Mutational analysis of the ligand-binding domain of the low-density lipoprotein receptor. J Biol Chem 263:13282–13290, 1988.)

Analysis of the gene has shown that the ligand binding domain is encoded by 5 exons (numbers 2–6), the EGF precursor homology region by the next 8 exons, the glycosylated portion of the molecule by a single exon, and the membrane-spanning region by exon 16 and part of 17 with the cytoplasmic tail being encoded by the remainder of exon 17 and part of exon 18.

Mutations in the LDL Receptor

Analysis of more than 135 homozygous patients has indicated a rich variety of mutations and a high degree of allelic heterogeneity in familial hypercholesterolemia (Fig. 7.9). More than 35 distinct mutations have now been defined including insertions and deletions as well as missense and nonsense mutations. Most families have unique mutations not found in other families, and in fact, many "homozygotes" have turned out to represent compound heterozygotes, heterozygous for different allelic mutations in the LDL receptor gene. The large 5′ deletion found in French-Canadian patients and the nonsense mutation in exon 14 in Lebanese patients are exceptions in that they have been found in several families within a population group. It is thought that this situation represents a founder effect (see Chapter 3).

Analysis of insertion and deletion mutations in the LDL receptor gene has yielded interesting information about the possible mechanism

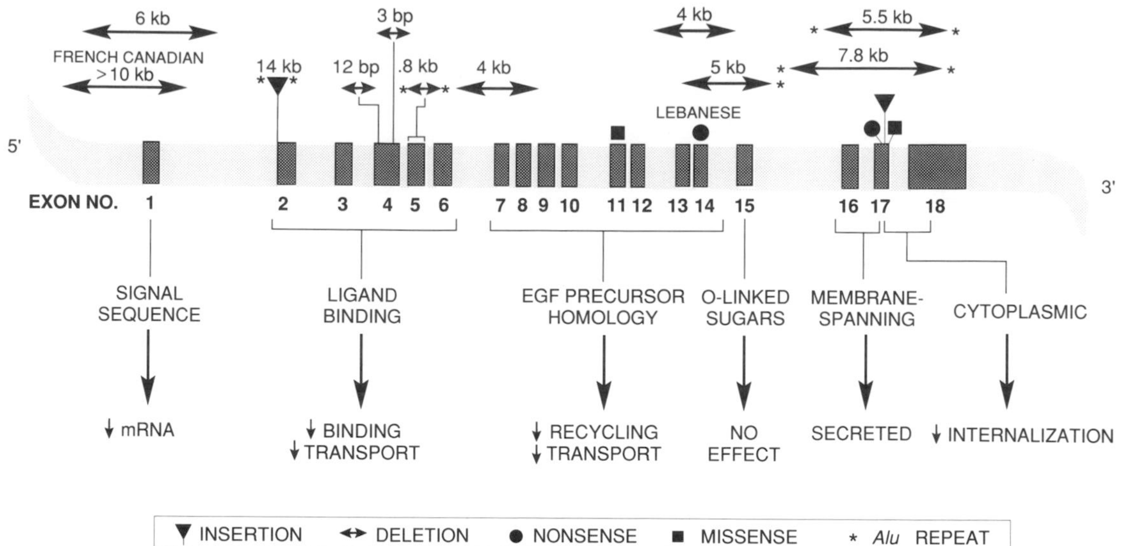

Figure 7.9. The location of missense, nonsense, insertion and deletion mutations in the LDL receptor gene. The size of the insertions and deletions is indicated in kilobases (kb), base pairs (bp) or nucleotides (nt). The functional consequences of mutations in the different domains is indicated below the gene. (From Goldstein JL, Brown MS: Familial hypercholesterolemia. In Scriver CR, Beaudet AL, Sly WS, Valle D: *The Metabolic Basis of Inherited Diseases.* 6th Ed. New York, McGraw-Hill, 1989, pp 1215–1250.)

of such mutations as well as about the evolution of the LDL receptor gene. Molecular analysis of a family with a 14-kb insertion in exon 2 revealed that this mutation causes a duplication of exons 2–8 and thus, of the entire binding domain. Sequence analysis of the ends of this insertion indicated the presence of *Alu* sequences at each end. *Alu* sequences are moderately repetitive sequences of approximately 150–300 bp in length containing a recognition site for the restriction enzyme *Alu.* There are approximately 500,000 copies of these sequences in the human genome, comprising about 5–10% of the genome (see Chapter 2). Because of the high degree of similarity of the sequences, it was proposed that unequal crossover events might occur between those homologous repetitive elements (Fig. 7.10). *Alu* sequences are found in introns 1 and 8 and might account for a homologous recombination event resulting in an unequal crossover and the duplication of exons to 2–8. A similar mechanism might explain the evolution of the exons encoding the 40 amino acid repeats comprising the ligand binding domain of this molecule. It is possible that an ancestral gene with a single 40-amino acid cysteine-rich sequence was duplicated several times by this mechanism of unequal crossing over to generate the current ligand binding domain of the molecule. Analysis of a family with a 7.8-kb deletion extending from the middle of intron 15 into exon 18 to a region encoding the 3′-untranslated end of the LDL receptor revealed that both deletion breakpoints have *Alu* sequences at each end, suggesting that this deletion also arose by an unequal crossover secondary to homologous recombination between *Alu* repeats. To date, several deletion mutations have been found to have *Alu* sequences at one or both ends, suggesting that this may be a common mechanism for the generation of deletion and insertion mutations in this and other genes (see Chapter 6).

The various mutations affecting the LDL receptor gene have been grouped into four functional classes (Fig. 7.11). The first and most common is a failure to synthesize the receptor; no cross-reacting protein is

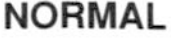

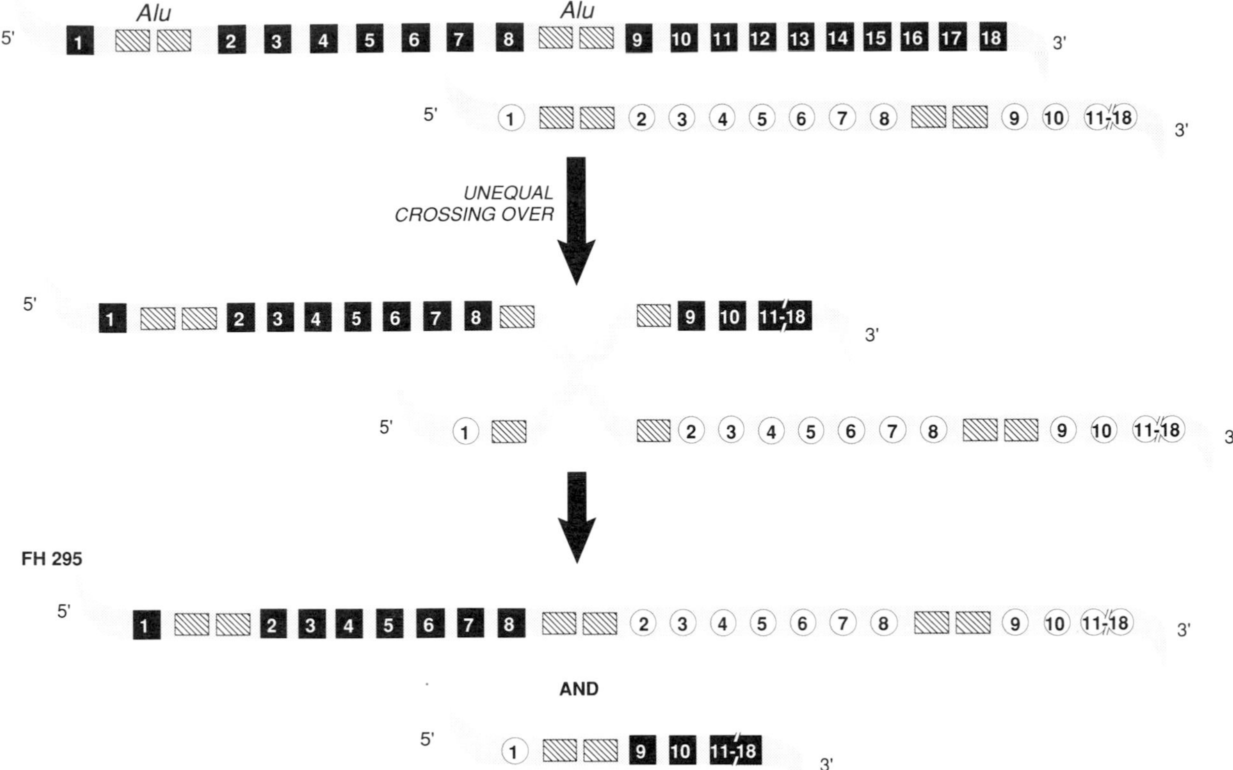

Figure 7.10. Unequal crossing over between two repetitive *Alu* elements in an LDL receptor gene from an FH homozygote. Two copies of the normal receptor gene, one with exons indicated by *bold rectangles* and the other with exons indicated by *light circles,* are aligned to illustrate the point of unequal crossing over in FH 295. The crossing over involved *Alu* elements in both genes that paired with each other. The recombination event is predicted to yield one gene with two copies of exons 2–8 and a hypothetical gene in which exons 2–8 are deleted. The exons are denoted by *numbered boxes;* exons and introns are not drawn to scale. (Redrawn from Lehrman LE, Goldstein JL, Russell DW, Brown MS: Duplication of seven exons in the LDL receptor gene caused by Alu-Alu recombination in a subject with familial hypercholesterolemia. Cell 48:827–835, 1987. © Cell Press.)

recognized immunologically in these mutants (null alleles). Thirteen different null mutations have been defined. A second class is characterized by failure to transport newly synthesized LDL receptor from the endoplasmic reticulum to the Golgi complex. Almost half of 128 fibroblast strains from FH homozygotes that have been analyzed carry at least one allele of this type. One example is the result of a missense mutation in exon 11 encoding a portion of the EGF precursor homology domain. A third class of mutations encodes a receptor that reaches the cell surface but is defective or deficient in binding LDL; affected individuals usually have 2–30% of normal binding. A fourth rare, but very interesting, class of mutations results in receptor mislocation.

In the last, the LDL receptor fails to be localized in coated pits and results in defective internalization of bound LDL. Three such mutations have been defined (Fig. 7.12), one each resulting from a missense mutation, a nonsense mutation, and a frameshift mutation, all in exon 17. The first receptor mislocation mutation was discovered because cultured fibroblasts from a boy with the clinical picture of homozygous familial hypercholesterolemia showed near normal binding of LDL but deficient internalization and, hence, deficient regulation of HMG-CoA

Figure 7.11. Four classes of mutations at the LDL receptor locus. See text for discussion. (Redrawn from Goldstein JL, Brown MS: Progress in understanding the LDL receptor and HMG-CoA reductase, two membrane proteins that regulate the plasma cholesterol. J Lipid Res 25:1450–1461, 1984.)

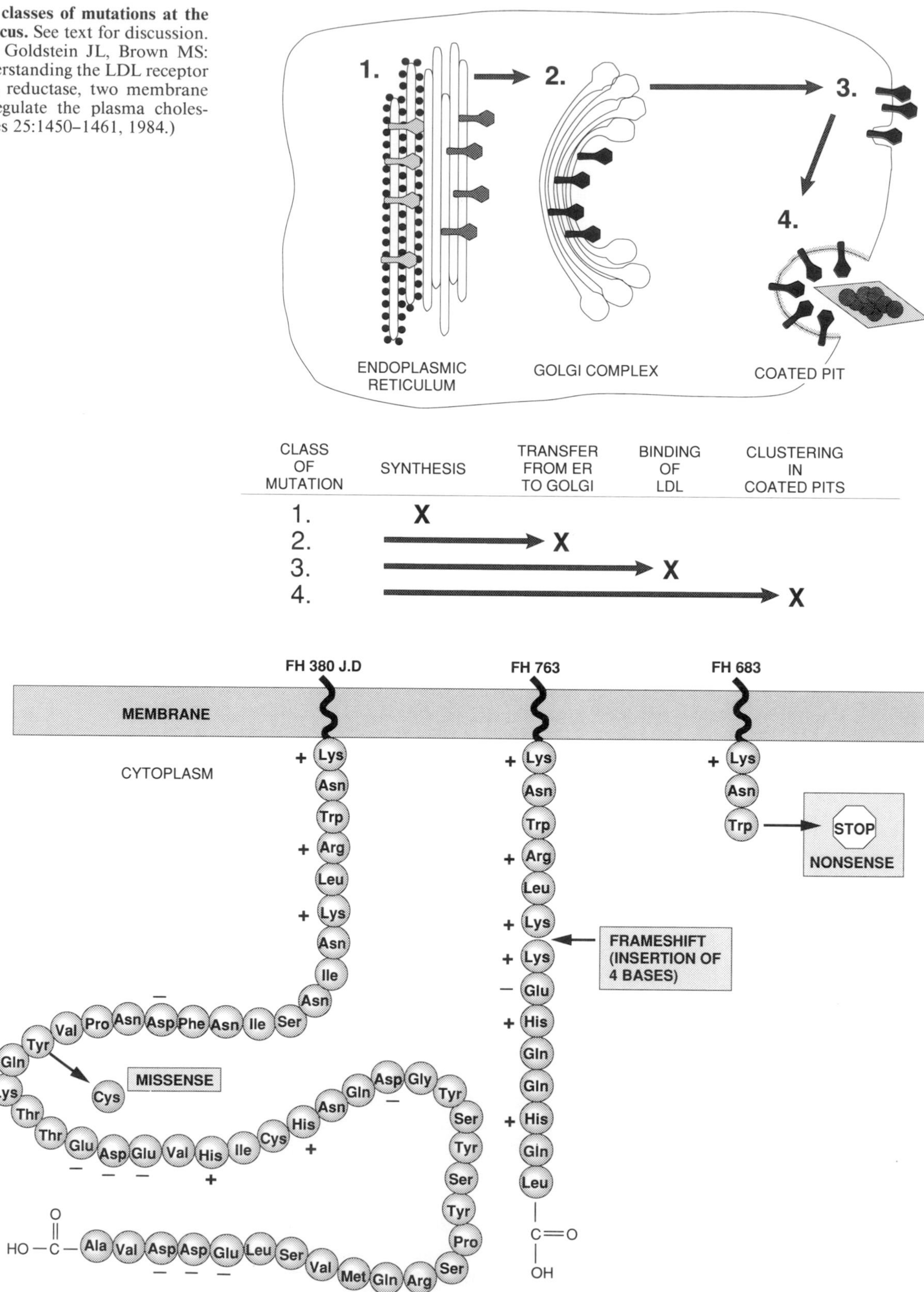

Figure 7.12. Mutations affecting the cytoplasmic domain of the LDL receptor in three FH homozygotes with the internalization-defective form of FH. (From Brown MS, Goldstein JL: A receptor-mediated pathway for cholesterol homeostasis. Science 232:34–47, 1986. © The Nobel Foundation, 1986.)

reductase. Analysis of fibroblasts from his parents indicated that no functional LDL receptor was encoded by his mother's mutant allele, whereas the LDL receptor encoded by his father's mutant allele was not found in coated pits but was inserted in the cell membrane at random; this LDL receptor was able to bind LDL but not to internalize it. In this mutation, a TAT/C encoding tyrosine was changed to TGT/C encoding cysteine (Fig. 7.12). Proof that this mutation caused the receptor mislocation phenotype was obtained by using oligonucleotide site-directed mutagenesis to mutate the normal LDL receptor cDNA so as to mimic the mutation in this patient. The mutated cDNA was transfected into a variant line of Chinese hamster ovary cells lacking LDL receptor. The transfected cells expressed LDL receptor randomly on the membrane but not in coated pits. Other mutations affecting the C-terminal end of the LDL receptor, such as the 7.8-kb deletion discussed above, result in a failure to anchor the receptor in the membrane and in secretion out of the cell of more than 90% of the newly synthesized receptor. Thus, analysis of a variety of mutations causing familial hypercholesterolemia has resulted in an understanding of the domain structure of this molecule and the functional properties of each structural domain.

Physiology of the LDL Receptor Pathway

Although the cellular and molecular defect in familial hypercholesterolemia was defined in cultured skin fibroblasts, the major site of cholesterol biosynthesis and uptake is the liver. Subsequent studies showed that liver contains the same LDL receptor system defined in fibroblasts and that 70% of hepatic LDL uptake is mediated by LDL receptor-dependent pathways. The pathophysiologic role of LDL receptor deficiency in familial hypercholesterolemia was further defined by studies on an animal model, the Watanabe heritable hyperlipidemic (WHHL) rabbit. The homozygous mutant rabbit lacks LDL receptors and has markedly elevated cholesterol, closely mimicking human familial hypercholesterolemia. LDL cholesterol levels are elevated because of a combination of increased production of LDL from intermediate density lipoproteins (IDL), which are normally taken up by hepatic LDL receptors, and reduced clearance of LDL secondary to the reduced number of LDL receptors.

Therapeutic Implications of the LDL Receptor Model

The studies of Brown and Goldstein predicted that one might be able to increase the number of hepatic LDL receptors in heterozygous deficient individuals by increasing hepatic demand for cholesterol. Decreasing exogenous cholesterol by decreasing dietary cholesterol and saturated fat does produce a modest and limited decrease in LDL cholesterol concentration in affected individuals. A more significant decrease in blood cholesterol is achieved by interfering with the enterohepatic circulation of bile acids using anion exchange resins such as cholestyramine (Fig. 7.13). Bile acids, containing significant amounts of cholesterol, are normally secreted into the bile and reabsorbed in the terminal ilium and returned to the liver. By interfering with the reabsorption of bile acids, cholesterol levels can be reduced by 25–30% in heterozygotes with familial hypercholesterolemia. This is presumably associated with an increased number of hepatic LDL receptors. Unfortunately, hepatocytes also respond to this decrease in cholesterol returning via the enterohepatic circulation by increasing the amount of HMG-

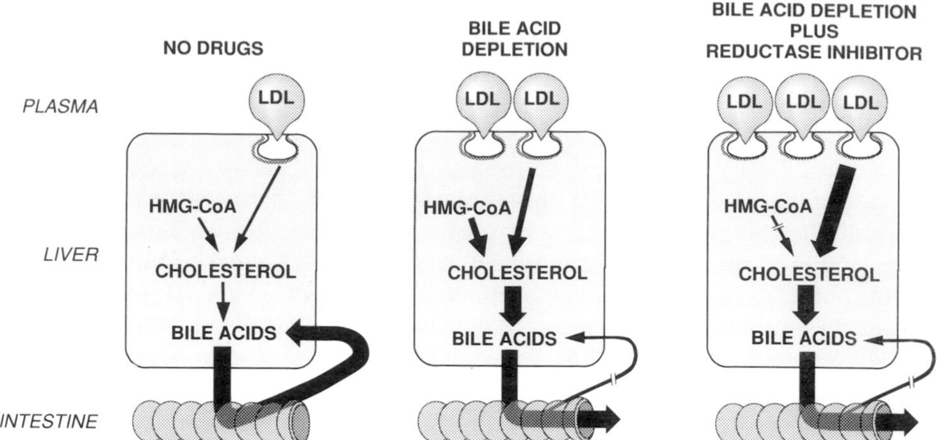

Figure 7.13. Rationale for the use of a bile acid-binding resin and an inhibitor of HMG-CoA reductase in the treatment of FH heterozygotes. (From Brown MS, Goldstein JL: A receptor-mediated pathway for cholesterol homeostasis. Science 232:34–47, 1986.© The Nobel Foundation, 1986.)

CoA reductase and endogenous cholesterol biosynthesis. Endogenous cholesterol biosynthesis can be inhibited by lovastatin, a potent competitive inhibitor of HMG-CoA reductase derived from the mold *Aspergillus.* Inhibition of endogenous HMG-CoA reductase results in an increase in LDL receptor number and, when used together with bile acid sequestering agents, can lower blood cholesterol to the normal range in heterozygotes with familial hypercholesterolemia. Under these conditions the amount of cholesterol available to the liver remains normal, but this is accomplished by increasing the number of LDL receptors in face of a decrease in blood LDL cholesterol concentration (Fig. 7.13). Thus, understanding the LDL receptor pathway has resulted in the development of rational and effective therapeutic approaches to this serious disease.

In homozygotes with familial hypercholesterolemia, LDL receptor number obviously cannot be increased. Such patients have been helped by a liver transplant, often coupled with a heart transplant because of the serious damage caused by the premature atherosclerotic coronary artery disease. Somatic gene therapy for this disease is under investigation. The LDL receptor cDNA has been successfully introduced into rabbit hepatocytes using a retroviral vector. Experiments are under way to assess the possibility of implanting such transfected hepatocytes into the livers of WHHL rabbits.

The LDL receptor model also may be relevant to hypercholesterolemia and cholesterol regulation in the general population not affected with familial hypercholesterolemia. Studies on the LDL receptor in several species including humans have suggested that the receptor has evolved in humans to function at a much lower blood LDL cholesterol concentration than is generally found in Western populations. Thus, the receptor is saturated at the usual concentrations of LDL cholesterol found in "normal" individuals, and LDL receptor synthesis is suppressed. Lowering dietary intake of cholesterol and saturated fats might be expected to increase modestly the synthesis of new LDL receptors in normal individuals. Furthermore, it is possible that polymorphism at the LDL receptor locus might account for different levels of functional LDL receptors in the population, possibly accounting for some of the variation in serum cholesterol.

The elucidation of the molecular pathology of familial hypercholesterolemia illustrates clearly the dynamic interface between medicine and genetics. Two medically trained investigators began by studying the problem of coronary artery disease, focusing their efforts on an inborn error of metabolism, an accident of nature, familial hypercholesterolemia. Astutely, they focused on a rare and pure mutant, homozygous familial hypercholesterolemia. Applying a succession of appropriate and state-of-the-art methods ranging from those of cell biology, biochemistry, and immunology to those of molecular biology, they made major contributions to the understanding of normal and abnormal cholesterol metabolism; they discovered and defined the role of the LDL receptor and developed a rational and successful therapy for familial hypercholesterolemia, a common and serious disease. Along the way, they defined and characterized receptor-mediated endocytosis, a mechanism of universal importance and significance for eukaryotic cells, and made major contributions to understanding molecular mechanisms of mutation and the role of unequal crossing over in the evolution of genes.

DISORDERS OF THE UREA CYCLE

The urea cycle (Fig. 7.14) catalyzes the metabolism of ammonia, the toxic end product of protein catabolism, to urea. Urea cycle activity occurs virtually only in the liver because the first two enzymes in the

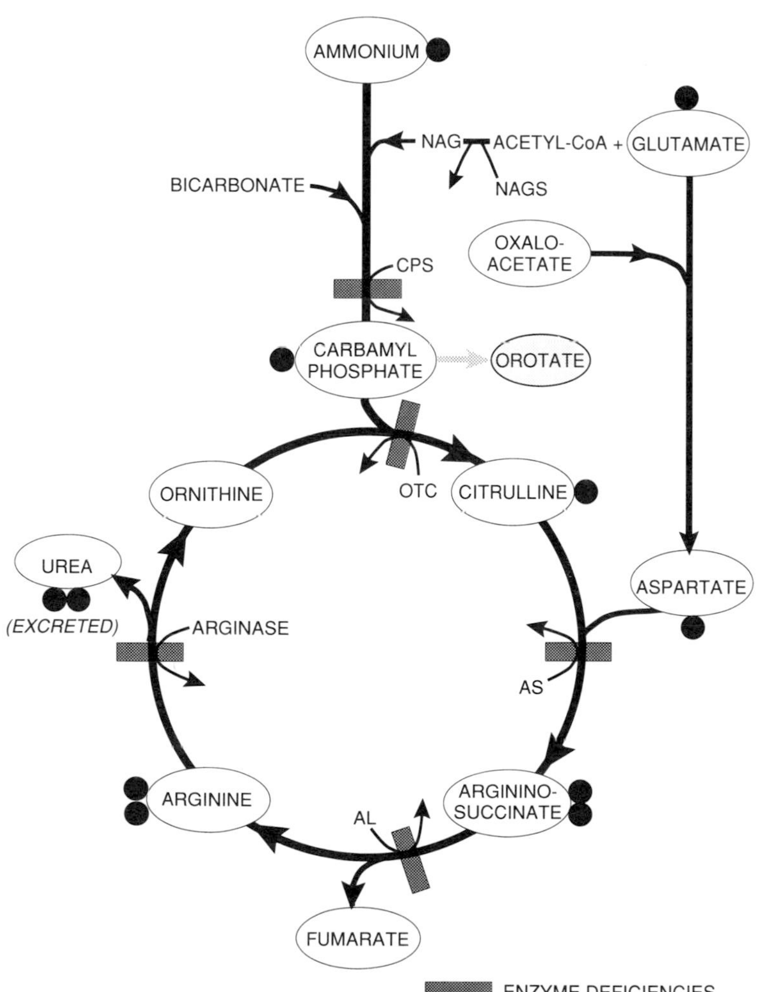

Figure 7.14. Schematic diagram of the urea cycle. The *red dots* indicate the source of the nitrogen atoms excreted as urea. *NAG, N*-acetylglutamate; *NAGS, N*-acetylglutamate synthase; *CPS,* carbamyl phosphate synthase; *OTC,* ornithine transcarbamylase; *AS,* argininosuccinate synthase; *AL,* argininosuccinate lyase. (From Brusilow SW: Disorders of the urea cycle. Hosp Pract 20:65–72, 1985.)

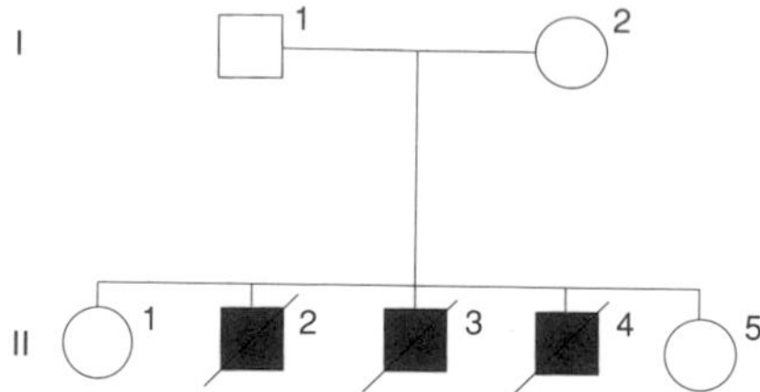

Figure 7.15. Pedigree of the D family. See text for details.

cycle, carbamyl phosphate synthase I and ornithine transcarbamylase (OTC), are effectively found only in hepatocytes. These two enzymes are also located in the mitochondrial matrix, whereas the other three enzymes of the cycle are cytoplasmic. The representation of the urea cycle shown in Figure 7.14 indicates the source of the two nitrogen atoms found in urea. One comes from ammonium and condenses with bicarbonate to form carbamyl phosphate; the second is contributed by aspartate, which condenses with citrulline to form argininosuccinate. It should be noted that carbamyl phosphate, if not used for citrulline formation, can leak out of mitochondria into the cytosolic compartment and be used for pyrimidine synthesis. Deficiency of the enzyme ornithine transcarbamylase is associated with high levels of urinary excretion of orotic acid, an intermediate in pyrimidine biosynthesis.

Severe deficiency of any of the first four enzymes in the urea cycle results in a similar clinical picture. The affected infant, usually the product of a normal full-term pregnancy and delivery, is normal at birth but becomes symptomatic after beginning protein feeding, usually milk. Clinical findings include vomiting, altered temperature regulation with profuse sweating, abnormal muscle tone, seizures, coma, and death. Laboratory examination reveals marked elevation of blood ammonia. This clinical picture is illustrated by the D family whose pedigree is shown in Figure 7.15. The couple, indicated by I-1 and I-2, sought medical consultation because they had three sons, each of whom was normal at birth but after beginning milk feedings developed profuse sweating, labored grunting respirations, seizures and coma, and died on the 2nd or 3rd day of life. Autopsy revealed no structural pathology that could account for their demise. Combined with a history of a similarly affected sibling, such a clinical picture is classical for a severe inborn error of metabolism including disorders of the urea cycle.

Less severe deficiency of urea cycle enzymes may present in childhood with episodic vomiting, irritability, and seizures or even coma, often related to high protein loads or situations of increased protein catabolism such as infection or trauma. Finally, adults with milder deficiencies of urea cycle enzymes may be entirely normal or may only give a history of aversion to high-protein foods; on the other hand, they may show significant mental retardation or neurologic impairment from early episodes of brain damage secondary to high blood ammonia (hyperammonemic encephalopathy).

Ornithine Transcarbamylase Deficiency

In the 1960s several infant girls were described with vomiting, irritability, and neurologic impairment with associated deficiency of hepatic ornithine transcarbamylase activity. Seven of the first eight patients reported were female, and in one family a mother and daughter were affected; it was thought that ornithine transcarbamylase deficiency was an autosomal dominant, sex-limited trait. Then several pedigrees were described in which there were severely affected males with virtually complete deficiency of ornithine transcarbamylase, suggestive of X-linked recessive inheritance. Further support for X-linked inheritance came from the pedigree shown in Figure 7.16. An 18-month-old girl with mental and physical retardation and hyperammonemic coma was found to have a partial ornithine transcarbamylase deficiency. Family history indicated that three maternal uncles had died in the neonatal period as had one brother. Subsequently, another brother was born who

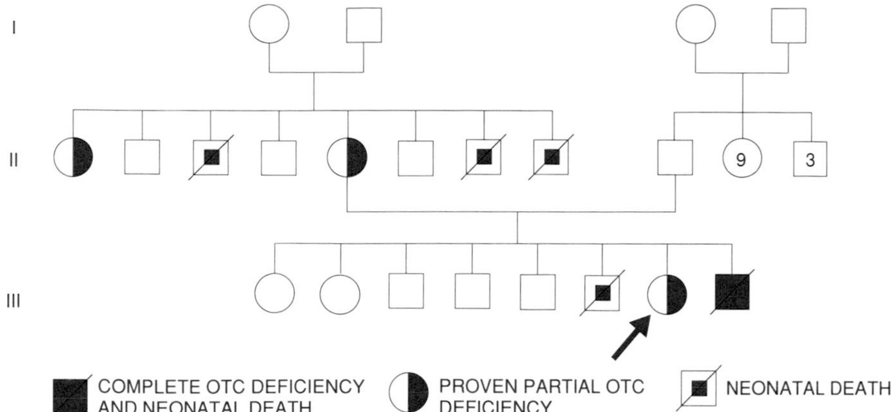

Figure 7.16. Pedigree of the C family with ornithine transcarbamylase deficiency in males and females in two generations. See text for details. (From Ricciuti FC, Gelehrter TD, Rosenberg LE: X-chromosome inactivation in human liver: Confirmation of X-linkage of ornithine transcarbamylase. Am J Hum Genet 28:332–338, 1976. © University of Chicago Press.)

also died in the neonatal period and was found to have complete OTC deficiency. The proband's mother was found to have abnormal ammonia tolerance and diminished OTC activity on liver biopsy. This pedigree could be consistent either with autosomal dominant, sex-influenced inheritance, with more severe disease in males than in females, or with X-linked inheritance, with more severe and stereotyped disease in hemizygous males and with variable clinical signs in heterozygous females.

Proof of X-linkage of OTC deficiency came from the demonstration of cellular mosaicism for OTC activity in hepatocytes of the mother of the proband in this family. Using histochemical staining to demonstrate OTC activity in liver biopsy samples, it was found that the liver of this obligate heterozygote showed patches of hepatocytes with fully normal OTC activity and patches of cells completely devoid of OTC activity (Fig. 7.17). This finding is consistent with X-linkage of OTC and X-chromosome inactivation (discussed in Chapter 8), but not with autosomal dominant sex-influenced exprcssion in which one might expect uniformly reduced OTC activity in all hepatocytes. X-chromosome inactivation also probably accounts for the considerable variation

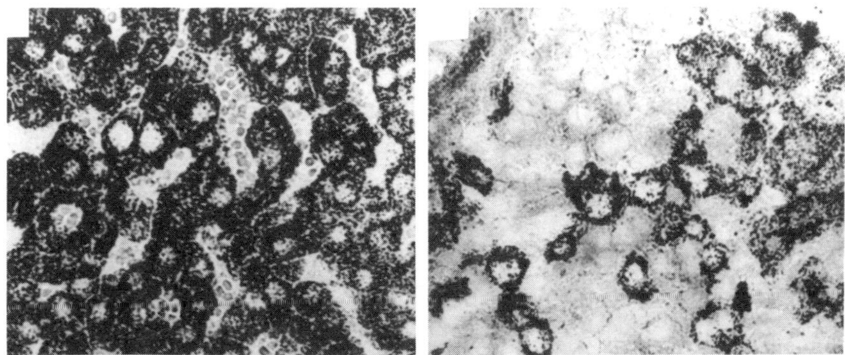

Figure 7.17. Histochemical staining of ornithine transcarbamylase activity in a liver biopsy from a normal woman *(left)* and a woman heterozygous for OTC deficiency *(right)*. The latter had 21% of normal OTC activity as assayed biochemically in this liver biopsy; however, individual cells have either normal activity *(dark staining)* or are devoid of activity. (From Ricciuti FC, Gelehrter TD, Rosenberg LE: X-chromosome inactivation in human liver: Confirmation of X-linkage or ornithine transcarbamylase. Am J Hum Genet 28:332–338, 1976. © University of Chicago Press.)

in OTC activity in heterozygous females. It is important to note that females heterozygous for OTC deficiency can develop significant clinical illnesses. In 17 OTC pedigrees with 61 heterozygotes, 11 (18%) had episodes of hyperammonemic encephalopathy, and 9 of these 11 died during such an episode.

Further support for the X-linkage of OTC deficiency came from the finding that the sparse fur (spf) mouse has a structurally abnormal OTC, indicating the presence of a structural gene mutation for OTC. Because the sparse fur mutation was known to be X-linked in the mouse and because there is evolutionary conservation of X-linkage among mammals, this provided further evidence for the X-linkage of the OTC gene. Subsequent cloning of the human OTC gene and mapping by in situ hybridization to the short arm of the X chromosome confirmed the X-linkage of the OTC gene.

Biogenesis of Nuclear-encoded Mitochondrial Proteins

Ornithine transcarbamylase is composed of a trimer of identical 36-kDa subunits. The primary translation product of the OTC gene has a 4-kDa amino-terminal leader peptide. This peptide is highly basic, containing 4 arginine residues, and is similar to the basic leader peptide found in the other mitochondrial proteins encoded by nuclear genes. By using in vitro mutagenesis techniques, it was shown that these basic residues are necessary for the targeting of OTC to the mitchondrion. It is believed that OTC is synthesized on cytoplasmic ribosomes and binds specifically to the mitochondrial membrane through which it is translocated by an energy-dependent process. The N-terminal peptide is then proteolytically removed and the OTC monomer inserted into the mitochondrion where it is further processed, assembled as a trimer, and localized in the mitochondrial matrix (Fig. 7.18). Although no human OTC mutants have been defined with an abnormality in the leader peptide, the mouse mutant spf^{ash} has a splicing mutation that results in the production of an abnormally long precursor that is not normally processed.

Prenatal Diagnosis and Therapy of OTC Deficiency

Using probes for the OTC gene, RFLPs have been defined that allow prenatal diagnosis in informative pedigrees. Twenty years after the D family (Fig. 7.15) first sought genetic counseling, their younger daughter, II-5 in Figure 7.19, sought counseling because she was pregnant. Her older sister, II-1, had had a son who died in the neonatal period of hyperammonemia secondary to OTC deficiency, thus confirming our clinical suspicion that his three maternal uncles had also died of this condition. Carrier detection testing demonstrated that II-5 excreted large amounts of orotic acid (10 times the normal level) in response to a protein load, strongly suggesting that she is a carrier of OTC deficiency. Her mother, I-2, an obligate carrier, excreted three times the normal level of orotic acid upon protein loading. RFLP haplotyping of the OTC gene was performed on I-1 and I-2 and II-5 and II-6 using the enzyme *Msp*I, which defines four haplotypes, A–D. II-5 has inherited the X chromosome marked by the B haplotype from her mother. Because both I-2 and II-5 appear to be carriers of OTC deficiency, the X-chromosome carrying the B haplotype presumably carries the mutant OTC allele. Prenatal diagnostic studies in this couple indicated that the male fetus, III-2, inherited the X chromosome carrying

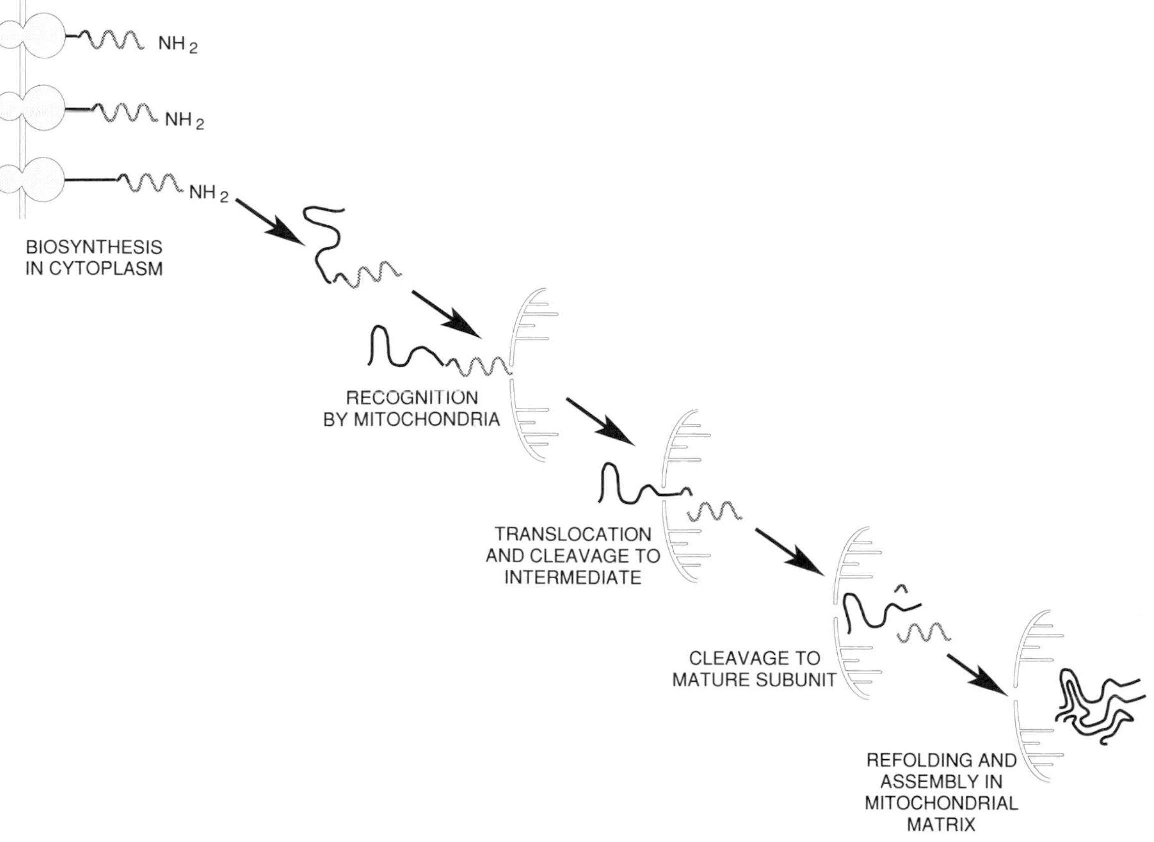

Figure 7.18. Model of the biogenesis of nuclear-encoded mitochondrial matrix enzymes. The amino-terminal leader peptide is denoted by the *wavy red line;* the mature portion by the *solid straight line.* (Redrawn from Rosenberg LE, Fenton WA, Horwich AL, Kalousek F, Kraus JP: Targeting of nuclear-encoded proteins to the mitochondrial matrix: Implications for human genetic defects. Ann NY Acad Sci 488:99–108, 1987, and from a figure courtesy of Dr. W. A. Fenton, Yale University).

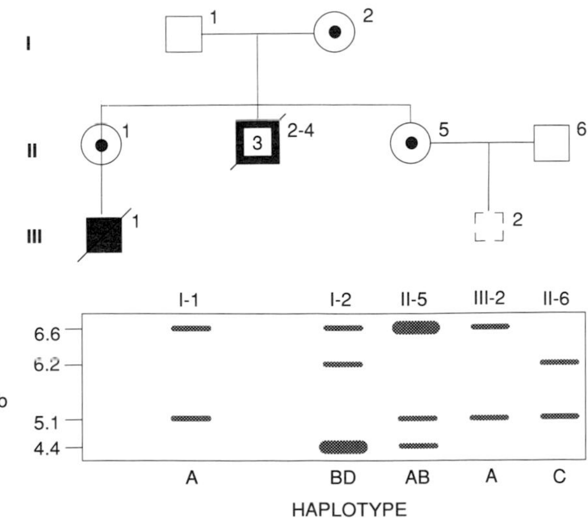

Figure 7.19. Prenatal diagnosis of OTC deficiency in the D family. Shown below the pedigree is RFLP haplotyping of DNA digested with *Msp*I and probed with the OTC cDNA. See text for details.

the A haplotype from his mother, II-5, and thus was not affected with OTC deficiency.

In the past, attempted therapy of severe OTC deficiency was heroic but unsuccessful. More recently it has been shown that the dietary administration of large amounts of sodium benzoate can conjugate glycine to form hippuric acid, which is secreted efficiently into the urine carrying with it one amino group per molecule. Phenylacetate, which is conjugated with glutamine and excreted as phenylacetyl glutamine, is even more effective because two amino groups are excreted in this conjugate (Fig. 7.20). Thus one can circumvent, at least partly, the metabolic block. Together with the provision of exogenous arginine, the administration of sodium benzoate and sodium phenylacetate has proved to be lifesaving even in cases of severe ornithine transcarbamylase deficiency. If patients are treated prospectively, i.e., before they have experienced hyperammonemic encephalopathy, the survival rate is at least 50% at 1 year, a significant improvement over the past. In many cases there appears to be preservation of neurological and mental function. Unfortunately, these children are in a very delicate metabolic balance and can be tipped into severe illness during periods of protein catabolism triggered by such trivial events as viral infections.

Thus, in the course of one generation, as indicated by the D family, our knowledge of congenital hyperammonemia, and especially of ornithine transcarbamylase deficiency, has progressed from the absence of any diagnostic or therapeutic measures to the molecular understanding of OTC deficiency, the availability of biochemical and molecular diagnostic tests including prenatal diagnosis, and a rational and potentially effective biochemical therapy to remove excess ammonia in patients with complete OTC deficiency. Along the way, these studies have generated information about X-linked inheritance and about the biogenesis of mitochondrial proteins encoded by nuclear genes. Clinically, the views expressed by Leon Rosenberg in 1972 are even more true in 1990:

> The rarity of any one of these disorders is no longer an acceptable explanation for failure to consider them, particularly when a simple battery of laboratory studies and a safe form of therapeutic trial should be available in almost every hospital. I have yet to see bereaved parents comforted by the knowledge that their child died of a rare disease. Nor, I maintain, do physicians gain succor from

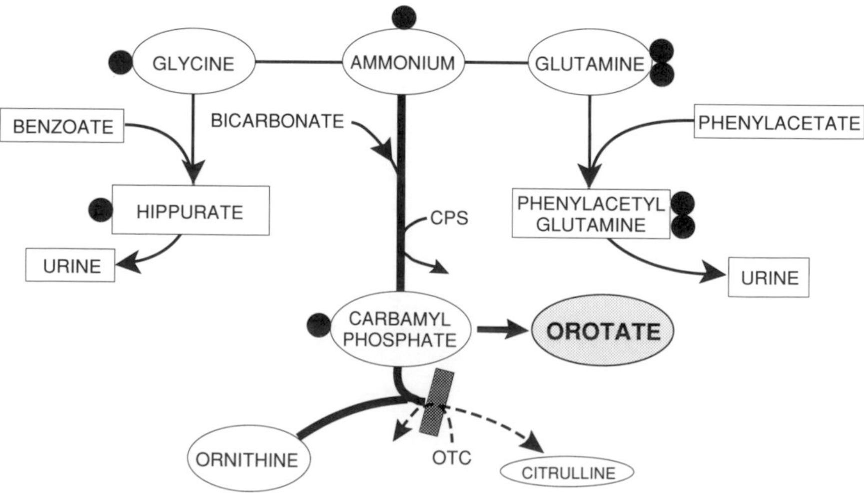

Figure 7.20. Therapy of ornithine transcarbamylase deficiency. See text for details (Redrawn from Brusilow SW: Disorders of the urea cycle. Hosp Pract 20:65–72, 1985.)

such information, particularly when life-saving intervention is at hand (1).

COLLAGEN AND ITS DISORDERS

The majority of inborn errors of metabolism, representing mutations in the genes for specific enzymes, are inherited in an autosomal recessive fashion. The quantity of most enzymes is sufficient that a reduction to 50%, as would occur in a heterozygote, does not cause any phenotypic abnormality. In the example of familial hypercholesterolemia, however, where the mutation is in a cell surface receptor gene, a reduction to 50% of the normal amount of receptor does lead to significant metabolic derangement. Mutations in nonenzymatic proteins including receptors, carrier proteins, and structural proteins are capable of creating disease in the heterozygous state and, hence, exhibiting a dominant inheritance pattern. Except for the LDL receptor, the most thoroughly worked-out dominant genetic defects are the "heritable disorders of connective tissue," at least some of which arise from mutations in the genes for human collagen.

Structure of Collagen

Collagen is not only the most abundant structural protein, but also the most abundant protein of any sort in the human body. In some tissues such as bone and cartilage, it constitutes as much as 60% of the protein present. While there are several types of collagen (see below), the basic structure common to all of them is a triple helix composed of three very long polypeptide chains. When initially assembled, this trimer includes globular domains at the amino and carboxy termini (Fig. 7.21), with the majority of the molecule being a tightly wound triple

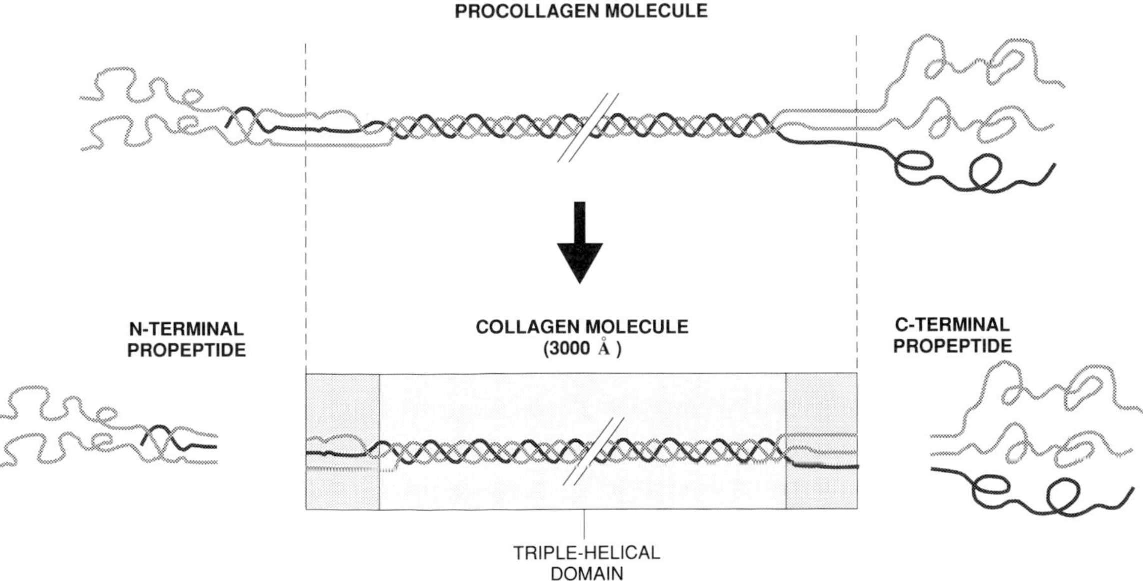

Figure 7.21. Schematic representation of the structure of the procollagen and collagen molecules. Procollagen is formed by the assembly of three collagen polypeptide monomers. The *two light strands* are $\alpha 1(I)$, and the *one dark strand* is $\alpha 2$. Once the molecule is secreted, cleavage of the N-terminal and C-terminal domains occurs, generating a 3000-Å long triple helical collagen molecule.

Table 7.3. Major Types of Collagen[a]

Collagen Type	Chains	Chromosomal Location	Procollagen Molecule	Tissue Distribution
I	$\alpha 1(I)$	17	$[\alpha 1(I)]_2\alpha 2$	Bone, tendon, skin
	$\alpha 2$	7		
II	$\alpha 1(II)$	12	$[\alpha 1(II)]_3$	Cartilage, vitreous
III	$\alpha 1(III)$	2	$[\alpha 1(III)]_3$	Skin, arteries, uterus, intestine

[a]This is only a partial listing; at least 12 types of collagen are known.

helical domain. This precursor molecule, called procollagen, is then modified in the extracellular space by proteolytic cleavage of the globular domains and self-assembly of the triple helical segments into an ordered array, which makes up a collagen fibril. Additional stability results from the covalent cross-linking of adjacent collagen molecules.

At least 12 different types of collagen have been identified in the human body, which differ in their structure and their tissue distribution. Table 7.3 provides information on the three most abundant and best characterized forms. Type I, which is ubiquitous but especially important in bones, tendons, and ligaments, is a trimer made up of two $\alpha 1(I)$ chains and one $\alpha 2$ chain. Type II and type III collagens are made up of homotrimers of their respective $\alpha 1$ chains, called $\alpha 1(II)$ and $\alpha 1(III)$. (The nomenclature for these polypeptides is a bit unwieldy but is now standardized.) Type II collagen is particularly abundant in cartilage, whereas type III plays a significant role in the structural integrity of large blood vessels.

The collagen genes are distributed throughout the human genome and are represented on several different chromosomes (Table 7.3). These genes are large and contain as many as 50 exons.

The central triple helical region of collagen is a remarkable protein structure. In this domain, each polypeptide chain consists of repeats of an amino acid sequence which can be written $(Gly\text{-}X\text{-}Y)_n$. The X position is frequently occupied by proline, and the Y position by the unusual amino acids hydroxyproline or hydroxylysine, which are generated by posttranslational modification of proline and lysine. This repeating triplet of amino acids is extremely crucial for the stability of the molecule. Mutations in this region tend to cause destabilization of the triple helix with a failure of collagen fibers to attain their normal configuration and strength.

Inherited Disorders of Collagen

The molecular genetics of two disorders that fall in the category of "heritable disorders of connective tissue," namely osteogenesis imperfecta and Ehlers-Danlos syndrome, is beginning to be defined. Another important disorder in this category is the Marfan syndrome, which has already been discussed in Chapter 3. The molecular basis of the Marfan syndrome remains to be elucidated; with the exception of one unusual patient, there is no direct evidence for involvement of the collagen genes in Marfan syndrome.

OSTEOGENESIS IMPERFECTA

The term osteogenesis imperfecta (OI) is used to describe a heterogenous group of disorders characterized by brittle bones. Table 7.4 presents the four clinical subtypes, but this classification undoubtedly represents a major oversimplification. Progress in the molecular genetics of

Table 7.4. Clinical Classification of Osteogenesis Imperfecta[a]

Type	Clinical Features	Inheritance[b]
I	Frequent fractures, but with normal height and little deformity. Sclerae are blue; 50% have hearing loss	AD
II	Perinatal lethal form, with multiple fractures at birth, poor mineralization of bones	New mutation AD Rarely AR
III	Progressively deforming form, with short stature, hearing loss common	AD Less commonly AR
IV	Mild to moderate bone deformity, normal sclerae	AD

[a]Modified from Sillence DO, Senn A, Danks DM: Genetic heterogeneity in osteogenesis imperfecta. J Med Genet 16:101–116, 1979.
[b]AD, autosomal dominant; AR, autosomal recessive.

these disorders makes it clear that each subtype can be further divided, as a result of both allelic heterogeneity and locus heterogeneity.

Type I OI is the most common, and it is inherited in an autosomal dominant fashion. Affected individuals are subject to frequent fractures, have a blue color to their sclerae, and may develop conductive deafness due to fixation of the bones of the middle ear. Given the distribution of collagens, as shown in Table 7.3, it might have been predicted that the defect in type I OI would reside within the type I collagen genes. In several families that prediction has been borne out. A frequently observed defect is inactivation of one allele of the $\alpha 1$(I) gene, such that only half of the normal amount of $\alpha 1$(I) protein is being produced. Since type I collagen requires a 2:1 ratio of $\alpha 1$(I) to $\alpha 2$ protein chains for triple helix formation, there is an excess of $\alpha 2$ chains, which are degraded. Thus, as shown in Figure 7.22, only half of the normal amount of type I collagen is produced. This presumably accounts for the fragility of bones that characterizes this disorder. Thus, unlike the situation in which the protein product is an enzyme, a reduction in amount of a structural protein to 50% has significant phenotypic consequences.

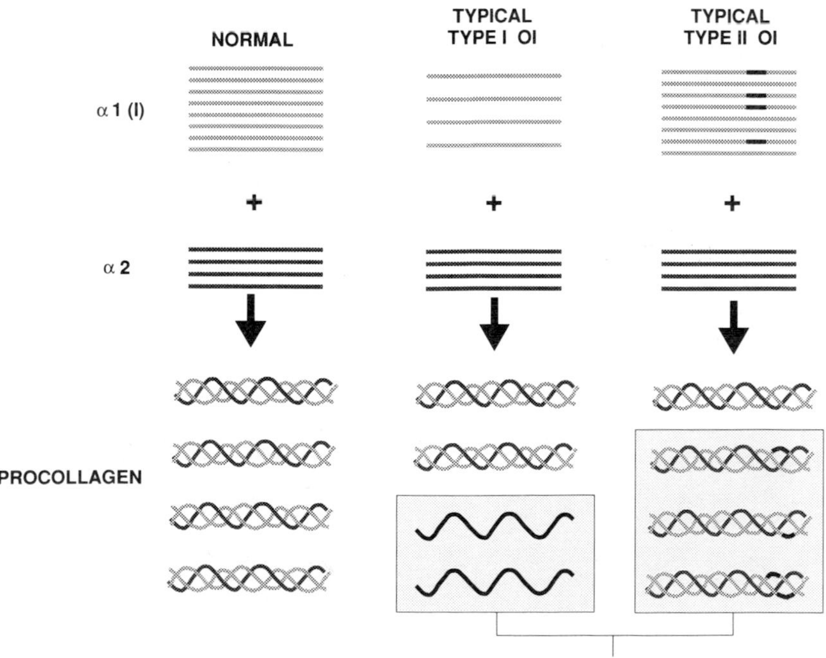

Figure 7.22. The mechanism for collagen deficiency in type I and type II osteogenesis imperfecta. The molecular cause of these two disorders is heterogenous; shown here are typical examples. In type I OI, the example shown reflects an inactivation of one allele of the $\alpha 1$(I) gene, resulting in only 50% of the normal amount of this polypeptide. The outcome is a 50% reduction in procollagen molecules, with degradation of the excess $\alpha 2$ chains. In type II OI, however, typically there is a qualitative defect in one of the α chains, as in this example in which an amino acid substitution in the $\alpha 1$(I) chain is indicated in *red*. If this substitution inhibits proper triple helix formation, then three quarters of the trimers will be abnormal and will undergo degradation, and only one quarter will survive.

Type II OI is a much more severe disorder, with innumerable fractures present at birth, and death normally occuring in the first few weeks or months of life. Figure 7.23 shows an x-ray of an affected individual, demonstrating the large number of congenital fractures and the telescoping of the long bones that occurs as a result of greatly reduced structural support. Here, the collagen deficiency is much more marked. The mineralized bone, lacking the protein scaffolding, which functions in a similar fashion to steel rods in reinforced concrete, is easily crumpled by routine movements of the fetus in the womb. The molecular basis of type II OI turns out to be a bit of a surprise. While the mutations that give rise to the milder type I disease are, in general, "knock-out" mutations that completely inactivate one allele of the $\alpha 1$(I) gene, the muta-

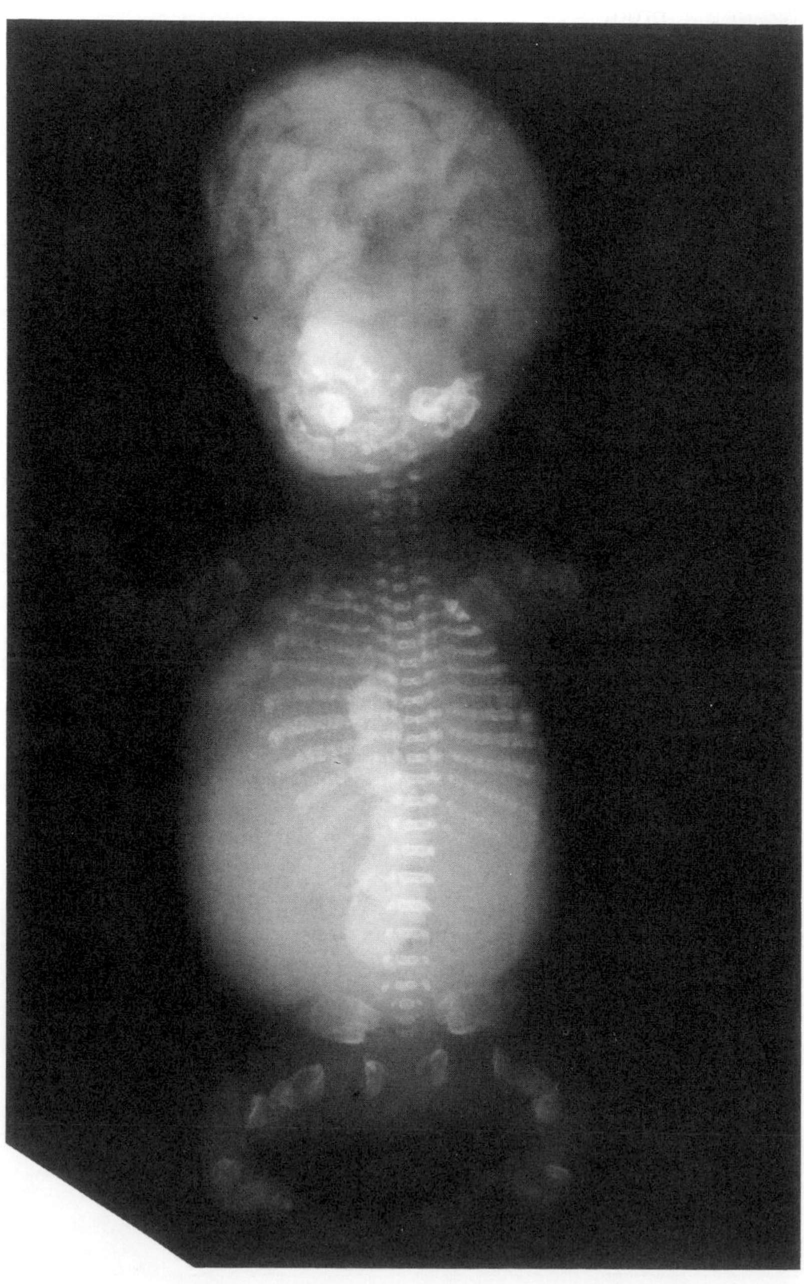

Figure 7.23. X-ray of an infant with the perinatal lethal form of osteogenesis imperfecta (OI type II). Note the compressed femurs which include multiple fractures.

tions in type II disease are much more subtle. Typically, these involve point mutations or rearrangements in the $\alpha 1(I)$ or $\alpha 2$ genes, which are compatible with production of a relatively normal amount of qualitatively abnormal protein from the affected allele. The fact that such subtle mutations cause such severe disease presents a challenging paradox, but one that has now been resolved. The mutant collagen peptide, present in normal or near normal amounts, can still be incorporated into a nascent procollagen triple helical molecule. As shown in Figure 7.22, the effect of a mutant $\alpha 1(I)$ gene is that *half* of the $\alpha 1(I)$ polypeptide chains but *three-quarters* of the collagen triple helices will be abnormal. These abnormal trimers tend to assemble poorly, may be difficult to export out of the cell, and may be degraded prematurely. The net result is a profound deficiency of normal collagen. Thus, a qualitative abnormality in the protein product of the $\alpha 1(I)$ gene leads to a more severe phenotype than a quantitative abnormality. This mechanism, aptly denoted "protein suicide," provides a general explanation for the dominant phenotype of a mutation affecting a subunit of a multimeric protein, provided that one abnormal subunit leads to loss or decreased function of the entire multimer.

Type II OI is a lethal disorder incompatible with reproduction. By molecular analysis, the vast majority of neonates with this disorder represent new dominant mutations and carry one mutant and one normal allele (Table 7.4). In rare situations, however, an affected individual may represent an autosomal recessive disorder; therefore, the possibility of recurrence in a future pregnancy cannot be confidently excluded.

EHLERS-DANLOS SYNDROME

Like OI, Ehlers-Danlos syndrome (EDS) has been classified into a large number of clinical subtypes. The hallmark of this set of disorders is increased tissue elasticity and fragility, but additional features vary widely from one type to another (Table 7.5). Figure 7.24 shows an individual with type I EDS, which is an autosomal dominant disorder characterized by dramatic hyperextensibility of skin and joints. The skin is thin and heals poorly, resulting in so-called "cigarette paper" scars after relatively minor trauma. The strength of major blood vessels, however, is in general preserved. The molecular defect in type I EDS remains to be defined. Also undefined are the molecular defects in type II EDS (a

Table 7.5. Ehlers-Danlos Syndromes[a]

Type	Clinical Features	Inheritance[b]	Defect
I, Gravis	Hyperextensible skin, hypermobile joints, cigarette paper scars	AD	Unknown
II, Mitis	Similar to type I but milder	AD	Unknown
III, Familial hypermobility	Marked hypermobility of joints	AD	Unknown
IV, Arterial	Thin translucent skin, marked bruising, arterial and intestinal rupture	AD	Abnormal type III collagen
V, X-linked	Similar to type II	XLR	Unknown
VI, Ocular	Soft, velvety skin, ocular fragility	AR	Lysyl hydroxylase deficiency

[a]Only a partial list is shown; at least 10 types of Ehlers-Danlos syndrome have been described.
[b]AD, autosomal dominant; AR, autosomal recessive; XLR, X-linked recessive.

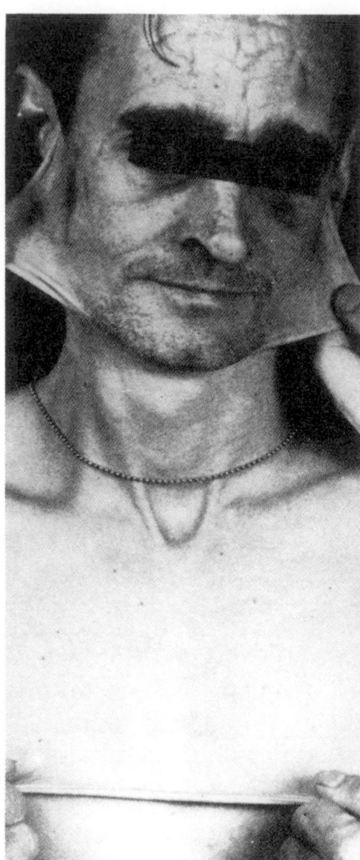
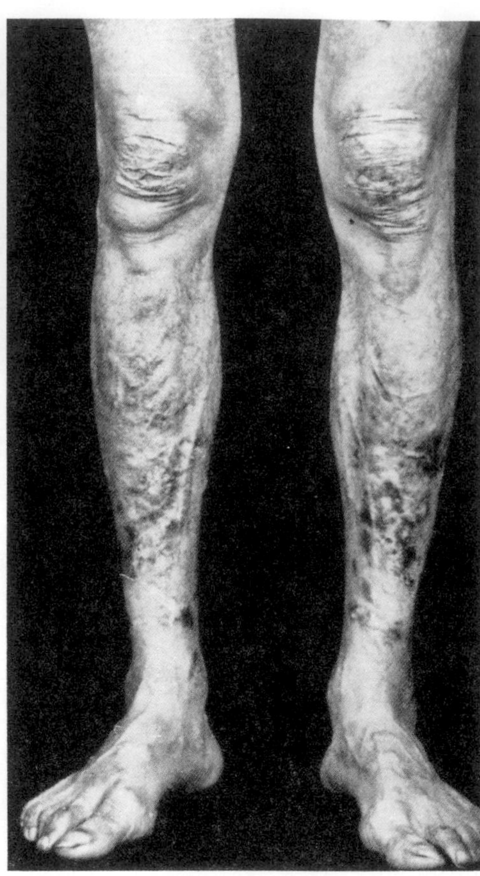

Figure 7.24. **Typical appearance of an individual with Ehlers-Danlos syndrome type I.** Note the hyperextensible skin and the cigarette paper scars over the lower legs. (Reproduced by permission from McKusick VA: *Heritable Disorders of Connective Tissue.* 4th Ed. St. Louis, 1972, The C. V. Mosby Co.)

milder version of type I) and type III EDS (benign familial hypermobility of joints).

The best understood and most dangerous form of EDS, type IV, displays less skin and joint hypermobility and is characterized by thin, almost translucent, skin and easy bruising. The major serious consequences, however, arise from the dramatic fragility of major arteries, with sudden death from rupture of the aorta, the splenic artery, or a renal artery. Spontaneous rupture of the colon is also common. Surgical attempts to repair these catastrophes are often extremely difficult, as the supporting tissues are found to be fragile and hold sutures poorly.

Virtually all families with type IV EDS, which is usually inherited in an autosomal dominant fashion, have been shown to have quantitative or qualitative abnormalities of type III collagen. (One must be careful to avoid confusing the roman numerals associated with the various types of EDS with the roman numerals used to designate the various collagen subtypes.) In some instances of EDS IV, one allele of the $\alpha 1$(III) gene has been completely inactivated, leading to a 50% reduction in the amount of the type III collagen triple helix. In other instances, qualitative abnormalities occur in this gene product as a result of more subtle mutations, and such mutations result in abnormal structure of ⅞ of the resulting triple helices (by the protein suicide mechanism diagrammed in Fig. 7.22). Since the defect is expressed in cultured fibroblasts, it is now possible to establish the diagnosis in affected family members prior to the onset of symptoms, or even prenatally.

Of the other types of EDS, the molecular mechanism of two others deserves mention. In type VI, a deficiency of the enzyme lysyl hydroxylase has been identified. This enzyme is required for the posttranslational hydroxylation of the lysines located in the Y position of the Gly-X-Y repeat mentioned above. Without that hydroxylation, stabilization and cross-linking of the triple helix are reduced and the collagen fibers lack appropriate strength. In type IX EDS, a deficiency of a different enzyme, lysyl oxidase, has been documented. This enzyme oxidizes lysine and hydroxylysine and is responsible for further cross-linking of collagen. This particular form is inherited as an X-linked recessive disorder. Thus, the Ehlers-Danlos syndromes show evidence of both allelic heterogeneity (different mutations in the α1(III) gene in EDS IV) and locus heterogeneity (mutations at different loci causing EDS IV, EDS VI, and EDS IX).

Lessons from the Collagen Disorders

Our purpose in discussing this category of disorders is partly to introduce an important group of human genetic diseases, but also to draw some general conclusions about the molecular basis of disease. First, categorization of disease based on clinical criteria, even if elaborate, often underestimates the degree of genetic heterogeneity that is recognized after the molecular basis of the disease has been defined. This is particularly true of the collagen disorders because a number of genetic loci are involved, the genes are large, and the number of potential mutations almost infinite. A natural consequence of this high degree of genetic heterogeneity is that some mutations are likely to cause intermediate phenotypes that do not fit conveniently into any of the clinical classifications. Second, even with a reasonable amount of information about the collagen proteins, it is still not entirely possible to predict the clinical phenotype based on the mutation. Thus, at least at present, accurate prediction of severity is often possible only by reference to other affected family members. Third, the protein suicide mechanism for dominant disorders, whereby one mutant subunit leads to loss of an entire multimeric protein, has emerged clearly from this analysis of collagen disorders and is likely to appear in other contexts. Finally, the great variation in severity of phenotype demonstrated by these disorders (OI is a good example) suggests that even milder phenotypes may turn out to have their basis in subtle alterations of the collagen genes. There is, in fact, some evidence that collagen gene abnormalities may contribute to more common disorders of older adults such as osteoporosis ("thinning of bones") and osteoarthritis (degenerative joint disease).

REFERENCE

Rosenberg LE: Diagnosis and management of inherited aminoacidopathies in the newborn and unborn. In *Genetics and the Perinatal Patient.* Mead Johnson Symposium on Perinatal and Developmental Medicine, No. 1, 1972, pp 45–49.

SUGGESTED READINGS

Inborn Errors of Metabolism

Beadle GW: Genes and chemical reactions in neurospora. Science 129:1715–1719, 1959.

Garrod AE: The Croonian lectures on inborn errors of metabolism. Lancet 2:1–7, 73–79, 142–148, 214–200, 1908. The classic publication defining the concept of the inborn errors of metabolism.

Harris H: *The Principles of Human Biochemical Genetics.* 3rd Ed. New York, Elsevier Scientific Publishing Co., 1980. A beautifully written exposition of the subject in the "premolecular" era.

LaDu BN: Alcaptonuria. In Scriver CR, Beaudet AL, Sly WS, Valle D: *The Metabolic Basis of Inherited Diseases.* 6th Ed. New York, McGraw-Hill, 1989, pp. 775–790.

Luzzatto L, Mehta A: Glucose-6-phosphate dehydrogenase deficiency. In Scriver CR, Beaudet AL, Sly WS, Valle D: *The Metabolic Basis of Inherited Diseases.* 6th Ed. New York, McGraw-Hill, 1989, pp. 2237–2265.

Scriver CR, Beaudet AL, Sly WS, Valle D: *The Metabolic Basis of Inherited Diseases.* 6th Ed. New York, McGraw-Hill, 1989. Encyclopedic and authoritative; the standard reference on inborn errors of metabolism and inherited metabolic diseases.

Valle DL, Mitchell GA: Inborn errors of metabolism in the molecular age. Prog Med Genet 7:100–129, 1988.

α_1-Antitrypsin Deficiency

Brantly M, Nukiwa T, Crystal RG: Molecular basis of alpha-1-antitrypsin deficiency. Am J Med 84 (suppl 6A):13–31, 1988.

Carrell RW: α1-Antitrypsin: Molecular pathology, leukocytes, and tissue damage. J Clin Invest 78:1427–1431, 1986. Short, current, critical, and provocative.

Cox DW: α_1-Antitrypsin deficiency. In Scriver CR, Beaudet AL, Sly WS, Valle D: *The Metabolic Basis of Inherited Diseases.* 6th Ed. New York, McGraw-Hill, 1989, pp. 2409–2437.

Familial Hypercholesterolemia

Brown MS, Goldstein JL: A receptor-mediated pathway for cholesterol homeostasis. Science 232:34–37, 1986. The Nobel Prize acceptance lecture; an elegant, detailed account of the molecular pathology and genetics of familial hypercholesterolemia.

Goldstein JL, Brown MS: Familial hypercholesterolemia. In Scriver CR, Beaudet AL, Sly WS, Valle D: *The Metabolic Basis of Inherited Diseases.* 6th Ed. New York, McGraw-Hill, 1989, pp. 1215–1250.

Motulsky AG: The 1985 Nobel Prize in physiology or medicine. Science 231:126–129, 1986. An excellent perspective on the importance of the familial hypercholesterolemia story to both genetics and medicine.

Disorders of the Urea Cycle

Brusilow SW: Disorders of the urea cycle. Hosp Pract 20:65–72, 1985. A clear description of the biochemistry and clinical aspects of the urea cycle disorders and a discussion of current methods of treatment.

Brusilow SW, Horwich AL: Urea cycle enzymes. In Scriver CR, Beaudet AL, Sly WS, Valle D: *The Metabolic Basis of Inherited Diseases.* 6th Ed. New York, McGraw-Hill, 1989, pp. 629–663.

Collagen Disorders

Byers PH: Disorders of collagen biosynthesis and structure. In Scriver CR, Beaudet AL, Sly WS, Valle D (eds): *The Metabolic Basis of Inherited Disease.* 6th Ed. New York, McGraw-Hill, 1989, pp. 2805–2842.

McKusick VA: *Heritable Disorders of Connective Tissue.* 4th Ed. St. Louis, CV Mosby, 1972.

Prockop DJ, Kivirikko KI: Heritable diseases of collagen. N Engl J Med 311:376–386, 1984.

7/ Study Questions

1/ Why would a mutation affecting stability of an enzyme expressed in both red and white blood cells be more likely to cause a detectable phenotype in red blood cells than in white blood cells?

2/ Suppose an enzyme were a tetramer consisting of four identical peptides encoded on an autosome. What would you predict to be the impact of the following mutations on the function of this enzyme in an individual *heterozygous* for each mutation?

a. Nonsense mutation in the first exon, resulting in premature termination of translation
b. Missense mutation in the first exon, resulting in a subunit that can participate in tetramer formation but, if present in the tetramer, destroys the active site

If less than 10% of normal activity of this enzyme is sufficient to cause disease, what would you expect to be the inheritance pattern or patterns of disease caused by the two mutations described above?

3/ G6PD A^- has two base changes when compared to the wild-type gene: A → G at nucleotide 376 and G → A at nucleotide 202. The enzyme has an altered mobility and decreased stability. How might you determine experimentally which alteration or combination of alterations is responsible for the altered mobility and decreased stability?

4/ Using the data in Table 7.2, calculate the allele frequencies for Pi^Z and Pi^S. What fraction of the population will be Pi^{MS}?

5/ What two therapeutic interventions have been shown to be effective in lowering blood cholesterol to normal levels in heterozygotes for LDL-receptor defects?

8

Cytogenetics

"It is inconceivable that particles of chromatin or any other substance, however complex, can possess the powers which must be assigned to our factors (genes). The supposition that particles of chromatin, indistinguishable from each other and almost homogeneous under any known test, can by their material nature confer all the properties of life surpasses the range of even the most convinced materialism."

—William Bateson, 1916
(From Borek E: *The Code of Life.* New York, Columbia University Press, 1964)

Chromosome abnormalities are responsible for at least half of spontaneous abortions or miscarriages and are an important cause of congenital malformations (1–3). More than 0.5% of newborns are born with significant abnormalities of autosomes or sex chromosomes. Among these, the most common and best known serious chromosomal disorders are trisomy 21, or Down syndrome, and the fragile X syndrome. The structure of chromosomes and their behavior has been described in Chapter 2. In this chapter we will examine these topics in more detail and discuss some of the more common abnormalities affecting chromosomes.

Until the 1950s, two salient facts about human chromosomes were recognized, both of them wrong. First, it was believed that human cells contained 48 chromosomes, and second, it was believed that sex was determined by the number of X chromosomes present in the mammalian cell as it is in the fruit fly *Drosophila.* Chromosomes could be examined only in actively dividing cells such as tumor cells, cells from the male gonad, cells growing in tissue culture, and bone marrow preparations. The quality of chromosome preparations was nowhere near that which we expect today (perhaps accounting for Bateson's skepticism) (4). In 1956, Tijo and Levan clearly demonstrated that human embryonic fibroblasts in culture contained 46 rather than 48 chromosomes. Within 3 years, three major disorders due to altered numbers of chromosomes were defined, including trisomy 21 Down syndrome, Turner syndrome, and Klinefelter syndrome, which are discussed later in this chapter.

The major advance that facilitated rapid development of the field of cytogenetics was the development of techniques for examining chromosomes in peripheral blood lymphocytes. In this technique, now standardly used for examining human chromosomes, a small amount of anticoagulated blood is added to tissue culture medium. Phytohemagglutinin, extracted from the red bean, is added to agglutinate red blood cells and stimulate lymphocytes to divide. These dividing cells can be blocked in mitosis using microtubule inhibitors and preparations of metaphase chromosomes stained and examined microscopically for alterations in number and structure (Fig. 8.1). Techniques for radioactively labeling DNA with tritiated thymidine during the S or synthetic phase of the cell cycle allowed investigators to examine the timing of chromosome replication. In the 1970s, newer staining and banding techniques were introduced that significantly improved the resolution of chromosome morphology (5).

The currently most widely used technique, Giemsa banding, or G-banding, involves gentle trypsin treatment of chromosome preparations followed by staining with Giemsa. This results in a pattern of light and dark bands that is unique for each human chromosome and allows the unequivocal definition of each chromosome (Fig. 8.2). By this technique approximately 350–550 bands per haploid set are observed. One band represents approximately $5–10 \times 10^6$ bp of DNA, and because one gene may range from 10^3 bp (e.g., α-globin) to more than 2×10^6 bp (e.g., Duchenne muscular dystrophy) each band represents a few to very many individual genes. Newer techniques allow examination of chromosomes in prometaphase, at which time the chromosomes are more extended than in metaphase, allowing even higher degrees of resolution (Fig. 8.3). More than 850 bands per haploid set can be distinguished by this technique (2, 3, 6).

Chromosome morphology is defined by the position of the centromere, or central constriction, that divides the chromosome into a short

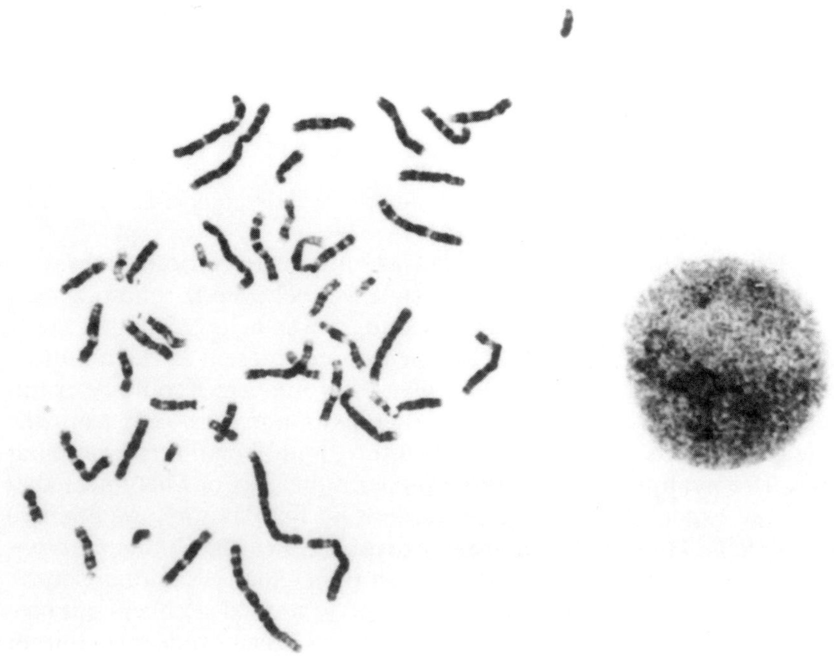

Figure 8.1. A metaphase spread prepared from a human peripheral blood lymphocyte culture and stained by the Giemsa banding method. An intact, nonmitotic lymphocyte nucleus is shown on the *right*. (Courtesy of the University of Michigan Clinical Cytogenetics Service.)

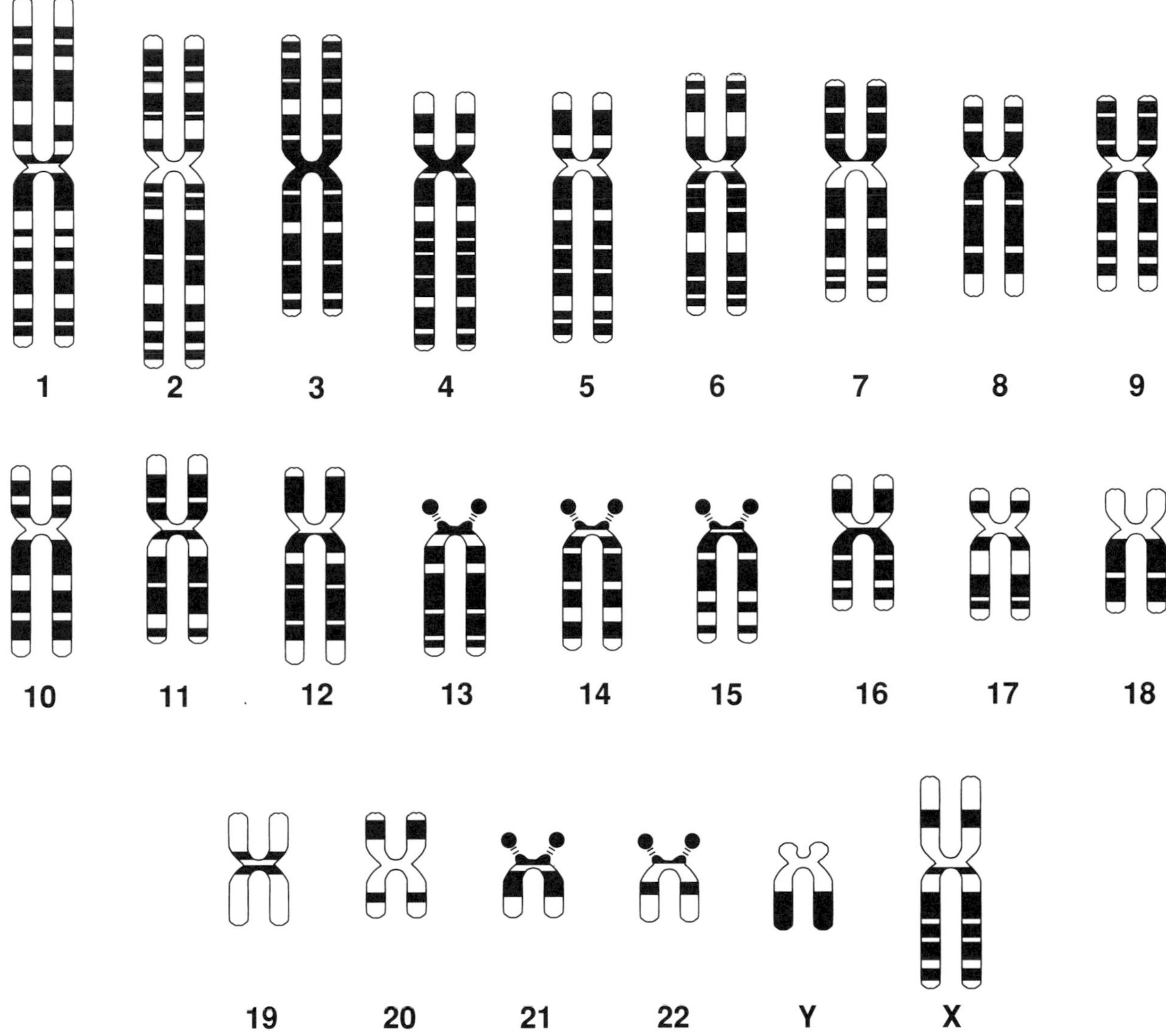

Figure 8.2. Ideogram of human chromosomes showing the Giemsa banding patterns, arranged and numbered according to the Paris classification of 1971. (From deGrouchy J, Turleau C: *Clinical Atlas of Human Chromosomes.* 2nd Ed. New York, John Wiley & Sons, 1984.)

arm designated **p** for petite and a long arm designated **q** (Fig. 8.4). Chromosomes are metacentric if the centromere lies in the middle of the chromosome, submetacentric when the centromere is somewhat distant from the center, and acrocentric when the centromere lies near the end of the chromosome. The human acrocentric autosomal chromosomes (chromosomes 13–15, 21, 22) have short arms that consist mainly of a satellite and a thin stalk, regions which form the nucleolus of the resting cell and contain multiple tandemly repeated copies of the genes for ribosomal RNA. The pattern of bands on each chromosome is numbered according to convention from the centromere to the terminal portion of the short and long arms, as indicated in Figure 8.5. Thus, chromosomes can be defined on the basis of their size, their morphology with respect to the position of their centromere, and the pattern of banding.

Chromosomes are arranged according to these criteria in a karyotype (Fig. 8.6). A karyotype is standardly described by first listing the

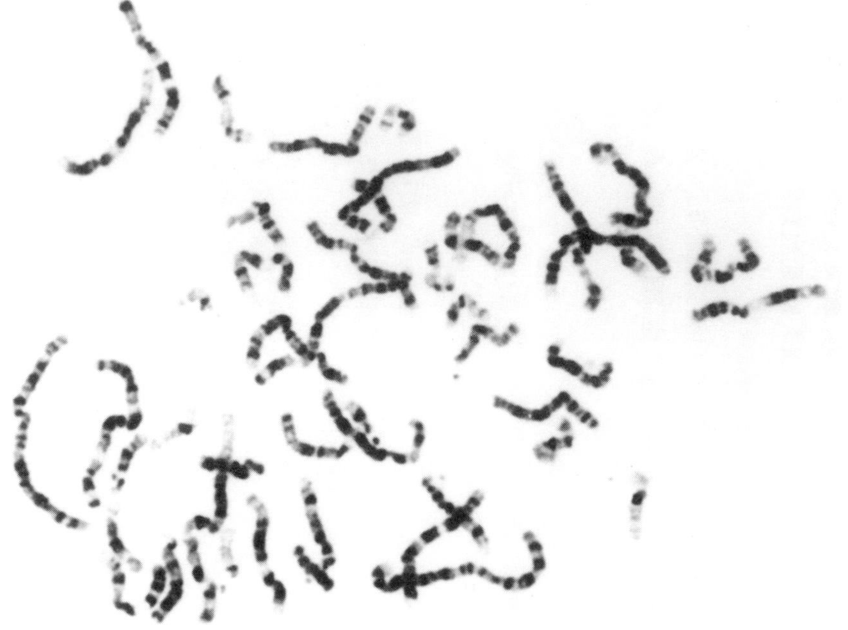

Figure 8.3. Human chromosomes from a peripheral blood lymphocyte culture arrested in prometaphase and stained by the Giemsa banding technique. (Courtesy of the University of Michigan Clinical Cytogenetics Service.)

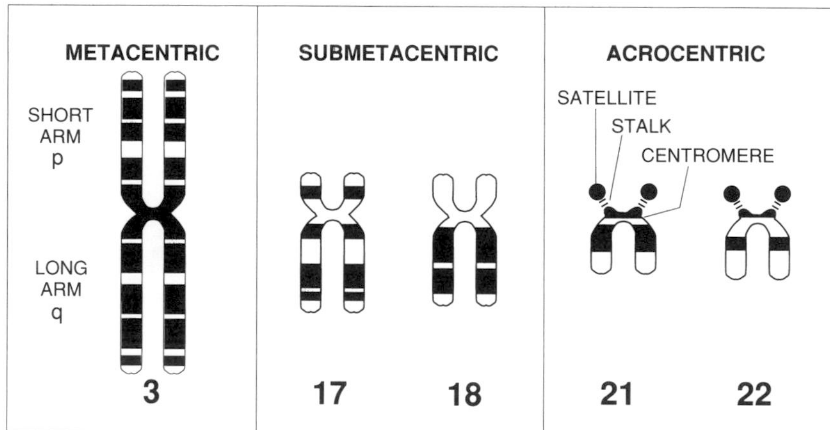

Figure 8.4. Human chromosome morphology as classified by variation in chromosome size and centromere position.

number of chromosomes followed by the sex chromosome constitution, followed by any abnormalities in number of morphology of chromosomes. The nomenclature used for describing chromosomes is shown in Table 8.1. For example, 45,XY,−14,−21,+t(14q21q) indicates an XY male with 45 chromosomes who is missing a normal 14 and a normal 21, but has an additional chromosome that is a translocation chromosome consisting of the long arm (q) of chromosome 14 attached to the long arm of chromosome 21.

CHROMOSOME ABNORMALITIES

Chromosome abnormalities may be numerical or structural. In discussing numerical chromosome abnormalities it is important to define ploidy. **Euploid** refers to any exact multiple of N, the number of chromosomes in a normal haploid gamete. The number of chromosomes in a normal somatic cell is **diploid** or 2N. Euploid chromosome

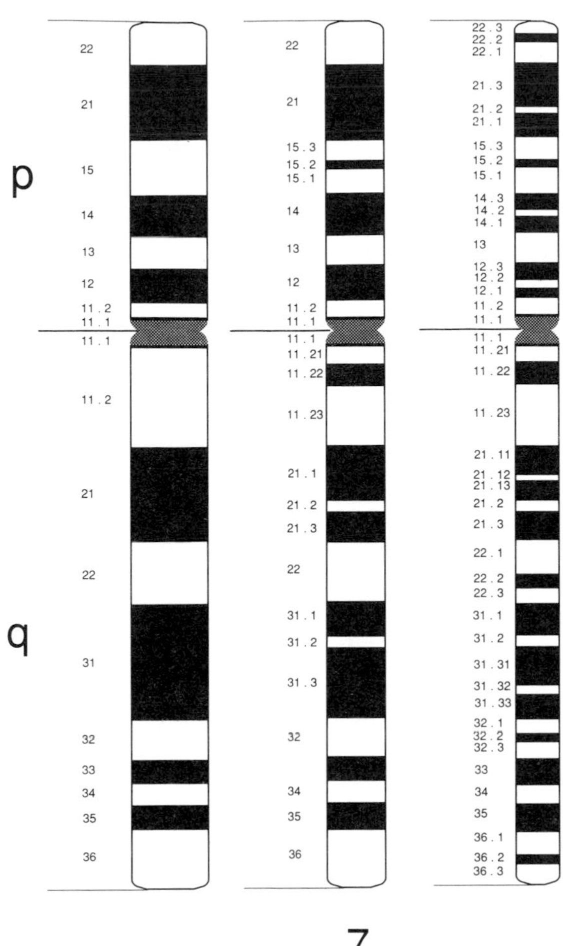

Figure 8.5. High resolution G banding pattern of chromosome 7. The level of resolution is 450 bands per haploid set *(left)*, 550 bands *(center)*, and 850 bands per haploid set *(right)*. (From An International System for Human Cytogenetic Nomenclature. Cytogenet Cell Genet 34:53, 1985. © S Karger, Basel.)

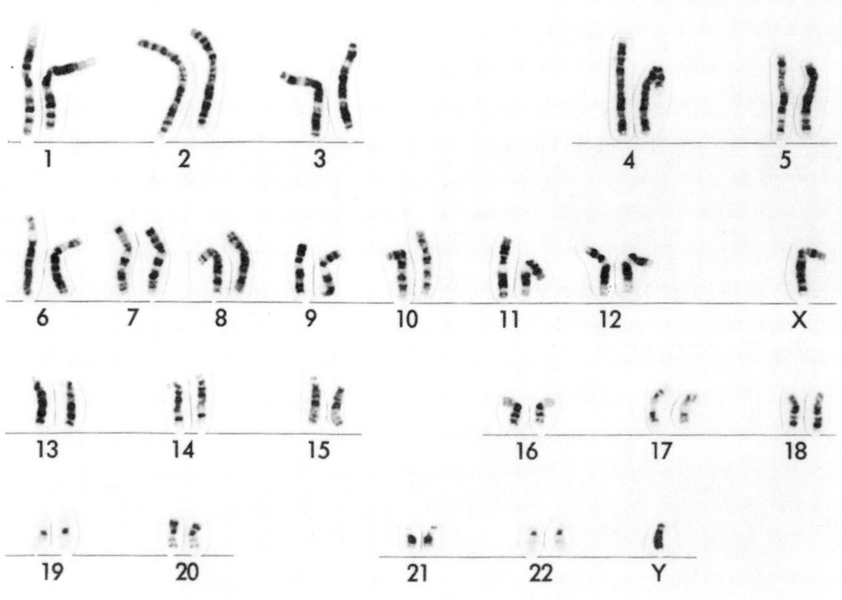

Figure 8.6. A human karyotype of G banded chromosomes. Chromosomes are placed in groups based on size and position of the centromere. (Courtesy of the University of Michigan Clinical Cytogenetics Service.)

Table 8.1. Chromosome Nomenclature

A–G	Chromosome groups
1–22	Autosome numbers
X, Y	Sex chromosomes
/	Diagonal line indicates *mosaicism,* e.g., 46/47 designates a mosaic with 46-chromosome and 47-chromosome cell lines
p	Short arm of chromosome, "petite"
q	Long arm of chromosome
del	Deletion
der	Derivative of chromosome
dup	Duplication
i	Isochromosome
ins	Insertion
inv	Inversion
r	Ring chromosome
t	Translocation
ter	Terminal (may also be written as pter or qter)
+ or −	Placed *before* the chromosome number, these symbols indicate addition (+) or loss (−) of a whole chromosome; e.g., +21 indicates an extra chromosome 21, as in Down syndrome. Placed *after* the chromosome number, these symbols indicate gain or loss of a chromosome part; e.g., 5p− indicates loss of part of the short arm of chromosome 5, as in cri-du-chat syndrome.

constitutions need not be normal; for example, triploidy (69 chromosomes) is a euploid chromosome abnormality commonly found in spontaneous abortions (Fig. 8.7). **Aneuploid** refers to any number of chromosomes that is noneuploid and, in practice, usually refers to an extra copy of a single chromosome, i.e., **trisomy** (as in trisomy 21 Down syndrome), or the absence of a single chromosome, i.e., **monosomy** (as in 45,X Turner syndrome).

Numerical Abnormalities

Aneuploidy is the result of **nondisjunction,** or failure of chromosomes to separate normally during cell division, and can occur during meiosis or mitosis. Although the causes of nondisjunction are not known, it is appreciated that the risk of meiotic nondisjunction increases with increasing maternal age. When nondisjunction occurs

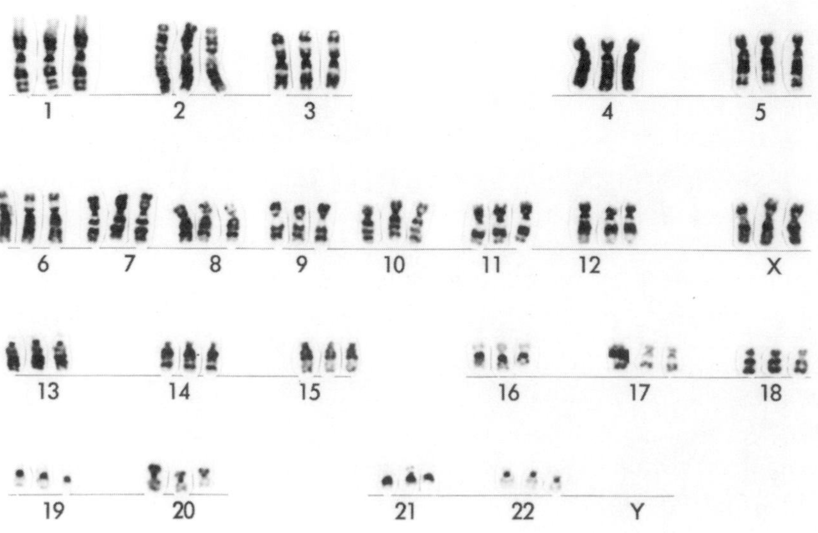

Figure 8.7. Peripheral blood lymphocyte karyotype from a newborn with triploidy. This abnormality is usually the result of fertilization of the egg by two sperm. (Courtesy of the University of Michigan Clinical Cytogenetics Service.)

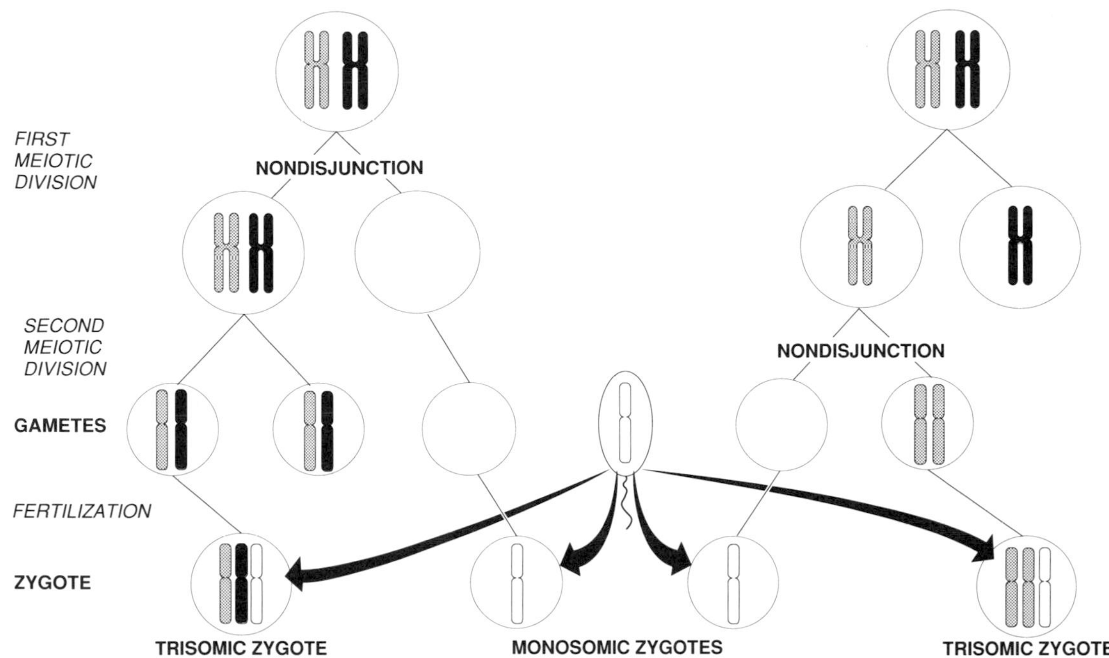

Figure 8.8. Chromosomal consequences of nondisjunction occurring in the first or second meiotic division. See text for details.

after fertilization, that is, mitotic nondisjunction, one expects to see mosaicism, or two or more populations of chromosomally different cells.

Meiotic nondisjunction can occur in either the first or second meiotic divisions with quite different consequences, as indicated in Figure 8.8. If nondisjunction occurs during the first meiotic division, the gametes formed will contain *both* the parental chromosomes that failed to separate or neither. When nondisjunction occurs in the second meiotic division, the gametes will contain two *identical* copies of the same chromosome or neither. Thus, the resulting offspring from a mating in which one of the gametes has undergone meiotic nondisjunction in the first meiotic division will have a copy of both the grandpaternally and grandmaternally derived chromosomes. In contrast, when meiotic nondisjunction has occurred in the second meiotic division there will be two identical copies of either the grandpaternally or grandmaternally derived chromosome. Note that monosomic zygotes can also arise from nondisjunction occurring in either the first or second meiotic division.

Structural Abnormalities

Structural abnormalities of chromosomes may involve either one or two (or more) chromosomes (Fig. 8.9). When only one chromosome is involved, it may have a deletion or duplication of a portion of the chromosome, a pericentric (involving the centromere) or paracentric inversion, or the formation of a ring chromosome or isochromosome. Structural abnormalities involving two or more chromosomes may result in insertions of material from one chromosome into another, or translocation or exchange of chromosomal material between two or more chromosomes. Two major forms of chromosome translocation are recognized: reciprocal translocation (Fig. 8.10) and Robertsonian translocation or centric fusion (Fig. 8.11). In both of these cases, if no essential chromosome material is lost and no genes are damaged by the

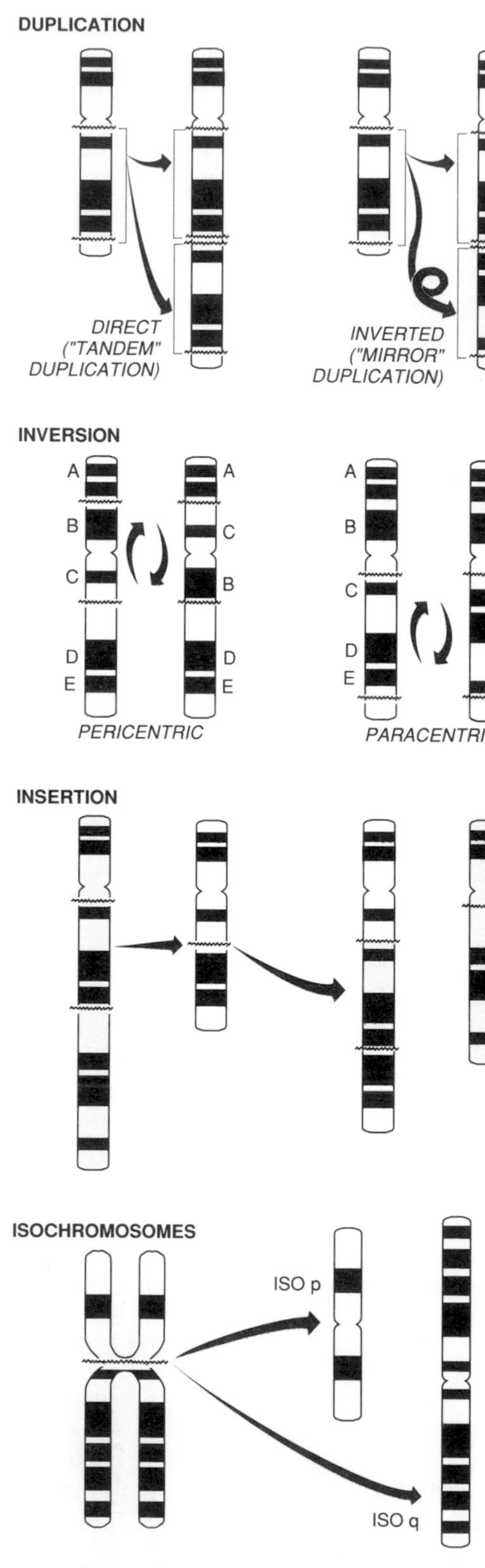

Figure 8.9. Structural abnormalities of chromosomes. *Inversions* involve two breaks in a single chromosome. If the breaks bracket the centromere, this is a pericentric inversion; if they do not, it is paracentric. *Isochromosomes* arise from abnormal centromere division and result in either duplication of the short arm and deletion of the long arm *(ISO p)*, or duplication of the long arm and deletion of the short arm *(ISO q)*. The latter does occur for the X chromosome. *Insertions* result from at least three breaks in at least two chromosomes. Karyotypically unbalanced offspring have pure duplications or pure deletions of the inserted region.

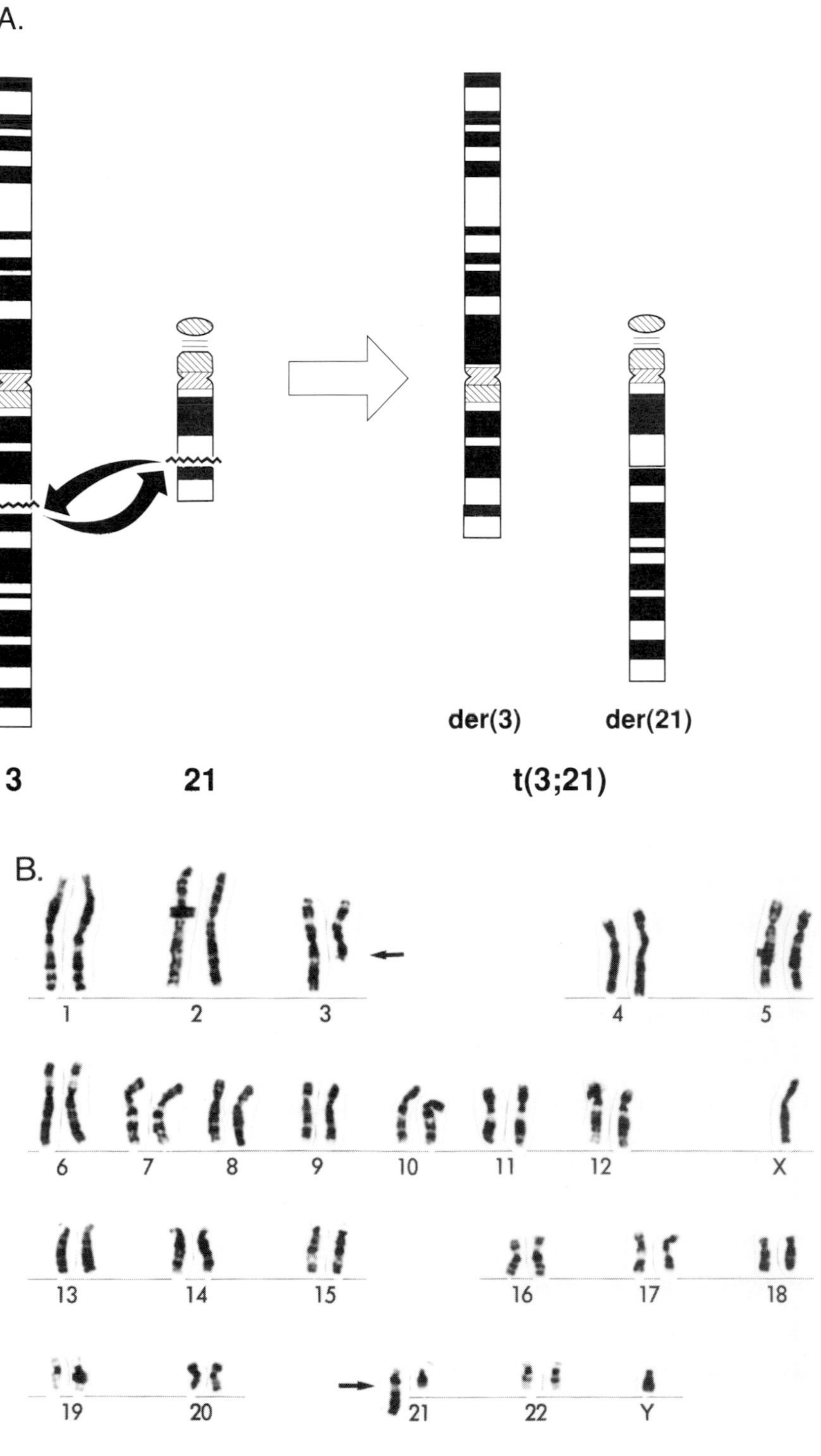

Figure 8.10. Reciprocal translocation between chromosomes 3 and 21. The breakpoints on the long arm of each chromosome are indicated by the *red wavy line* in the diagram (**A**). Chromosome 21 material is shown in *red.* The translocation chromosomes (der (3) and der (21)) are indicated by *arrows* on the karyotype (**B**).

breakage and reunion, the individual carrying such a balanced translocation will be genetically normal and thus clinically normal. However, such individuals are at increased risk of having chromosomally unbalanced offspring. This is illustrated in Figures 8.12 and 8.13.

In the example shown in Figures 8.10 and 8.12, there has been a reciprocal translocation between chromosomes 3 and 21 involving a portion of the long arm of each chromosome. At meiosis, a cross-shaped or quadriradial structure is formed (Fig. 8.12) and the homologous chro-

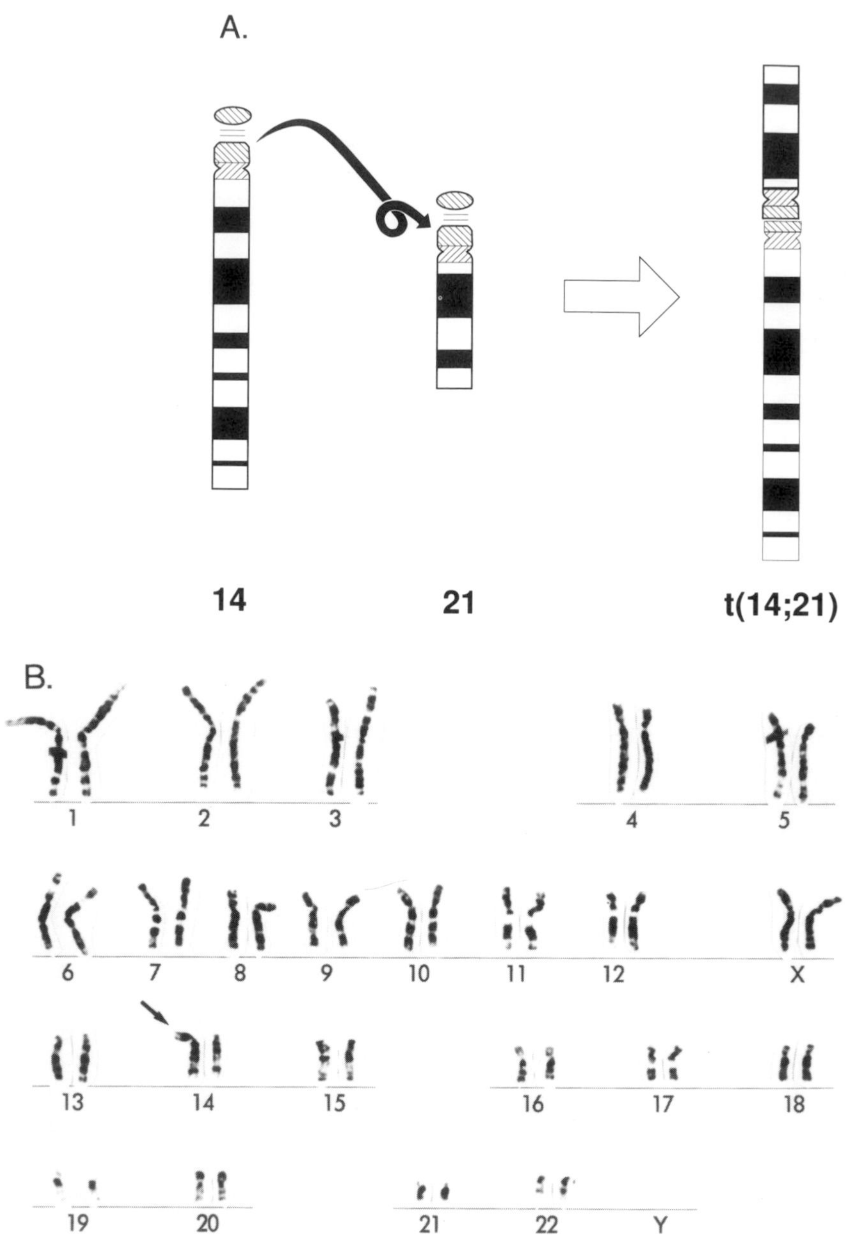

Figure 8.11. Robertsonian translocation or centric fusion involving the long arms of chromosomes 14 and 21. Chromosome 21 material is shown in *red* in the diagram (**A**). The translocation chromosome is indicated by the *arrow* on the karyotype (**B**).

mosomes can separate in several different ways. In alternate segregation, the two normal chromosomes go to one daughter cell and the translocation chromosomes to the other. In this case, two kinds of gametes are formed: normal gametes and those carrying a balanced reciprocal translocation. Fertilization of the normal gamete results in a normal offspring, whereas fertilization of the gamete with the balanced translocation results in an offspring with a balanced reciprocal translocation who should be clinically normal just as is the parent. However, if separation of the chromosomes at meiosis results in the production of gametes containing one normal chromosome and one translocation chromosome as in the so-called adjacent 1 or adjacent 2 segregation, then an unbalanced chromosome constitution is transmitted by that gamete.

In adjacent 1 segregation, homologous centromeres segregate from one another. Fertilization of an unbalanced gamete results in an offspring who has an extra copy of the end of the long arm of chromosome

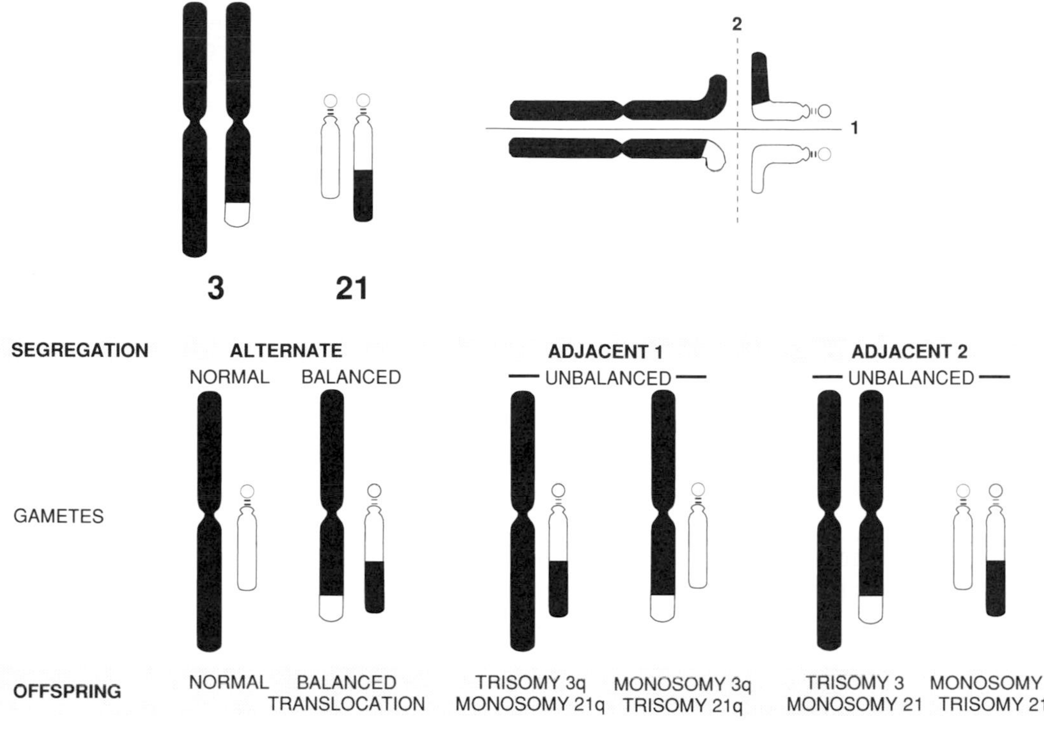

Figure 8.12. Meiotic segregation in a reciprocal translocation involving chromosome 3 and 21. See text for details.

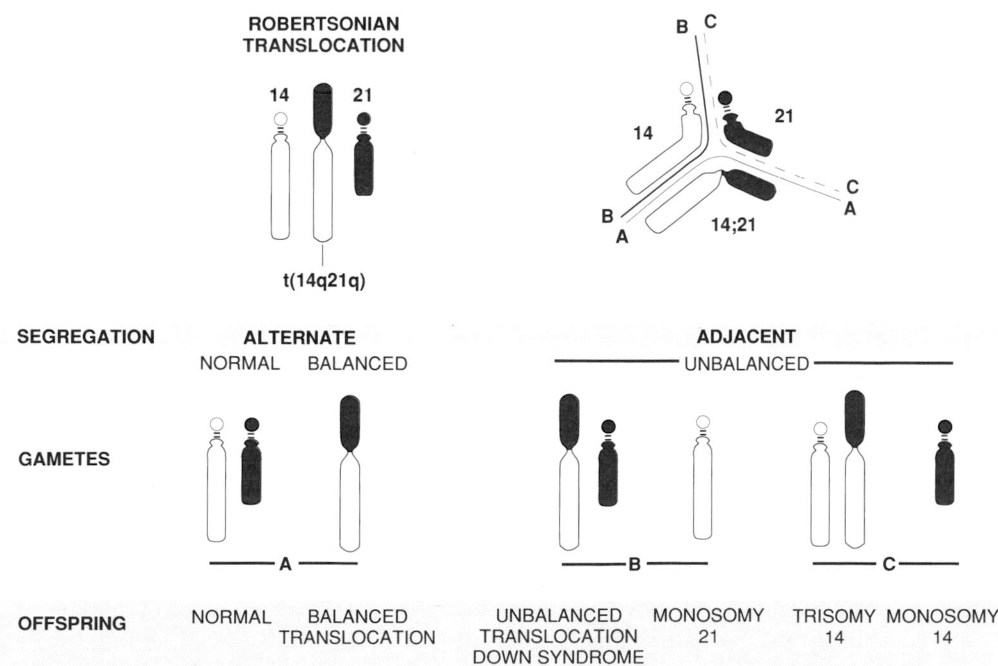

Figure 8.13. Meiotic segregation in Robertsonian translocation involving chromosomes 14 and 21. See text for details.

3 and is missing a portion of the long arm of chromosome 21, or an individual with the reciprocal arrangement, that is, the absence of a portion of the long arm of chromosome 3 and the addition of material from the long arm of chromosome 21. Fertilization of gametes produced by adjacent 2 segregation, in which homologous centromeres do not segregate, results in this example in virtually total monosomy for one of the two chromosomes and a partial trisomy of the other. This degree of chromosome abnormality is generally incompatible with viability even in early embryonic life and results in spontaneous abortion, so that this outcome is rarely seen. In certain translocations, e.g., t(11;22), 3 to 1 segregation (three chromosomes to one pole and one to the other) is usually seen, but this is otherwise rare.

It is clear that certain segregation patterns (e.g., adjacent 2) usually produce a greater degree of chromosomal imbalance than others and are thus observed less frequently in liveborn offspring or even fetuses because they are less likely to survive. However, it appears that the different segregations also do not occur with equal frequency in meiosis. Using the technique of in vitro fertilization of hamster oocytes with human sperm, it is possible to examine karyotypes of sperm from men heterozygous for balanced translocations. Approximately 50% of sperm karyotypes were found to be balanced, resulting from alternate segregation, with the expected equal frequency of normal and balanced translocation complements. Adjacent 1 segregation was responsible for the majority of chromosomally unbalanced gametes. Unbalanced karyotypes were more frequent in sperm than in fetuses and liveborns, again indicating intrauterine selection against chromosomally abnormal zygotes (7).

Figure 8.11 shows a typical Robertsonian translocation or centric fusion between chromosome 14 and chromosome 21. Such translocations tend to involve only chromosomes in the D and G groups, that is, chromosomes 13, 14, 15, and 21 and 22. These are acrocentric chromosomes with short arms consisting of a satellite and stalk containing the nucleolar organizing region and tandemly repeated ribosomal RNA genes. These chromosomes tend to cluster during meiosis and will more often than other chromosomes undergo breakage and recombination with loss of the short arms and fusion of the long arms of the involved chromosomes. The loss of the short arms is apparently not clinically significant because individuals with balanced Robertsonian translocations are clinically normal. However, they are at significant risk for having offspring with an unbalanced translocation. In the example, shown in Fig. 8.13, of an individual with 45 chromosomes and a fusion of the long arm of 14 with the long arm of 21, the involved chromosomes line up in a triradial configuration at meiosis. There are three possible ways the chromosomes can segregate during meiosis and these are shown in Figure 8.13.

During alternate segregation at meiosis (indicated by the *line* marked *A*), one gamete will receive one copy each of the normal chromosome 21 and normal chromosome 14, whereas the other gamete will receive the translocation chromosome carrying the long arms of 14 and 21. Fertilization of these gametes by a normal gamete will result, respectively, in a normal karyotype with 46 chromosomes, and a balanced translocation karyotype with a total of 45 chromosomes like that of the translocation carrier parent. These offspring are clinically normal.

If, on the other hand, adjacent segregation occurs as indicated by *line B,* one gamete will receive a normal chromosome 14 but no chromosome 21. Fertilization by a normal gamete will result in a karyotype with 45 chromosomes but only a single copy of chromosome 21 and hence, monosomy 21, which is generally not viable. The other gamete formed will contain the normal copy of chromosome 21 plus the translocation chromosome. Upon fertilization with a normal gamete, this zygote will contain 46 chromosomes including two copies of the normal chromosome 21, one copy of the normal 14, and the translocation chromosome containing the long arms of chromosomes 14 and 21. Functionally, this individual has three copies of the long arm of chromosome 21, and hence will have the clinical phenotype of Down syndrome.

Finally, in the adjacent segregation indicated by *line C,* one gamete will receive the normal copy of chromosome 14 plus the translocation chromosome. Fertilization of such a gamete by a normal gamete results in a zygote containing 46 chromosomes and functionally trisomic for chromosome 14, which is not viable. The other gamete will receive the normal chromosome 21 but no chromosome 14. Upon fertilization by a normal gamete, this zygote will contain only 45 chromosomes and be lacking one copy of chromosome 14. Monosomy 14 is also not viable.

Because monosomy 21 and monosomy 14 as well as trisomy 14 are not viable, one might expect three possible outcomes in the offspring of a 14q21q translocation parent: normal, balanced translocation, and unbalanced translocation causing Down syndrome. These three types of progeny do not occur with the expected equal frequency, however. Instead, when the mother is the carrier of the 14q21q translocation, approximately 10–15% of offpsring are affected with Down syndrome because they carry two copies of the normal chromosome 21 plus the translocation chromosome, approximately half are balanced translocation carriers like the mother, and 40% are chromosomally normal. For reasons that are not known, when the father is the carrier of the translocation, the risk that a child will be affected is considerably lower, less than 5%. The lower-than-expected frequency of trisomy 21 among liveborn offspring is thought to reflect the high frequency of spontaneous abortion of trisomic fetuses.

CLINICAL CONSEQUENCES OF CHROMOSOME ABNORMALITIES

Spontaneous Abortions

Numerous studies have shown that approximately 50% or more of spontaneously aborted fetuses have major chromosomal abnormalities (1). Because approximately 15% of recognized pregnancies end in spontaneous abortion or miscarriage, this indicates that at least 7.5% of conceptions have major chromosome abnormalities. Furthermore, it is estimated that as many as 50% of conceptions end in spontaneous abortion (many of which are so early as to be unrecognized), suggesting that 25% of all conceptions are afflicted with major chromosome abnormalities.

The major types of chromosome abnormalities found in abortuses are indicated in Table 8.2. The most common are 45,X, triploidy, and trisomy 16. It is interesting that while trisomy 16 is never seen in liveborn infants and triploidy is only rarely seen in liveborns who tend to die very early in infancy, 45,X is seen in liveborn females with a frequency of approximately 1 in 7000 and is the cause of Turner syndrome. Trisomy 13, 18, and 21 are found in about 9% of chromosomally abnormal abortuses but in only 0.1% of liveborns, indicating a high rate of loss of chromosomally abnormal zygotes. Most of this loss occurs early in gestation, as indicated by the much higher frequency of chromosome

Table 8.2. Relative Frequencies of Different Abnormalities in Chromosomally Abnormal Abortuses[a]

Type		Frequency (%)
Trisomy		52
16	15	
13,18,21	9	
XXX,XXY,XYY	1	
All others	27	
45,X		18
Triploidy		17
Tetraploidy		6
Other		7
Total		100

[a]Modified from Hassold TJ: Chromosome abnormalities in human reproductive wastage. Trends Genet 2:105–110, 1986.

abnormalities among spontaneous abortuses (50%) than among stillborns (5%).

Birth Defects

The second major consequence of chromosome abnormalities is birth defects. The frequency of various chromosome aberrations found in newborn surveys is indicated in Table 8.3. Balanced rearrangements, which usually cause no clinical abnormality but which may predispose a carrier adult to bearing a chromosomally unbalanced offspring, are the most common, affecting 1 in 500 individuals. However, various unbalanced chromosome constitutions are not uncommon and the burden of chromosome abnormalities is clearly a significant one, with more than

Table 8.3. Incidence of Chromosomal Abnormalities in Newborn Infants[a]

	Number	Approximate Incidence
Sex chromosome abnormalities *in 28,580 males*		
XXY	30	1/1000
XYY	26	1/1100
Other	17	1/1700
Total	73	1/400
Sex chromosome abnormalities *in 14,976 females*		
45,X	2	1/7500
XXX	13	1/1200
Other	5	1/3000
Total	20	1/750
Autosomal abnormalities *in 43,556 babies*		
+D (trisomy 13)	3	1/15,000
+E (trisomy 18)	4	1/11,000
+G (trisomy 21)	45	1/900
Other trisomies	2	1/22,000
Total	54	1/800
Structural rearrangements		
Balanced	81	1/500
Unbalanced	21	1/2100
Total	102	1/400
Total chromosomal abnormalities	249	1/170

[a]Data from six surveys in Scotland, Denmark, Canada, and the United States. From Jacobs PA, Melville M, Ratcliffe S, Keay AJ, Syme J: A cytogenetic survey of 11,680 newborn infants. Ann Hum Genet 37:359–376, 1974. © Cambridge University Press.

0.5% of all newborns affected with serious chromosome abnormalities. Although the clinical findings in chromosome abnormalities can vary considerably, the general features are a triad of growth retardation, mental retardation, and specific somatic abnormalities.

DOWN SYNDROME

One of the best recognized and most common serious chromosomal disorders is Down syndrome, which is usually caused by an extra copy of chromosome 21 or trisomy 21. The clinical features of this condition include growth retardation, varying degrees of mental retardation, and a spectrum of somatic abnormalities including head and facial features, which resulted in this condition being given the unfortunate designation of mongolism in the past. These features include a flattened face and occiput, upward slanting of the eyes, an extra skin fold at the medial aspect of the eyes (epicanthal folds), and small ears (Fig. 8.14). In addition, Down syndrome babies are often very floppy or hypotonic, and 40% have significant congenital heart disease. There is a markedly increased risk of leukemia and an increased frequency of cataracts and signs of premature aging. Virtually all individuals with Down syndrome who live beyond 35 years show pathologic features of Alzheimer's disease. The most serious health problem faced by children with Down syndrome is congenital heart disease. With improved medical and surgical care for these problems, and with changed attitudes toward the care of children with Down syndrome, the average life expectancy has increased from approximately 9 years in 1930 to more than 30 years by 1980.

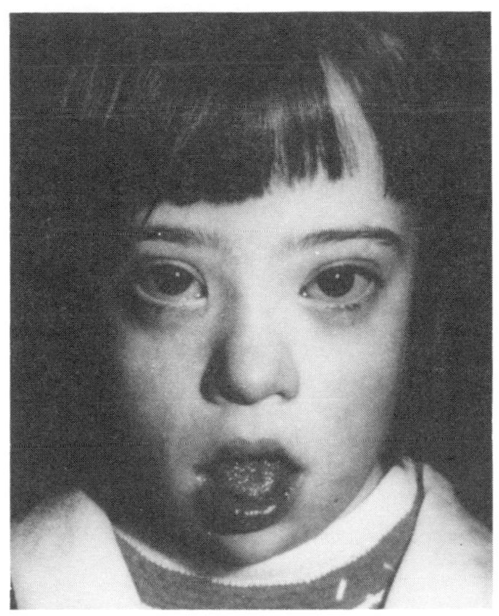

Figure 8.14. A girl with Down syndrome. Note the straight hair, flattened face, open mouth with large tongue, and upward slanting eyes with epicanthal folds.

The chromosomal basis for Down syndrome in approximately 95% of affected individuals is trisomy 21 secondary to nondisjunction during meiosis. By using cytogenetic heteromorphisms (variations in the size or staining intensity of the chromosome 21 satellite) and RFLP markers (8), it is possible in some families to determine in which parent and at which meiotic step nondisjunction has occurred (Fig. 8.15). In cases in which it has been possible to determine where the meiotic error occurred, more than 80% occur in the first meiosis, and more than ¾ of the total during maternal rather than paternal meiosis (9). It has long been recognized that there is a strong association between maternal age

	MOTHER	FATHER	CHILD	
CYTO	A, B	A, A	A, A, B	IF MATERNAL, THEN I
p21-4U	2, 2	1, 2	2, 2, 2	IF PATERNAL, THEN II
SOD1	1, 1	1, 2	1, 2, 2	PATERNAL II

Figure 8.15. Determination of the site of nondisjunction in Down syndrome using chromosome heteromorphisms and RFLP markers. *Cyto A* and *B* refer to variation in the size of the satellite; *p21-4U* is an anonymous probe mapping to the proximal part of 21q; *SOD1* is superoxide dismutase. The chromosomal heteromorphisms are consistent with nondisjunction in paternal meiosis I or II, or in maternal meiosis I. The RFLP recognized by p21-4U is consistent with nondisjunction in material meiosis I or II, or paternal meiosis II. The RFLP recognized by SOD1 is compatible *only* with nondisjunction in paternal meiosis II, establishing the division in which nondisjunction must have occurred. (Redrawn from Stewart GD, Hassold TJ, Berg A, Watkins P, Tanzi R, Kurnit DM: Trisomy 21 (Down syndrome): Studying nondisjunction and meiotic recombinations by using cytogenetic and molecular polymorphisms that span chromosome 21. Am J Hum Genet 42:227–236, 1988.)

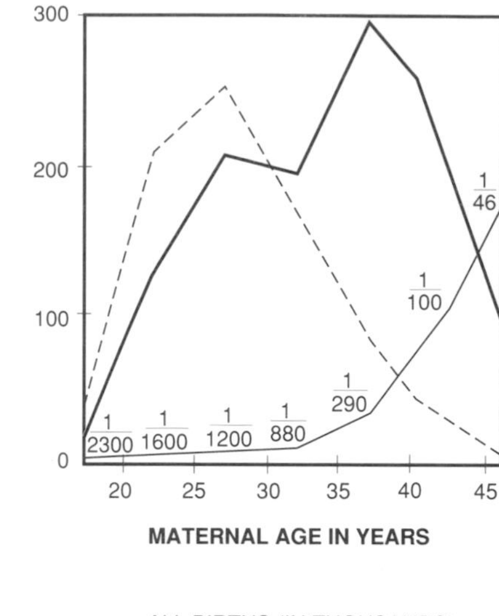

Figure 8.16. The relationship between maternal age and incidence of Down syndrome due to trisomy 21. (Redrawn from Hamerton JL: Human Cytogenetics. Vol. II, New York, Academic Press, 1971.)

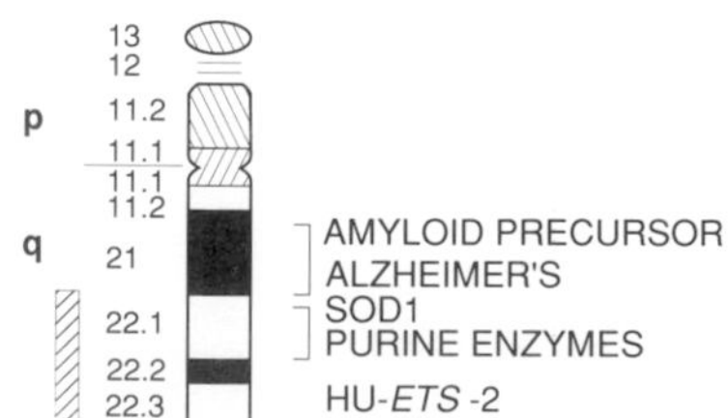

Figure 8.17. Partial gene map of chromosome 21. *rDNA*, ribosomal RNA genes; *SOD1*, superoxide dismutase; *Hu-ets-2*, human homolog of *ets*-2 oncogene. The *cross-hatched bar* at the *left* indicates the region of 21q thought to be important in the etiology of Down syndrome.

and the risk of bearing a child with trisomy 21 but not Down syndrome secondary to translocation (Fig. 8.16); the basis for this association, however, remains unknown.

Approximately 4% of cases of Down syndrome are the result of an unbalanced translocation; 9% of Down syndrome babies born to mothers under 30 years of age have an unbalanced translocation, whereas fewer than 2% of those born to mothers over 30 years do. Approximately 60% of such translocations involve the long arm of a D group chromosome (chromosome 13, 14, or 15) fused to the long arm of 21; two-thirds of these involve chromosome 14. Although more than half of such unbalanced translocations represent de novo events occurring during gametogenesis in a parent of the affected child, the remainder are the result of inherited translocations. This latter fact is important because it indicates that other family members may also be translocation carriers and at significant risk of bearing a child with Down syndrome. Approximately 40% of translocations involve only the G group chromosomes, 21 and 22. Eighty percent of these are 21q21q translocations and nearly all of these represent de novo events. In those rare circumstances where the parent is a carrier of a 21q21q translocation, the only viable offspring such an individual could have would necessarily have Down syndrome. Finally, approximately 1% or fewer of individuals with Down syndrome are mosaics in that they have a 47,+21 line of cells in addition to a normal euploid line. These individuals usually have milder manifestations of the Down syndrome.

The empirical recurrence risks to parents who have had a child with trisomy 21 are approximately 1%, although these risks are somewhat higher among older women. The reasons for this increased risk are unknown. For carriers of a balanced translocation, the risks that a child will be affected are approximately 10% if the mother is a carrier but less than 5% if the father is carrier. Again, it is important to recognize that there is a similar risk to other relatives if the translocation is inherited. Each first degree relative of a balanced translocation carrier has approximately a 50% chance of also being a carrier of that same translocation.

From studies of individuals with trisomy for only a part of chromosome 21, it is thought that only the distal one-third of the long arm of chromosome 21 must be present in an extra copy to cause Down syndrome. Chromosome 21 is one of the smallest of the chromosomes, containing approximately 1.5% of the total cellular DNA or approximately 1500 genes. A number of genes have now been mapped to the long arm of chromosome 21, including the genes for familial Alzheimer's disease and the amyloid precursor, both of which map closer to the centromere than the region involved in the causation of Down syndrome. In the distal end of the chromosome 21, however, are genes for superoxide dismutase-1, for certain purine synthetic enzymes, for a human oncogene Hu-*ets*-2, and for alpha-A crystallin, a protein found in the lens (Fig. 8.17). All of these are of interest in that patients with the Down syndrome develop Alzheimer's disease relatively early in life, and they frequently have increased levels of purines, an increased risk of acute leukemia, and a higher frequency of cataracts. Whether any of these findings can be correlated with the presence of the specific genes on the long arm of chromosome 21 remains to be determined (10).

OTHER AUTOSOMAL ABNORMALITIES

Other serious chromosome abnormalities include a number of trisomies and partial trisomies (2, 3). One example is trisomy 13 with a

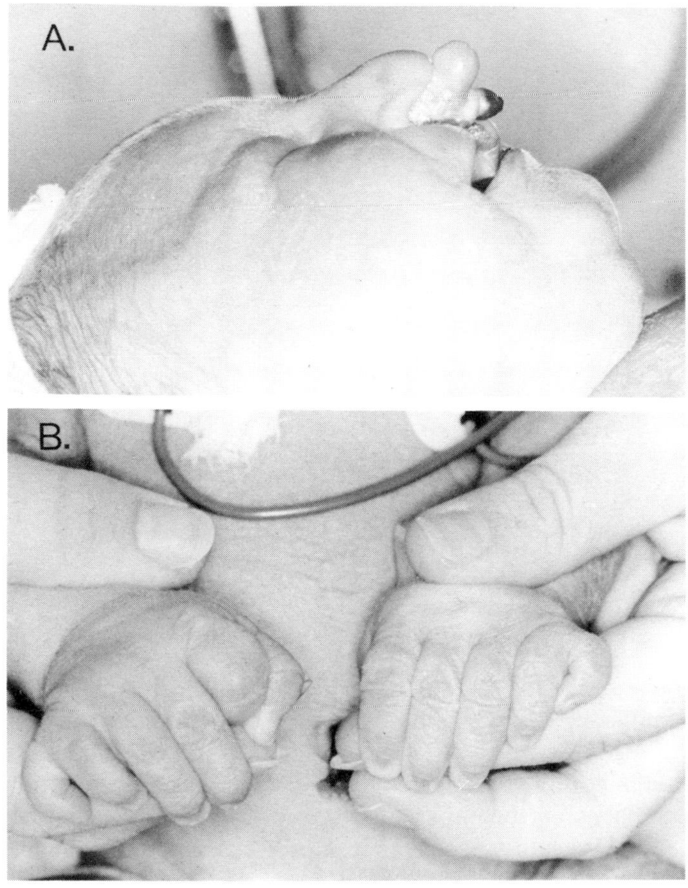

Figure 8.18. An infant with trisomy 13. Note the facial malformation and severe cleft lip and palate (**A**) and polydactyly (**B**).

frequency of approximately 1 in 15,000 live births. Approximately one-half of these babies die within the 1st month of life. Characteristically they have a failure of normal brain development called holoprosencephaly, in which there is an absence of normal formation of the frontal cortex. There are associated abnormalities of the skull and face including severe cleft lip and palate and midfacial abnormalities (Fig. 8.18). Peculiar punched-out scalp defects are characteristic of this syndrome, as is polydactyly (extra fingers and toes). As is the case with other major chromosome abnormalities, these babies are growth retarded and severely developmentally retarded.

Other chromosome abnormalities include structural defects such as partial trisomies or partial monosomies; that is, extra pieces or missing pieces of a chromosome. A typical example is the 5p− syndrome, or cri-du-chat, so-called because of the weak mewing cry reminiscent of a cat's cry (Fig. 8.19).

Chromosomal Changes in Neoplasia

In addition to germ line chromosome abnormalities, there is a growing recognition of chromosome abnormalities in a variety of cancers. The early observation that such changes were not random, together with newer developments in gene mapping, have resulted in a better understanding of the possible causation of a number of malignancies. One particularly well-understood example is the Burkitt lymphoma in which there is frequently a reciprocal translocation of a piece of the long

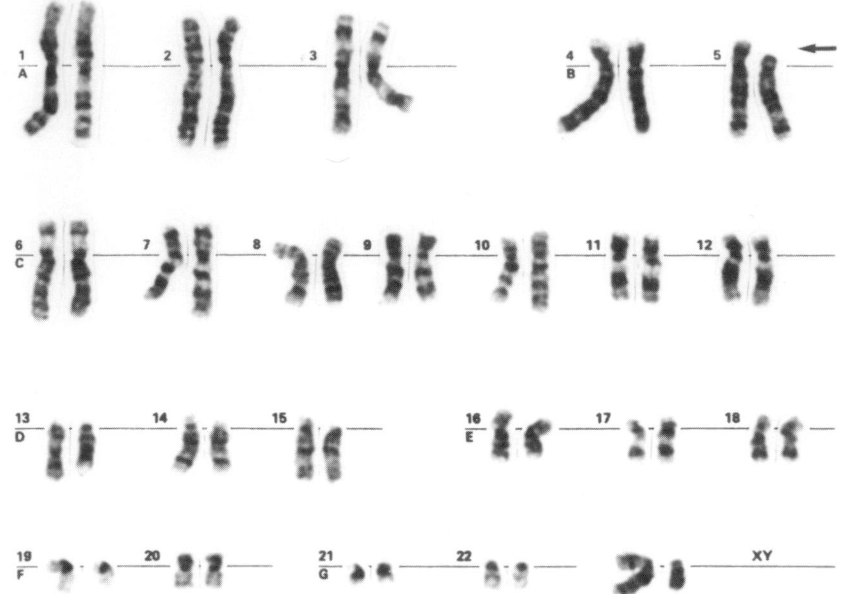

Figure 8.19. Karyotype of a child with 5p−, cri-du-chat syndrome. The *arrow* indicates the deletion on 5p. (Courtesy of the University of Michigan Clinical Cytogenetics Service.)

arm of chromosome 8 with the long arm of chromosome 14. Less frequently the exchange involves the long arm of chromosome 8 with the long arm of chromosome 21 or 2. In chronic myelogenous leukemia, a form of leukemia in adults, there is frequently a reciprocal translocation between the long arms of chromosome 9 and 22 (Ph^1 or Philadelphia chromosome). The mechanisms by which these translocations might cause malignancy is discussed in Chapter 10.

SEX CHROMOSOMES

It is as if in the evolution of sex a fragment at one time broke away from an X chromosome . . . and thereafter in relation to the other chromosomes was helpless to prevent them from expressing themselves in the form of an incomplete female, the creature we call the male! It is largely to this original X-chromosome deficiency of the male that almost all the troubles to which the male falls heir may be traced. . . .

—Ashley Montagu
(From *The Natural Superiority of Women* by Ashley Montagu.© 1952, 1953, 1968, 1974 by Ashley Montagu. Reprinted with permission of Macmillan Publishing Company)

Sex Chromosomes and Sexual Differentiation

It has been noted (11) that "of all life's inequities, the contrast between the X and Y chromosomes is one of the most fundamental and certainly one of the most intriguing." The X chromosome is large, containing 6% of the total DNA in contrast to the small Y chromosome. More than 100 diseases have been shown to be X-linked, but only one to be Y-linked. More than 50 genes and 200 DNA markers have been mapped to the X chromosome, with most of the genes encoding somatic functions. In contrast, although there are several DNA markers now mapped to the Y chromosome, only two genes thus far have been assigned to this chromosome. One of these, the testis-determining factor (TDF) plays the critical role of determining gonadal sex.

In early embryonic life, the human fetal gonad is undifferentiated. Germ cells migrate from the yolk sac into the gonad during the 4th week of development, and at approximately 6–7 weeks of development, the gonad undergoes sexual differentiation (Fig. 8.20). In the presence of a Y chromosome the central portion, or medulla, of the gonad develops to become the testis. The testis elaborates two inducers. One is the androgen testosterone, which causes wolffian duct proliferation. These ducts become the male internal genitalia. The other inducer is a nonsteroid glycoprotein called müllerian inhibitory substance, which causes regression of müllerian duct structures. In the absence of a Y chromosome, as in the human XX female, the outer portion or cortex of the gonad develops into the ovary. There is no production of testosterone or of müllerian inhibitory substance. Therefore, there is regression of the wolffian duct structures and proliferation of müllerian duct structures, which form the female internal genitalia including the upper portion of the vagina, the uterus, and the oviducts or fallopian tubes. It is usually the presence or absence of the tesis that determines sexual differentiation rather than whether or not an ovary is present. Removal of the gonad in early mammalian fetuses results in development of female internal genitalia.

The mechanism of sex determination has been the subject of scientific speculation and investigation since antiquity. It was assumed that sex was determined in humans, as in *Drosophila,* by the number of X chromosomes. Only in 1959 was it realized that it is the presence or absence of a Y chromosome that determines sex. This was based on the discovery of 47,XXY Klinefelter syndrome individuals who were phe-

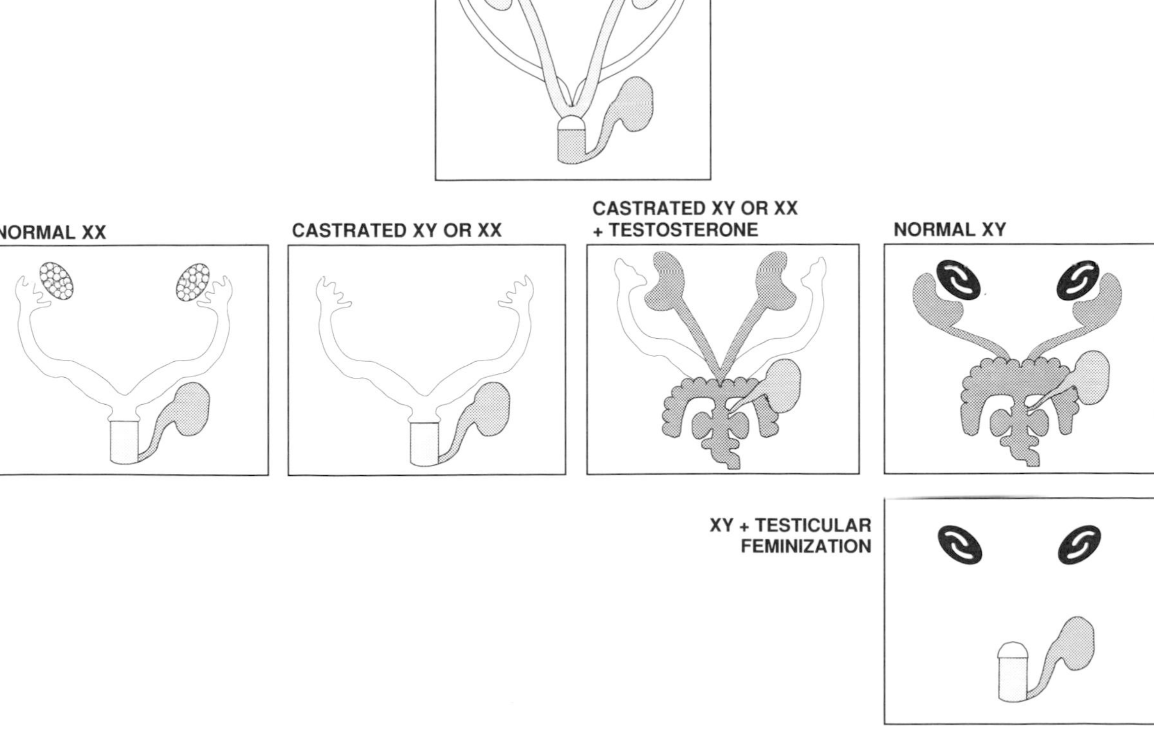

Figure 8.20. Human sexual differentiation. See text for details.

notypically male, and the finding that mice with only a single X chromosome were female (4).

The specific gene on the Y chromosome responsible for development of the testis was discovered by a study of rare exceptions to the rule that it is the Y chromosome that determines gonadal sex. Males with a 46,XX constitution and females with a 46,XY constitution were studied using a series of DNA probes mapped to various portions of the Y chromosome (Fig. 8.21). From such studies it was determined that the testis-determining factor gene must reside in a 230-kb segment of the Y chromosome near the end of the short arm. This DNA sequence has been highly conserved during evolution and is found in all mammals. The sequence of this region suggests that it encodes a transcription-activator protein of the "zinc finger" type, hence its designation as *zfy* for zinc finger Y (12). It is speculated that this protein may act upon a number of other genes encoded by autosomes whose expression is necessary for the orderly progress of sexual differentiation. Interestingly, similar DNA sequences occur on the X chromosome of humans and other mammals; their relationship to sexual differentiation remains unknown. It is assumed that XX males and XY females arise because of reciprocal exchange of genetic material between the X and Y chromosomes during male meiosis. Just distal to the testis-determining factor region is the so-called pseudoautosomal region at which the X and Y chromosomes pair during meiosis and in which extensive recombination occurs (13).

External sexual differentiation is the result of the infuence of an androgen derivative, 5α-dihydrotestosterone, which causes differentiation of male external genitalia. In individuals with the X-linked mutation testicular feminization, there is androgen insensitivity secondary to

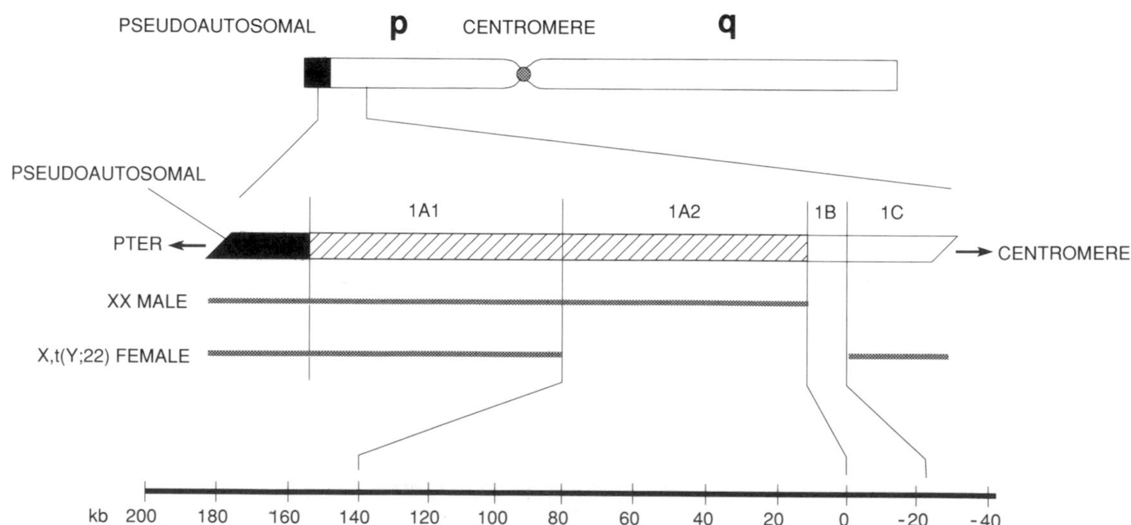

Figure 8.21. Deletion analysis of the distal short arm of the Y chromosome indicating the region containing the testis-determining factor (TDF). The pseudoautosomal region *(black)* undergoes recombination with the homologous region on the short arm of the X chromosome, Xpter, during male meiosis. Regions designated *1A1, 1A2, 1B,* and *1C* were mapped by deletion analysis, and show strictly Y-linked inheritance. The *red bars* indicate portions of the Y chromosome present in an XX male and an XY (actually X,t(Y:22)) female. At least part of TDF, the testis-determining gene, must lie in interval 1A2, which is present in the XX male and absent in the XY female. (Redrawn from Page DC, Mosher R, Simpson EM, Fisher EMC, Mardon G, Pollack J, McGillivray B, de la Chapelle A, Brown LG: The sex-determining region of the human Y chromosome encodes a finger protein. Cell 51:1091–1104, 1987. © Cell Press.)

an abnormal or deficient androgen receptor and these individuals fail to develop normal male external genitalia. They have testes and a normal female external phenotype (Fig. 8.22) but lack female or male internal genital structures. These women are often detected clinically when they fail to menstruate and investigation reveals a 46,XX karyotype and the presence of testes, usually found in the inguinal region.

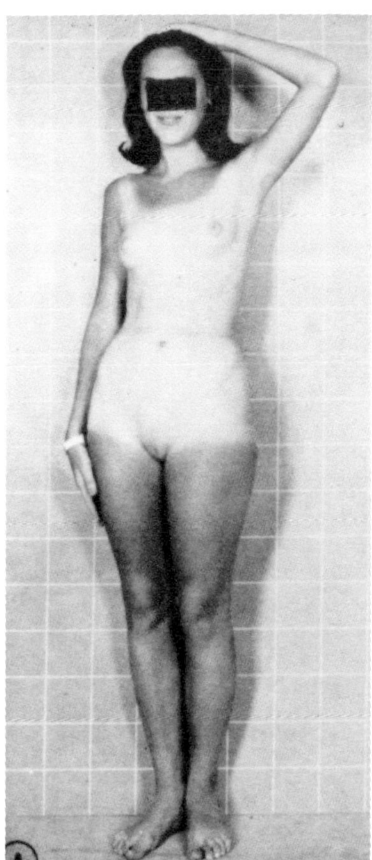

Figure 8.22. A patient with testicular feminization. Note the normal female phenotype except for decreased axillary and pubic hair. (From Grumbach MM, Van Wyk JJ: Disorders of sex differentiation. In Wilson JD, Foster DW (eds): *Textbook of Endocrinology.* 7th Ed. Philadelphia, WB Saunders, 1985.)

X-Chromosome Inactivation

Although males are hemizygous for the X chromosome (have only a single copy), the mean amounts of gene products of X-encoded genes such as red blood cell G6PD activity (Fig. 8.23) are the same as in females who have two X chromosomes. Therefore, there must be some mechanism of dosage compensation. The independent investigations of four geneticists, Mary Lyon, Lianne Russell, Ernest Beutler, and Susumo Ohno, resulted in an understanding of this mechanism that now is called the "Lyon hypothesis" after Mary Lyon a British geneticist. The Lyon hypothesis (Fig. 8.24) states that in ***somatic*** cells (*a*) X inactivation occurs **early** in embryonic life; (*b*) the inactivation is **random;** that is, either the paternal or maternal X chromosome may be inactivated; (*c*) X inactivation is **complete,** in that virtually all of the X chromosome is inactivated; and (*d*) X-chromosome inactivation is **permanent and clonally propagated;** that is, if the paternally derived X chromosome is inactivated in a given cell, all of the progeny of that cell will express an

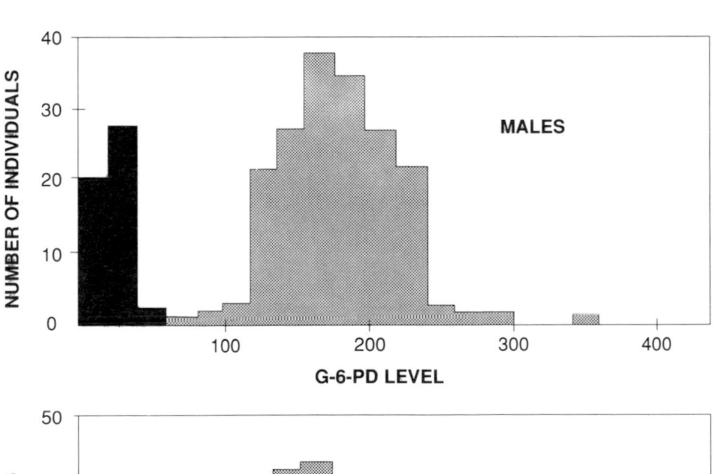

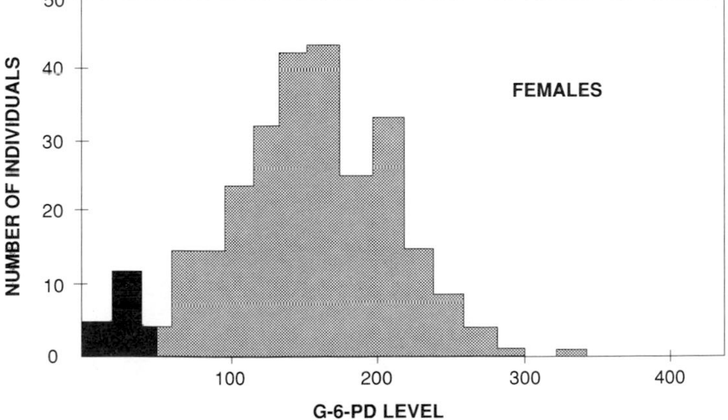

Figure 8.23. Distribution of red cell G6PD activity in a population of black male and female subjects from Nigeria. *Black bars* indicate G6PD-deficient individuals. Note that the distribution of G6PD activity in nondeficient individuals (*red-shaded area*) is essentially the same in males and females. (Redrawn from Harris H: *The Principles of Human Biochemical Genetics.* 2nd Ed. Amsterdam, North-Holland Publishers, 1975.)

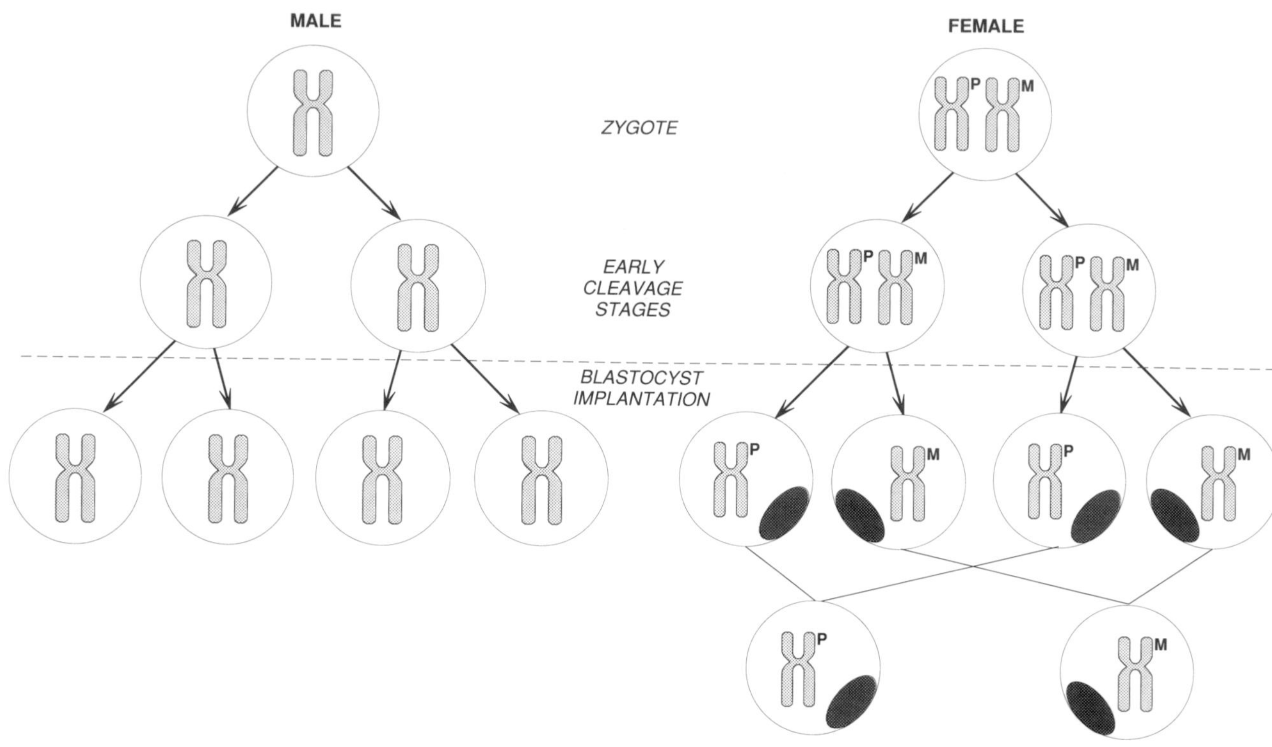

Figure 8.24. Schematic diagram of the Lyon hypothesis. *P* represents the paternally derived X chromosome, and *M*, the maternally derived X in the female; the single X in the male must be inherited from the mother. The inactive X is shown as the *dark mass.*

active maternally derived X whereas the paternally derived X remains inactive. The result of lyonization is that the female is a **mosaic** (Fig. 8.25) of cells, each functionally hemizygous for one or the other X chromosome.

It should be noted that there are exceptions to the above statements about X inactivation. Although X inactivation is usually random, a structurally abnormal X, e.g., an X chromosome bearing a deletion, is preferentially inactivated. On the other hand, in individuals with X-autosome translocations, it is usually the normal X chromosome that is preferentially inactivated (see Chapter 9). Although X inactivation is extensive, it is not entirely complete. At least two genes at the end of the short arm of the X, those encoding the Xg^a antigen and the enzyme steroid sulfatase, do not undergo inactivation. Furthermore, there is evi-

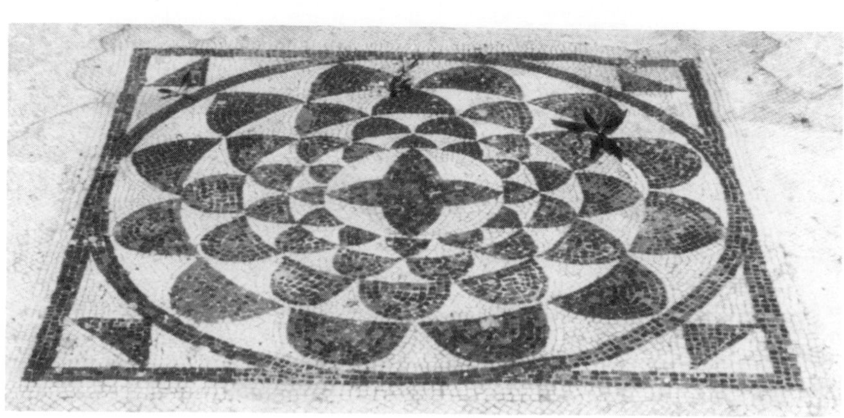

Figure 8.25. Mosaic from the floor of a Roman villa at Pompeii. Note patches of only black stones and patches of only white.

dence that some genes on the long arm of the X (Xq26) also must escape inactivation in order to maintain ovarian function until the normal age of menopause (11). Finally, it should be noted that while X inactivation is permanent in most somatic cells, it must be reversible in the development of germ cells.

Several lines of evidence support the Lyon hypothesis (14). The first came from genetic studies in mice. Female mice heterozygous for an X-linked coat color mutation, e.g., tortoiseshell, were always found to have a mottled coat; that is, they showed patches of tortoiseshell fur and of wild-type fur (Fig. 8.26). In contrast, males hemizygous for this mutant showed uniform tortoiseshell coat color. Calico cats are another familiar example of this phenomenon. Female mice heterozygous for two nonallelic, mutant coat color genes expressed patches of fur containing only one or the other mutant color when the genes were in repulsion (on opposite chromosomes), but patches containing a blend of both mutant colors or patches of wild-type fur when the genes were in coupling (on the same X chromosome).

The cytologic evidence for lyonization came first from the serendipitous discovery of sex chromatin, or the Barr body. The Canadian cytologist Murray Barr, studying the morphologic effects of repetitive electrical stimulation on neurons in the cat, noted that the nuclei of neurons from some cats contained an extra dark-staining chromatin body and that these chromatin bodies were found only in female cats. Subsequent studies in humans, using epithelial cells scraped from the buccal mucosa, indicated that the number of sex chromatin bodies is equal to the number of X chromosomes minus one. Normal males who have only one X chromosome have no sex chromatin, whereas normal females with two X chromosomes have one (Fig. 8.27). Individuals with three X chromosomes have two Barr bodies. Later studies showed that during prophase one of the two X chromosomes appeared to be heteropyknotic, i.e., dense and dark-staining, suggestive of inactive chromatin. Finally, studies using thymidine labeling of chromosomes in cultured cells indicated that one of the two X chromosomes replicated late during the S phase of the cell cycle. Examination of patients with X chromosome aneuploidy, e.g., 49,XXXXX, indicated the presence of four sex chromatin bodies, four heteropyknotic X chromosomes in prophase, and four late-replicating X chromosomes in S phase, suggesting that all three of these cytologic features indicated a genetically inactive X chromosome (Fig. 8.28).

The biochemical evidence supporting lyonization came initially from studies on the expression of G6PD in cultured skin fibroblasts from women heterozygous for Gd A, encoding a common electrophoretic variant of G6PD, and the wild-type Gd B allele. Mass cultures of

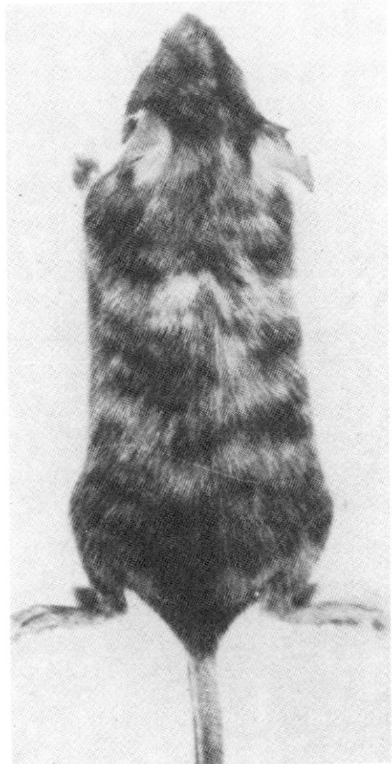

Figure 8.26. Female mouse heterozygous for the X-linked coat color mutation tortoiseshell. (From Thompson MW: Genetic consequences of heteropyknosis of an X chromosome. Can J Genet Cytol 7:202–213, 1965.)

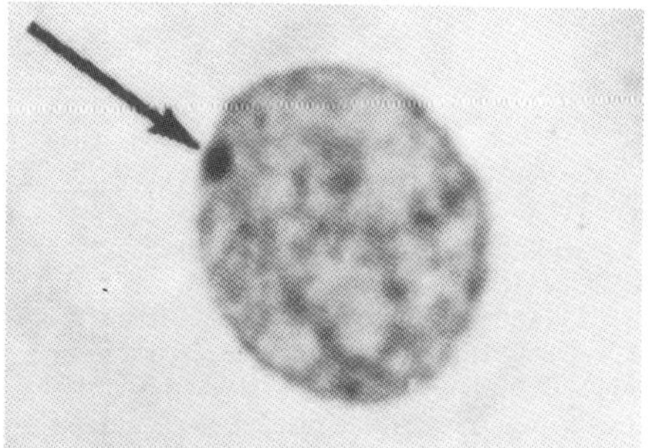

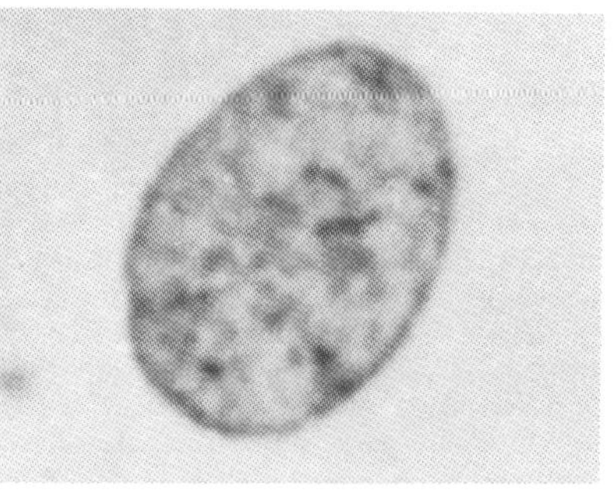

Figure 8.27. Sex chromatin body in human buccal mucosa cells. Note that a Barr body *(arrow)* is present in the nucleus of a cell from a female subject *(left)* but not from a male *(right)*. (From Grumbach MM, Van Wyk JJ: Disorders of sex differentiation. In Wilson JD, Foster DW (eds): *Textbook of Endocrinology*. 7th Ed. Philadelphia, WB Saunders, 1985.)

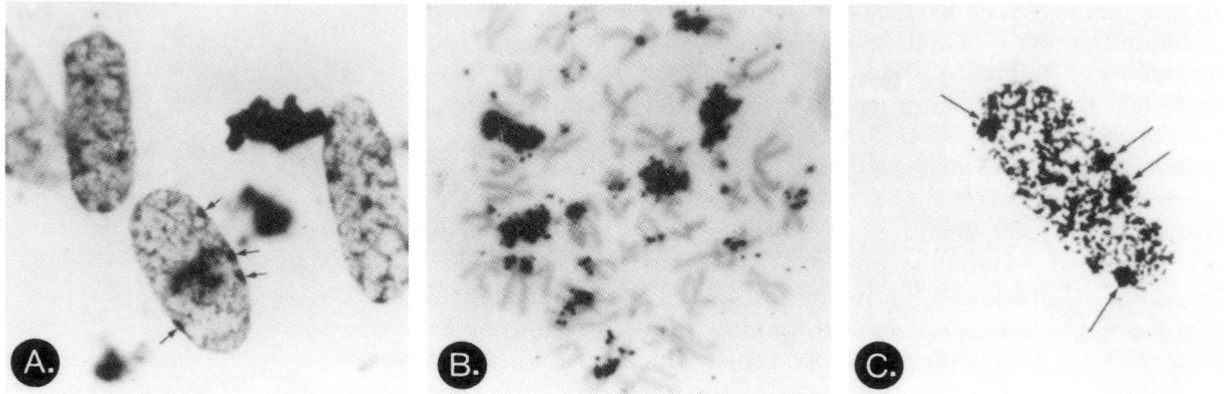

Figure 8.28. Sex chromatin and late-replicating X chromosomes in skin fibroblasts from a girl with a 49,XXXXX karyotype. Note that there are four sex chromatin bodies *(arrows)* in interphase nuclei (**A**) and four late-replicating X chromosomes detected by tritiated thymidine incorporation in S-phase cells (**B**). The radioactive late-replicating X chromosomes in **B** correspond to the radioactively labeled sex chromatin bodies *(arrows)* seen in interphase nuclei (**C**). (From Grumbach MM, Morishima A, Taylor JH: Human sex chromosome abnormalities in relation to DNA replication and heterochromatinization. Proc Natl Acad Sci USA 49:581–589, 1963, and Grumbach MM: Second International Congress of Congenital Malformations. Compiled and edited by the International Medical Congress, Ltd., New York, NY, 1964, p 63.)

fibroblasts expressed both the A and B forms of this enzyme, whereas clones of skin fibroblasts, that is, cell lines derived from a single cell precursor, expressed *either* A or B but never both (Fig. 8.29). Similar clonal expression of biochemical markers has been defined for other X-linked genes including ornithine transcarbamylase (see Fig. 7.17) and hypoxanthine phosphoribosyltransferase. The correlation of this biochemical evidence with cytologic evidence came from studies in mules, the female hybrid offspring of a cross between a horse and a donkey. Because horse and donkey X chromosomes can be distinguished cytologically and the G6PD activity differentiated electrophoretically, one could correlate, in individual lines of skin fibroblasts cultured from mules, the presence of the horse G6PD when the donkey X chromosome was inactive and vice versa. Taken together, the genetic, cytologic and biochemical evidence strongly supports the hypothesis that in every somatic cell in a female mammal, only one X chromosome is active.

The significance of the Lyon hypothesis is severalfold. First, it helps to understand the manifestations of X-linked genes and diseases in humans and it accounts for the much greater variability of clinical manifestations in heterozygous females than in hemizygous males. By the same token, it helps explain the considerable difficulties that arise in biochemical carrier detection techniques aimed at identifying female

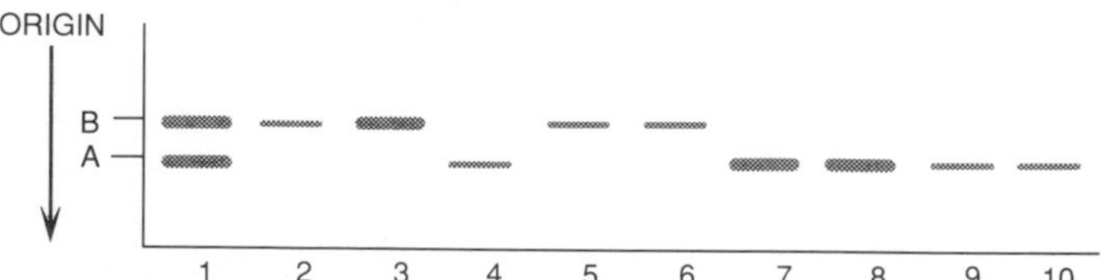

Figure 8.29. Electrophoretic analysis of G6PD in fibroblast cultures from a woman heterozygous for an electrophoretic variant (*A*) of G6PD. Note that in the mass culture of fibroblasts *(lane 1)* both G6PD and B are expressed. Clonal isolates of fibroblasts from this mass culture *(lanes 2–10)* express only G6PD A or only B but never both electrophoretic types. (Redrawn from Davidson RG, Nitowsky HN, Childs B: Demonstration of two populations of cells in the human female heterozygous for glucose-6-phosphate dehydrogenase variants. Proc Natl Acad Sci USA 50:481–485, 1963.)

carriers of X-linked diseases. Lyonization also helps in understanding the phenotype of X-chromosome aneuploidy as discussed below. Perhaps most importantly, X inactivation provides an interesting model for the study of gene regulation because it provides an example in which almost an entire chromosome is permanently inactivated (15). Thus far, there is no proven explanation for X inactivation, although DNA methylation has been suggested as a likely possibility. The timing of X inactivation during embryonic development is not firmly established, but is thought to occur in humans at approximately the 100-cell stage or blastocyst implantation. Finally, X-chromosome inactivation has been used as a marker for studies of differentiation and malignant transformation. For example, in a study of uterine fibroids (benign smooth muscle tumors arising in the uterus), it was shown that in women heterozygous for Gd A and B that each fibroid tumor expressed only A or B type G6PD but never both. This was interpreted to indicate that each tumor most likely arose from a single cell. The power of this technique has been markedly increased by the use of X-linked DNA markers.

Disorders of Sex Chromosomes

KLINEFELTER SYNDROME

The Klinefelter syndrome, which occurs in approximately 1 per 1000 male live births, is characterized by postpubertal testicular failure. The patient is a phenotypic male with small testes, hyalinized testicular tubules, and azoospermia (failure to produce normal amounts of sperm) resulting in infertility and variable signs of hypogonadism. These individuals are normal in appearance before puberty, but after puberty are recognized by their small testes and occasionally by enlargement of the breasts (gynecomastia) and abnormal body proportions (Fig. 8.30). Interestingly, individuals with this syndrome have a greater-than-expected frequency of social pathology, which can range from lack of normal social adjustment to actual difficulties with the law. Significant mental retardation is not usually part of this syndrome, although average IQ may be somewhat reduced. Individuals with the Klinefelter syndrome typically have a 47,XXY chromosome constitution. Their cells are chromatin-positive (that is, they contain a Barr body) and there are at least two X's and one Y in at least some of their cells. This form of X-chromosome aneuploidy is thought to arise from meiotic nondisjunction. When X-linked gene products or DNA markers are available, one can determine in which meiotic division the nondisjunction occurred. Some men with the Klinefelter syndrome have been found to have more than two copies of the X chromosome plus a Y. The more X chromosomes the patient has, the greater the likelihood that there is mental retardation associated with this syndrome. As described earlier, the discovery that Klinefelter syndrome men had a 47,XXY karyotype was the first demonstration that sex in humans was determined by the presence or absence of a Y chromosome rather than by the number of X chromosomes.

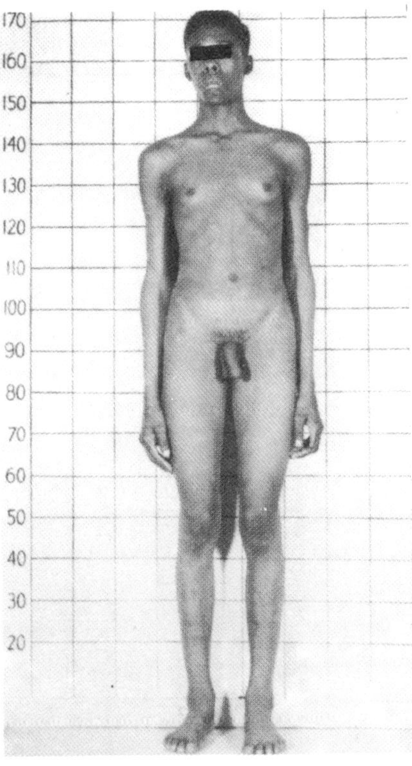

Figure 8.30. The Klinefelter syndrome. Note that the patient has a normal phallus but has gynecomastia (female-like breast development). (This photo appeared in *J Chronic Dis* (July 1960) Feinstein AR (ed), and in *Medical Genetics 1958–1960.* St. Louis, 1961, The C.V. Mosby Co. Reproduced by permission of the editors of the Journal of Chronic Diseases.)

XYY SYNDROME

Because of the social pathology associated with the Klinefelter syndrome, studies were undertaken in mental-penal institutions in the United Kingdom to asses the frequency of the 47,XXY karyotypes among inmates in such institutions (4). This led to the discovery of indi-

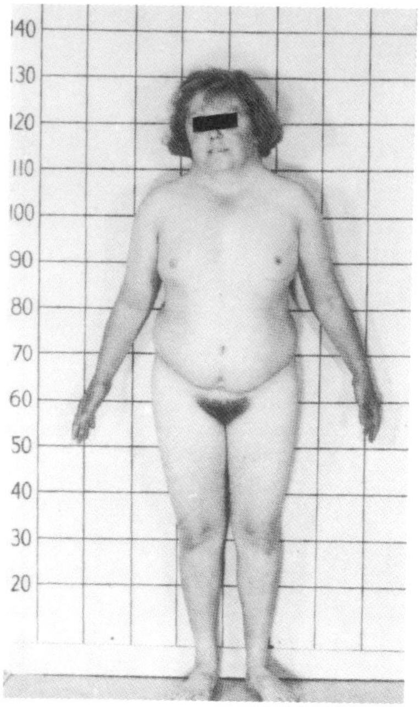

Figure 8.31. The Turner syndrome. The patient has short stature, webbed neck, shield-shaped chest with wide-spaced nipples and underdeveloped breasts, and an increased carrying angle of the arms. (This photo appeared in *J Chronic Dis* (July 1960) Feinstein AR (ed), and in *Medical Genetics 1958–1960*. St. Louis, 1961, The C.V. Mosby Co. Reproduced by permission of the editors of the Journal of Chronic Diseases.)

viduals with aneuploidy of the Y chromosome, for example 47,XYY and 48,XXYY. 47,XYY occurs in approximately 1 in 1000 male live births but was found in 4–20 per 1000 inmates of mental-penal institutions. The frequency of 48,XXYY, which is associated with the Klinefelter phenotype, was 50 times as high among inmates as in the newborn population. This has raised the question of whether the extra Y chromosome is causally associated with behavior abnormalities. The only phenotype uniformly associated with the XYY karyotype, however, is tall stature; the magnitude of the increased risk, if any, of social pathology associated with this syndrome is as yet unclear (16). Aneuploidy of the Y chromosome must arise from meiotic nondisjunction in the father.

TURNER SYNDROME

The Turner syndrome is characterized by a phenotypic female with gonadal dysgenesis and sexual immaturity. Characteristically, these women have primary amenorrhea (failure to menstruate) and infertility. The typical syndrome is also associated with short stature (usually under 5 feet) and a host of somatic abnormalities including webbing of the neck, increased carrying angle at the elbow, and cardiovascular and renal abnormalities (Fig. 8.31). Karyotypically, there is something wrong with the second sex chromosome in at least some of the cells of individuals with the Turner syndrome (Table 8.4). Slightly more than half of patients with the Turner syndrome are monosomic for the X, i.e., 45,X, and are chromatin negative. Approximately 15% have structural abnormalities of the X chromosome, including isochromosome X, deletions of portions of the X or ring chromosomes (2, 3). These individuals have 46 chromosomes and are chromatin-positive; i.e., a Barr body would be present. Another 15% are mosaic for 45,X/46,XX, and an additional 15% are mosaic for a 45,X cell line plus a 46,X, abnormal X cell line or a 47,XXX cell line. The presence of mosaicism indicates that nondisjunction must have occurred during mitosis following fertilization rather than during meiosis. Thus, the Turner syndrome can arise from either meiotic nondisjunction (in approximately 80%, the nondisjunction is in paternal meiosis (9)) or from mitotic nondisjunction, the latter resulting in mosaicism. It should also be noted that because a significant portion of patients with the Turner syndrome are chromatin-positive, the diagnosis cannot be made by looking for Barr bodies on a buccal smear, but must be made by karyotypic analysis.

Table 8.4. Abnormal Karyotypes in Turner Syndrome

45,X		
46,X, abnormal X		
Deletion	X,Xp−	
Isochromosome	X,i(Xq)	Monosomy short arm Trisomy long arm
Ring	X,r(X)	
Mosaicism		
X/XX		
X/XY		Virilization, gonadoblastoma
X/X, abnormal X		
X/XXX		
X/XX/XXX etc.		

From studies of patients with the Turner syndrome with an abnormal X chromosome it has been suggested that monosomy of the short arm of the X chromosome is responsible for the short stature and somatic abnormalities accompanying this syndrome. However, it is genes on the long arm of the X that are critical for ovarian development and maintenance. Because only one X chromosome is normally active in the somatic cells of the female, the question arises as to why Turner syndrome occurs at all. Apparently there must be two active X chromosomes during ovarian development and it would appear that certain genes on both X chromosomes must remain active for normal adult ovarian function (11). It is known that the inactive X chromosome is reactivated in oogonia when meiosis begins during fetal life.

The ovary is an unusual organ in that there is programmed destruction of its major product, eggs (11). The fetal ovary is thought to contain some 7 million oocytes, which have decreased in number to 3 million at the time of birth. By the time of menarche, or onset of menses, the number has fallen to approximately 400,000 and by menopause it is around 10,000. Individuals with the Turner syndrome have oocytes during fetal life but they are virtually gone by the age of 2 years; menopause has occurred before menarche. In addition, families have been described in which women have premature menopause and have been found to have a deletion of a portion of the X chromosome, particularly Xq26. This suggests that genes in this region of the X are necessary for the maintenance of ovarian function and the prevention of premature menopause. Furthermore, it suggests that these particular genes are not inactivated on the inactive X chromosome.

From the study of patients with Turner syndrome with mosaicism, it is known that the presence of a normal 46,XX cell line mollifies the disorder and there have been rare patients with 46,XX/45,X mosaicism who have had normal menses and even fertility. The presence of an XY cell line (found in approximately 5% of patients with the Turner syndrome) may be associated with virilization at birth and again at puberty, and more significantly, a 20% risk of malignancy of the dysgenic gonad. It is interesting to consider that women with 46,XY/45,X Turner syndrome mosaicism must have arisen as male zygotes who then underwent a mitotic nondisjunctional event resulting in the Turner syndrome.

X-LINKED MENTAL RETARDATION AND FRAGILE X

The fact that significant mental retardation is more common in males than in females has been recognized for many decades, and it has been known that there are families with X-linked mental retardation. In 1969, a family was described with X-linked mental retardation and the association of a marker X chromosome. When lymphocyte cultures are deprived of folate, or thymidine metabolism is perturbed, apparent breaks or gaps in chromosomes, so-called fragile sites, can be observed. Using these techniques, the fragile X or fraXq27 syndrome has been defined (17). It is characterized by moderate to severe mental retardation, large testes and large ears in some patients, and the presence of the fraXq27 (Fig. 8.32) in up to 60% of mitotic cells from affected males (less than 1% of mitotic cells from normal males show this abnormality). Approximately 20% of obligate heterozygous females have both the fragile X and some degree of mental retardation and another 15% have mental impairment but not the fragile X. It is now recognized that this

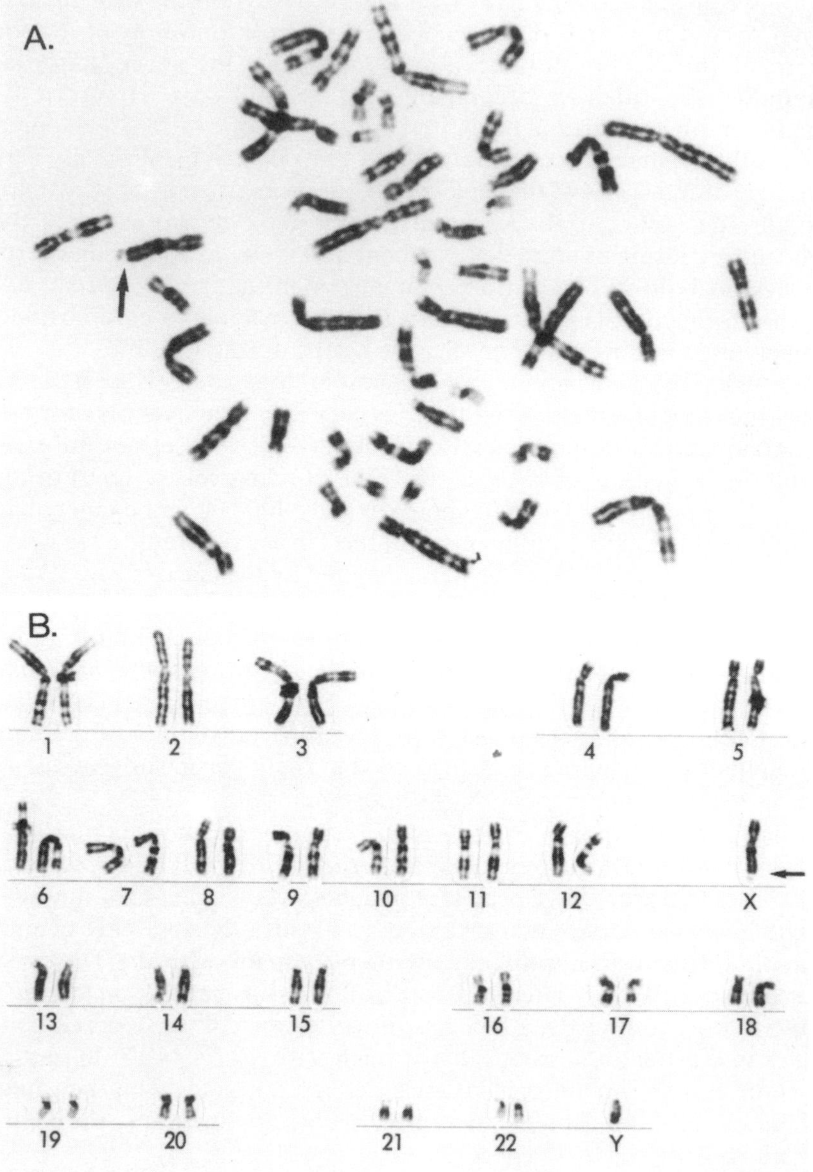

Figure 8.32. Metaphase spread (A) and karyotype (B) from a peripheral blood leukocyte culture of a patient with mental retardation and the fragile X syndrome. The *arrow* indicates the fragile X abnormality, which involves bands 27 and 28 on the long arm of the X chromosome. (Courtesy of the University of Michigan Clinical Cytogenetics Service.)

syndrome is second in frequency only to the Down syndrome as a cause of chromosomally determined severe mental retardation. It occurs in approximately 1 per 2000 males and approximately 0.4 per 2000 females. Curiously, affected males have never been proven to be the result of a new maternal mutation; thus, the mothers of all affected males are thought to be obligate fragile X carriers. Affected females receive the fragile X from their mothers and not from their fathers. However, some affected males, defined by the fact that they transmit the trait, may show neither mental retardation nor the fragile X chromosome marker. Active investigation and analysis of the DNA surrounding this fragile site hopefully will result in the identification of genes which, when mutated, can cause mental retardation. The awareness of this syndrome has significant implications for genetic couseling. The fragile X should be sought in any male with unexplained mental retardation and particularly in families in which there is X-linked mental retardation. One must request that the karyotype be done specifically for this diagnosis so that the appropriate culture conditions can be used; routine karyotypes will not detect the fragile X site.

X-AUTOSOME TRANSLOCATIONS

Occasionally, reciprocal translocation can occur between the X chromosome and one of the autosomes. These accidents of nature have turned out to be very useful for gene mapping (as discussed in Chapter 9 with respect to Duchenne muscular dystrophy) and in understanding karyotype-phenotype correlations. Presumably, during the breakage and rejoining of chromosomal segments there is either loss of some chromosome material or breakage within a gene on the X chromosome. Because the normal X chromosome is preferentially inactivated in cases of X-autosome translocation, females heterozygous for such a translocation may express X-linked recessive diseases otherwise observed only in hemizygous males.

Indications for Chromosome Analysis (Table 8.5)

1. Known or Suspected Chromosome Abnormality. It is imperative that any patient with a known or suspected chromosome abnormality have the diagnosis made or confirmed by a karyotypic analysis. Even experienced physicians may miss the diagnosis of Down syndrome in a newborn, for example. These serious disorders deserve the most accurate diagnostic procedures available and there is no reason not to perform such a study. As discussed above, it is also important in the case of Down syndrome to determine whether the individual has trisomy 21 or an unbalanced translocation that might be inherited from a carrier patient.

2. Multiple Congenital Anomalies, Especially When Associated with Growth and/or Mental Retardation. Because the characteristic phenotype of major chromosome abnormalities is the combination of growth retardation, mental retardation, and somatic abnormalities, this combination should always suggest the possibility of a chromosome abnormality and a karotype should be done.

3. Disorders of Sexual Differentiation. These conditions, discussed earlier in this chapter, require a definition of chromosomal sex for accurate diagnosis and management of the condition.

4. Familial Mental Retardation in Males. The frequency of the fragile X syndrome requires that this condition be sought in X-linked mental retardation

5. Hematologic Malignancies and Diseases Associated with Chromosome Instability. The frequent finding of specific chromosome abnormalities in certain hematologic malignancies has established the value of chromosome studies in diagnosis and in prognosis of these disorders. In addition there are certain genetic diseases associated with chromosome instability and a high risk of leukemia and other malignancies.

Table 8.5. Indications for Karyotype

1. Known or suspected chromosome abnormality
2. Multiple congenital anomalies and/or growth and mental retardation
3. Disorder of sexual differentiation
4. Familial mental retardation in males
5. Hematologic malignancy
6. Multiple miscarriages

6. Multiple Miscarriages. In approximately 5% of couples who have had two or more spontaneous abortions, one or the other parent carries a balanced translocation. The assumption is that the unbalanced state might account for the spontaneous abortions, although this has rarely been proven. Nevertheless, the detection of such couples would be an indication to monitor future pregnancies by amniocentesis.

Finally, chromosome studies are not indicated in cases of clear-cut Mendelian diseases. Genetic diseases do not necessarily have detectable chromosome abnormalities. However, it should be remembered that a small chromosomal deletion will segregate within a family in exactly the same fashion as a single gene, dominant, Mendelian trait. With the development of newer techniques for improved resolution of structural abnormalities of chromosomes, diseases not previously thought to be associated with chromosomal changes may indeed be found to have such changes. For example, the Prader-Willi syndrome, characterized by mental retardation, obesity, hypogonadism, and small hands and feet, has been found, in a majority of cases, to be associated with an interstitial deletion of chromosome 15 involving bands q11–q13 (Fig. 8.33). As discussed in Chapter 10, retinoblastoma, a dominantly inherited cancer of the eye, was found to be associated with an interstitial deletion of chromosome 13 and this finding was helpful in the eventual mapping of the gene for this cancer.

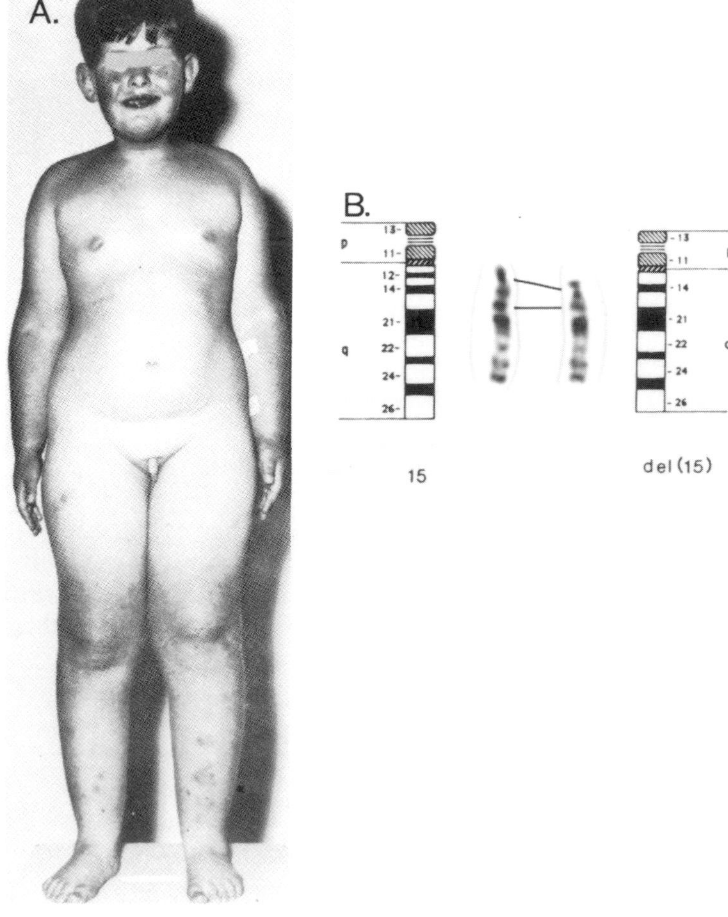

Figure 8.33. **A**, Prader-Willi syndrome. Note that the patient has obesity, small penis, and small hands and feet. (From Jones KL: *Smith's Recognizable Patterns of Human Malformations.* 4th Ed. Philadelphia, WB Saunders, 1988.) **B**, schematic diagram and a partial karotype from a patient with the Prader-Willi syndrome showing the interstitial deletion of bands 11 to 13 in the long arm of chromosome 15 (15q11-13-). (Courtesy of the University of Michigan Clinical Cytogenetics Service.)

REFERENCES

1. Hassold TJ: Chromosome abnormalities in human reproductive wastage. Trends Genet 2:105–110, 1986.
2. deGrouchy J, Turleau C: *Clinical Atlas of Human Chromosomes.* 2nd Ed. New York, John Wiley & Sons, 1984.
3. Gardner RJM, Sutherland GR: *Chromosome Abnormalities and Genetic Counseling.* New York, Oxford University Press, 1989.
4. Jacobs PA: Human population cytogenetics: The first twenty-five years. Am J Hum Genet 34:689–698, 1982.
5. Bickmore WA, Sumner AT: Mammalian chromosome banding—An expression of genome organization. Trends Genet 5:144–148, 1989.
6. Francke U: Elusive chromosome anomalies. Hosp Pract 21:175–193, 1986.
7. Martin RH: Segregation analysis of translocations by the study of human sperm chromosome complements. Am J Hum Genet 44:461–463, 1989.
8. Stewart GD, Hassold TJ, Berg A, Watkins P, Tanzi R, Kurnit DM: Trisomy 21 (Down syndrome): Studying nondisjunction and meiotic recombination by using cytogenetic and molecular polymorphisms that span chromosome 21. Am J Hum Genet 42:227–236, 1988.
9. Magenis RE: On the origin of chromosome anomaly. Am J Hum Genet 42:529–533, 1988.
10. Patterson D: The causes of Down syndrome. Sci Am 257:52–60, 1987.
11. Federman DD: Mapping the X chromosome. Mining its p's and q's. N Engl J Med 317:161–162, 1987.
12. Page DC, Mosher R, Simpson EM, Fisher EMC, Mardon G, Pollack J, McGillivray B, de la Chappelle A, Brown LG: The sex-determining region of the human Y chromosome encodes a finger protein. Cell 51:1091–1104, 1987.
13. de la Chapelle A: The complicated issue of human sex determination. Am J Hum Genet 43:1–3, 1988.
14. Davidson RG: The Lyon hypothesis. J Pediatr 65:765–775, 1964.
15. Grant SG, Chapman VM: Mechanisms of X-chromosome regulation. Annu Rev Genet 22:199–233, 1988.
16. Walzer S, Gerald PS, Shah SA: The XYY genotype. Annu Rev Med 29:563–570, 1978.
17. Nussbaum RL, Ledbetter DH: Fragile X syndrome: A unique mutation in man. Annu Rev Genet 20:109–145, 1986.

8/ Study Questions

1/ What is the difference between metacentric, submetacentric, and acrocentric chromosomes? What special structures and sequences are present in acrocentric chromosomes?

2/ Which of the following individuals have aneuploid karyotypes?

a. A female with a balanced translocation involving 11q and 22q
b. A female with trisomy 21 Down syndrome
c. A female with a balanced Robertsonian translocation involving chromosomes 13 and 21

What kinds of gametes can each of the individuals in a, b and c above produce? List the chromosomal makeup of the fertilized eggs when each of these types of gametes is fertilized by a normal sperm.

*** 3/** Why hasn't every human chromosome been found involved in chromosomal trisomy in newborns? Why might the types and frequencies of various chromosomal abnormalities seen in chorionic villus samples obtained at 8 weeks gestation be different from those seen in live newborns?

4/ A family with a child with Down syndrome due to trisomy 21 is studied for RFLPs on chromosome 21. One such RFLP has alleles of 7, 6, 5, or 4 kb. Shown below is a diagram of a Southern blot for the child, her father, and her mother. Can you tell in which parent the nondisjunction event occurred? Can you tell in which stage of meiosis it occurred?

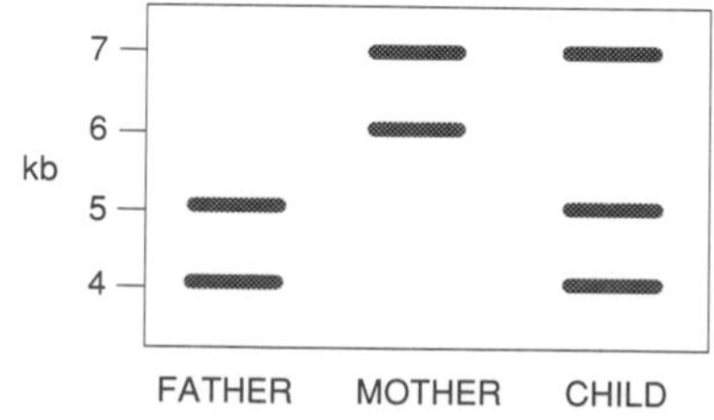

5/ What kind of gonad and what internal and external genitalia would you expect in the following disease states?

a. A 46,XY individual with a complete deletion of the testis-determining factor gene
b. A 46,XY individual homozygous for deficiency of an enzyme required for androgen biosynthesis
c. A 46,XY individual hemizygous for deficiency of the androgen receptor.

6/ Hemophilia A due to mutation of the X-linked gene for clotting Factor VIII is often thought of as a disease that affects males exclusively. However, there can be females with serious bleeding abnormalities due to hemophilia A. Describe four mechanisms by which females can have this disease.

7/ If an individual is a mosaic for a chromosome aneuploidy, what likely inference can you make about when the event causing the mosaicism occurred?

8/ What phenotype or phenotypes are likely to occur in an individual with a 46,XY/45,X mosaicism?

9/ Why is it important to obtain a karyotype in a child in whom a clinical diagnosis of Down syndrome is completely obvious?

10/ Why is it important to obtain a karyotype in a child in whom a clinical diagnosis of Turner syndrome is completely obvious? Will a buccal smear for Barr body count suffice?

9

Anatomy of the Human Genome: Gene Mapping and Linkage

"I am frequently asked, 'Why map genes?' There are many reasons, but three stand out. The first relates to the challenge. Many of us were motivated to develop methods of human gene mapping simply because the problem seemed insuperable at the outset. A second motivation is the aesthetic satisfaction. For some reason we gain gratification in placing a well-known gene in its correct position on the map. There is however, a third reason: the utilitarian reason. I believe that we can safely say, 'Gene mapping is good for you!'"

—Frank Ruddle
(From Reverse genetics and beyond. Am J Hum Genet 36:944, 1984)

As the above quotation from one of the leaders in the gene mapping field indicates, placing genes on their correct chromosomes began mostly as an intellectual exercise without immediate and obvious consequences for biology or medicine. However, that has rapidly changed over the course of the last decade. As we will see in this chapter, gene mapping is now even capable of leading to the cloning of previously unapproachable disease genes.

Gene mapping prior to 1950 was essentially limited to the X chromosome. In that instance the characteristic pattern of inheritance of an X-linked disease or trait allowed "gene mapping" by pedigree inspection. Autosomal loci were, however, far more difficult to approach. The first autosomal gene placed on a chromosome was the Duffy blood group locus, mapped by Donahue in 1968. This, in fact, is a wonderful example of the rule that "serendipity favors the prepared mind." Donahue was learning how to visualize metaphase chromosomes in the early days of cytogenetics and was practicing on his own white blood cells. He noticed that one of his chromosome 1's had a large heterochromatic region just below the centromere (Fig. 9.1). This is not associated with any disorder and simply represents a variable feature of this chromosome, commonly called a "heteromorphism." Being curious, he also studied other members of his family and was able to observe the Mendelian transmission of this chromosome variant. As part of this analysis he also derived blood type information for other members of the family. On inspection of the results, he noted that while the more famous red cell antigens for the ABO

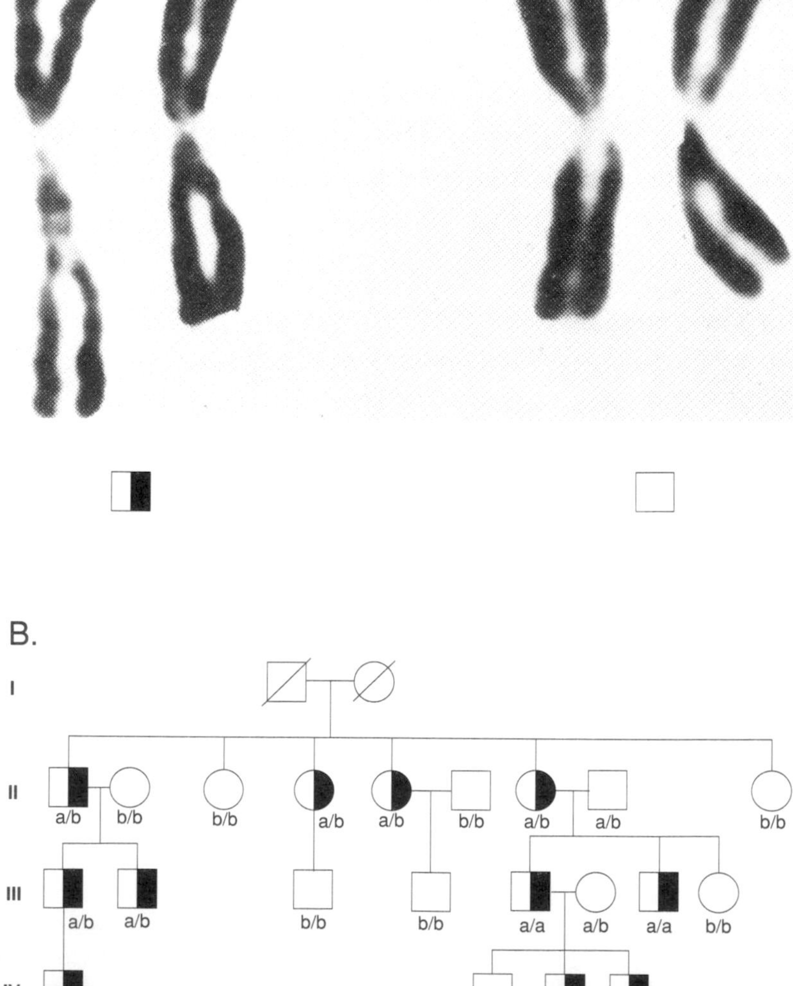

Figure 9.1. **A,** A pair of number 1 chromosomes from two different individuals. These studies, done prior to the advent of chromosome banding, show that in the pair on the *left* one chromosome shows a remarkable increase in length below the centromere, referred to as a heteromorphism. The chromosomes on the *right* show the more usual morphology. **B,** Pedigree demonstrating probable linkage of Duffy blood group to chromosome 1. The *half-solid symbols* indicate the presence of the heteromorphism on chromosome 1, and the *a* and *b* designations indicate the Duffy blood group genotypes. While the individuals in generation I are of unknown status, in the rest of the pedigree it can be seen that the chromosome with the heteromorphism universally travels with the a allele at the Duffy locus. (Modified from Donohue RP, Bias WB, Renwick JH, McKusick VA: Probable assignment of the Duffy blood group locus to chromosome 1 in man. Proc Natl Acad Sci USA 61:949, 1968.)

and Rh blood groups showed no relationship to this chromosome 1 finding, the Duffy blood group, which is a less commonly measured red blood cell antigen, had its inheritance entirely predicted in the family by the chromosome 1 heteromorphism. The pedigree, together with the chromosome findings and the Duffy blood group genotypes, is shown in Figure 9.1. Inspection of the pedigree shows that the chromosome 1 heteromorphism without exception travels with the a allele at the Duffy locus. Donahue correctly concluded that the gene for the Duffy blood group must reside on chromosome 1, thereby achieving the first success in autosomal gene mapping.

METHODS OF GENE MAPPING

While Donahue's achievement was truly impressive for the technology available at the time, this approach could hardly be generalized to the mapping of large numbers of genes, depending as it did on the occurrence of a visible chromosome heteromorphism that does not occur on most chromosomes. Over the course of the last 30 years a powerful set of mapping methods have been developed, which are far more generalizable, and we will consider these in some detail. These will not be presented in the chronological order in which they were developed, but rather beginning from the most direct and easily understood approaches to the more indirect and conceptually difficult.

In Situ Hybridization

One of the most direct means of mapping a gene, since it provides a direct visual signal, depends on molecular hybridization of a cloned DNA sequence to metaphase chromosomes spread out on a microscope slide. The probe is labeled in such a way that its presence can be detected, either by radioactivity (usually using tritium as the radioactive marker) or by fluorescence labeling. The metaphase chromosomes are denatured in place on the microscope slide, and the labeled probe is hybridized to them. The excess probe is washed off and the location of the probe is visualized by x-ray film or fluorescence. Figure 9.2*A* shows an example of such a procedure, where an insulin probe has been labeled with tritium. The small blob marked by the *arrow* indicates the location of the radioactive probe, on the tip of the short arm of chromosome 11. In general, a large number of metaphase spreads must be scored in order to be able to distinguish the true location from the background nonspecific probe localization. The band location of each radioactive grain is recorded, and a histogram is built up as shown in Figure 9.2*B*. The correct location of the gene can be deduced by the most highly represented region, in this instance 11p15.

More recently, the radioactive labeling procedure is being replaced by a fluorescence method. In a commonly used protocol, the probe DNA is labeled with a vitamin called biotin, hybridized to the metaphase chromosome spread, and then the probe is visualized using the very strong binding of fluorescence-labeled streptavidin to biotin (Fig. 9.2*C*).

The resolution of in situ hybridization often allows the localization of a specific DNA sequence to a chromosome band, which is one of the advantages of this approach. As must be obvious, however, this can be done only if the cloned DNA sequence is available; human diseases cannot be mapped this way unless their causative gene has already been identified.

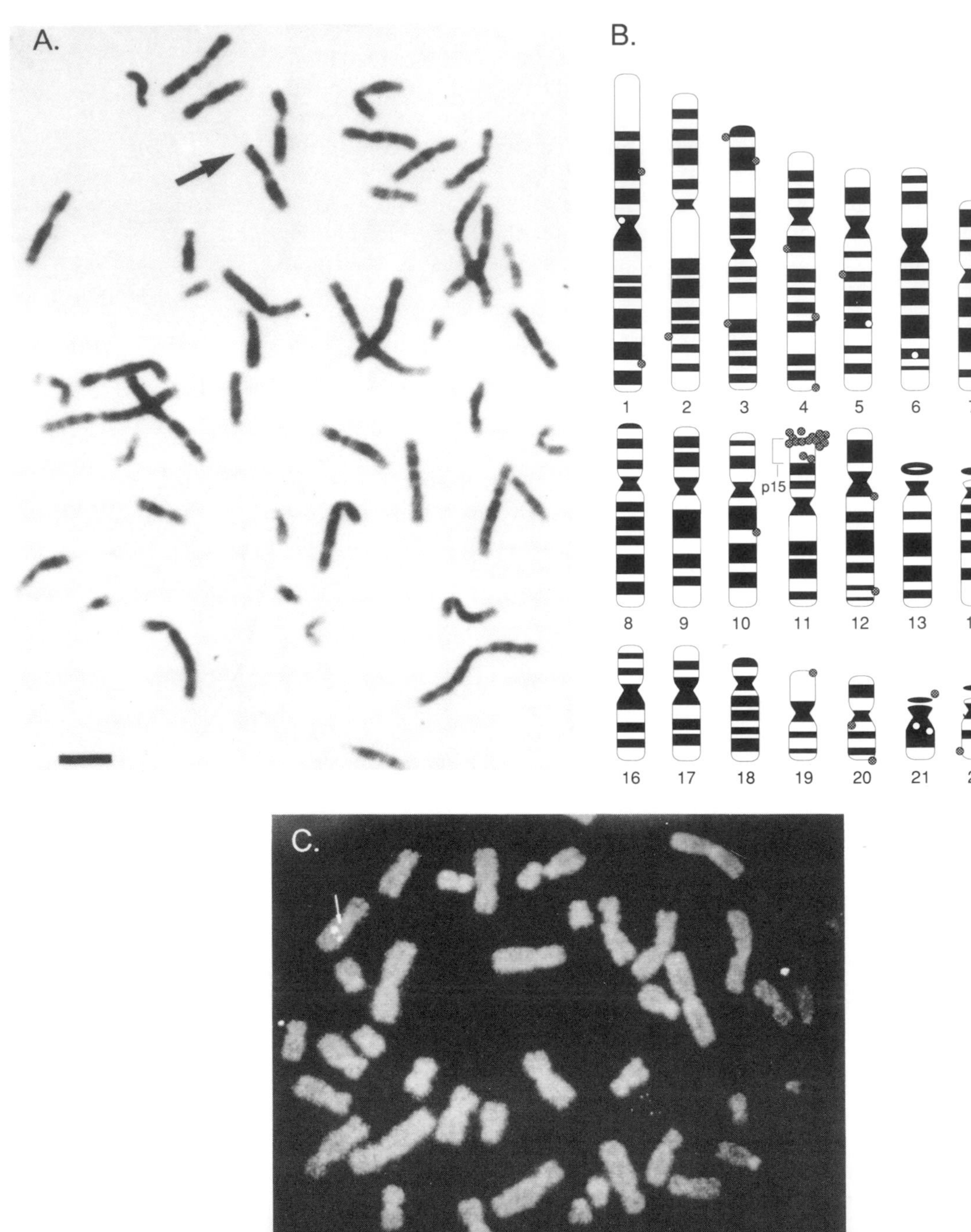

Figure 9.2. **A,** Human metaphase chromosomes hybridized with a tritium-labeled probe for the insulin gene. The *arrow* indicates a radioactive grain over the tip of chromosome 11. **B,** Composite from 35 cells that were scored for insulin probe localization. Each *dot* represents the location of a grain in a particular chromosome spread. It is apparent that, although there is a background of nonspecific hybridization, a significant accumulation of grains is found at 11p15. **C,** In situ hybridization using a nonradioactive biotin labeling system. The probe is a cloned DNA fragment that maps very close to the cystic fibrosis (CF) gene by genetic linkage (see Fig. 9.21). The bright spot of hybridization on chromosome 7 indicates the location of the probe, and, by implication, the location of CF. (A and B from Harper ME, Ullrich A, Saunders GF, et al.: Localization of the human insulin gene to the distal end of the short arm of chromosome 11. Proc Natl Acad Sci USA 78:4458, 1981; C is courtesy of Dr. Kathy Klinger.)

Somatic Cell Hybrids

The second approach for gene mapping arose out of years of experience in growing mammalian cells in culture flasks. A somatic cell is simply any cell of an organism not involved in the germ line, and somatic cell hybrids are made by fusing cells from different species together. Most somatic cell hybrids used for human gene mapping are created by fusing human and mouse or human and hamster cells, as shown in Figure 9.3. For reasons that are not entirely clear, such hybrids tend to lose many of the human chromosomes but retain the rodent chromosomes. After this has proceeded for several generations, a cell line often becomes fairly stable, maintaining a specific set of human chromosomes. The human chromosomes retained are rather random. Therefore, it is possible to create a panel of such hybrids, where each clonal hybrid line contains a different group of human chromosomes. For this panel to be useful, it is essential

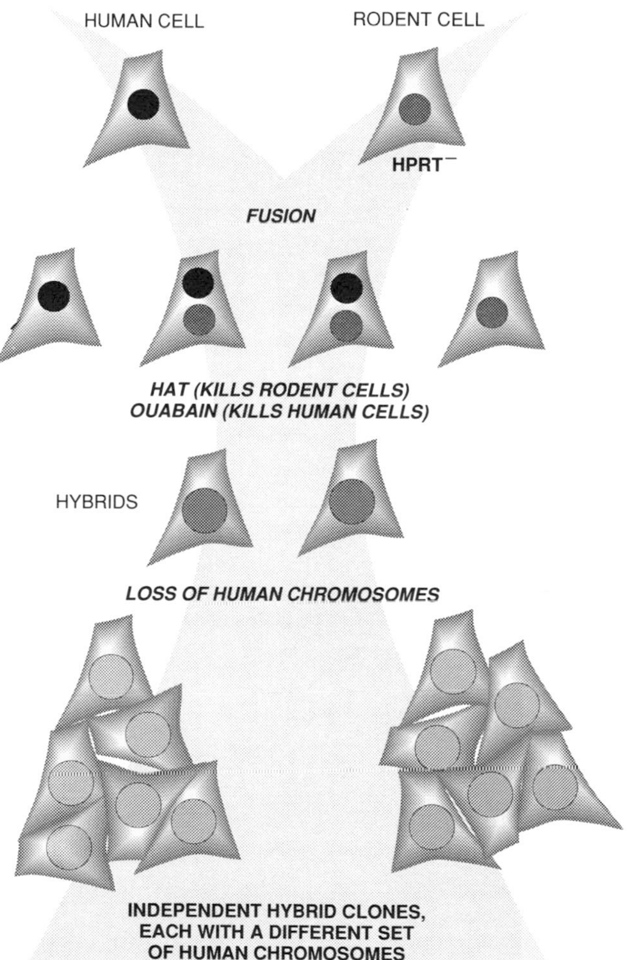

Figure 9.3. Scheme for generating human-rodent somatic cell hybrids. The rodent cell is usually chosen to contain a selectable genetic marker, in this example the absence of the enzyme hypoxanthine phosphoribosyltransferase (HPRT). This allows selection after fusing human and rodent cells in hypoxanthine/aminopterin/thymidine (HAT) medium, which allows only cells with a functioning HPRT gene to survive. Human cells that have not undergone fusion can also be killed by the use of the drug ouabain, which kills human cells but not rodent cells. As a result of this dual selection, only cells that contain both human and rodent chromosomes survive. Such hybrids tend to lose human chromosomes preferentially over the first several cell generations and then become relatively stable. If one starts off with a large population of cells, each clone of cells will contain a different set of human chromosomes, allowing the generation of a useful somatic cell hybrid panel.

Table 9.1. Mapping a DNA Probe Using Somatic Cell Hybrids[a]

HYBRID	HUMAN CHROMOSOMES																							
	1	2	3	4	5	6	7	8	9	10	11	12	13	14	15	16	17	18	19	20	21	22	X	Human *met*
A			■					■						■		■	■					■		−
B														■	■		■	■			■	■	■	−
C						■	■																	+
D		■			■			■				■							■					−
E								■																−
F	■		■		■			■	■				■	■				■		■			■	−
G	■				■			■	■					■				■		■			■	−
H	■		■		■			■	■	■				■				■		■			■	−
I	■		■		■			■	■	■			■	■				■		■			■	−
J				■			■								■		■			■				+
K				■			■				■	■				■				■		■		+
L														■										−

[a] A panel of somatic cell hybrids (A–L), each of which contains 1–11 human chromosomes in a rodent background, has been used to score for the presence of the cloned human *met* oncogene. The *met* probe is positive in hybrids C, J, and K, which could occur only if the *met* gene is on chromosome 7. (Reprinted by permission from Cooper CS, Park M, Blair DG, et al.: Molecular cloning of a new transforming gene from a chemically transformed human cell line. Nature 311:29. © 1984, Macmillan Magazines Ltd.)

for the user to know which human chromosomes are present in each hybrid. This is accomplished by cytogenetic techniques, taking advantage of the fact that there are sufficient differences between rodent and human chromosomes that they can be individually recognized. An example of a chromosome spread from a somatic cell hybrid is shown in Figure 9.4.

Once such a panel of hybrids has been generated, it can be used for gene mapping of both cloned DNA fragments and expressed proteins. A diagram of this procedure is shown in Figure 9.5. To map DNA fragments, Southern blots can be carried out. Each *lane* of the blot contains DNA from a different hybrid, whose human chromosome complement has been determined previously. By considering which chromosomes are present in those cell lines that give a positive signal on the Southern blot, it is possible to deduce the chromosomal location of that probe. Table 9.1 shows an example, in this case indicating that the cancer-related gene called *met* is on chromosome 7. Note that in the table, all hybrids containing chromosome 7 were found to be positive with the *met* probe and all hybrids not containing chromosome 7 were negative. This was not true for any other chromosome.

To do regional mapping on a chromosome, somatic cell hybrids can still be used as long as fragments of particular chromosomes rather than the entire thing are present in the hybrids. Often times, one can take advantage of translocation chromosomes (see Chapter 8) to construct such hybrids, if it is desirable to do mapping to specific regions.

As shown in Figure 9.5, this same procedure can be used to localize the gene for an identifiable protein, as long as that protein is actually expressed in the hybrid cells themselves. This is true for proteins involved in many "housekeeping" functions, such as the genes that specify many of the enzymes involved in intermediary metabolism. For both DNA and protein mapping, it is important to be sure that one can distinguish the rodent and the human signal.

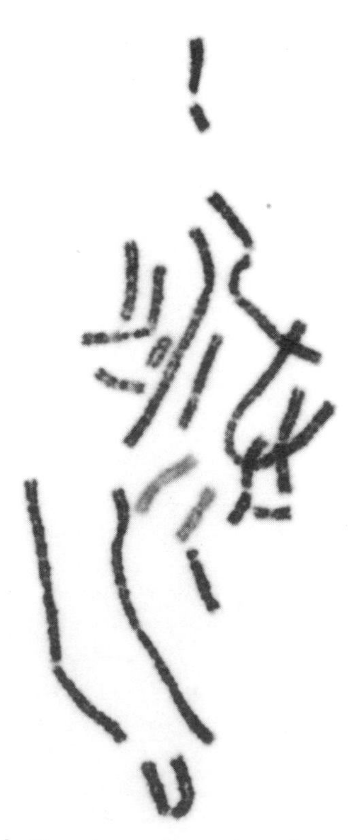

Figure 9.4. Karyotype of a mouse-human hybrid. The metaphase chromosomes are visualized with G-11, which stains the mouse chromosomes more darkly than the human ones. A human chromosome 3 and X are present in this hybrid near the center of the spread. (Courtesy of Drs. C. Stein and T. Glover.).

Dosage

It is also possible to map a gene to a specific chromosome if cell lines are available that have varying numbers of that particular chromosome. This is most commonly done for the X chromosome, by taking advantage

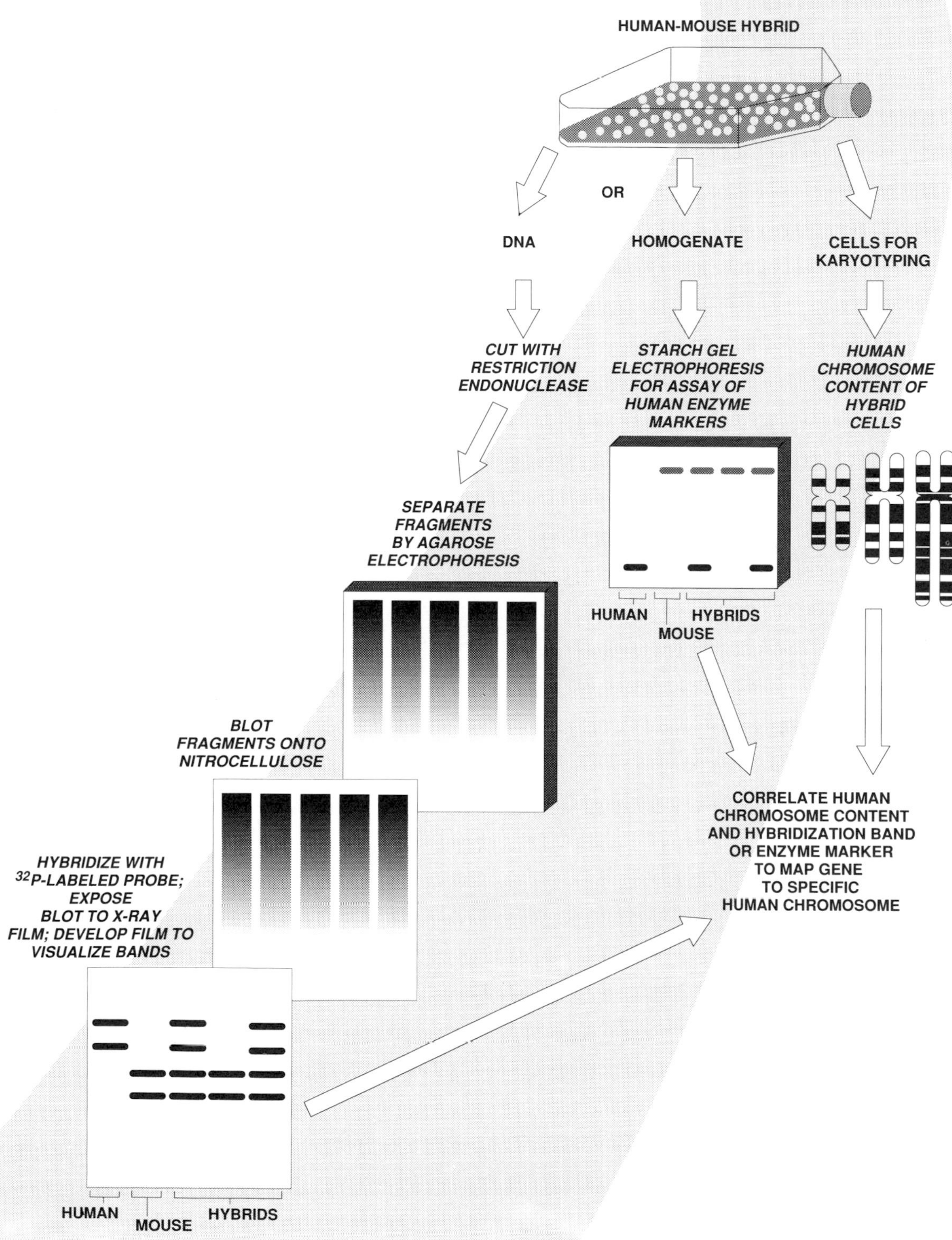

Figure 9.5. Use of human-rodent somatic cell hybrids for gene mapping a collection of somatic cell hybrids, each of which contains different human chromosomes as identified by karyotyping. These can then be used to map a given DNA sequence by Southern blotting or a given protein by starch gel electrophoresis. Those hybrids giving a positive signal for the human DNA sequence or protein must contain the chromosome from which this is derived. (From Shows TB, Sakaguchi AY, Naylor SL: Mapping the human genome, cloned genes, DNA polymorphisms, and inherited disease. Adv Hum Genet 12:341, 1982. Published by Plenum.)

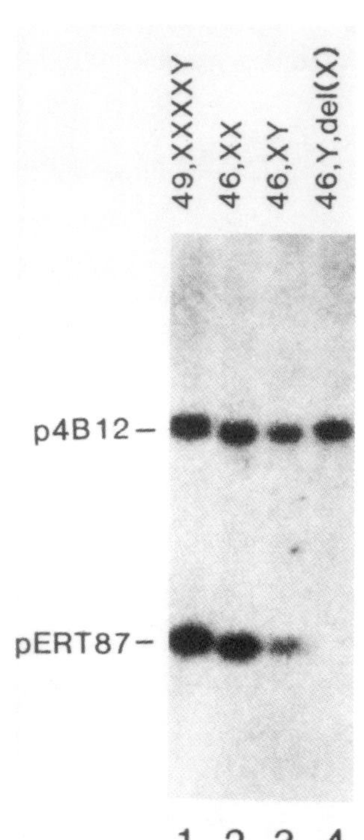

Figure 9.6. Use of dosage to map a DNA probe to the X chromosome. DNA in *lane 1* was obtained from an individual with a 49,XXXXY karyotype, whereas that depicted in *lane 2* is from a normal female, and that in *lane 3* is from a normal male. *Lane 4* contains DNA from a male (BB) with a small deletion within the short arm of the X chromosome (see Fig. 9.9). Probe p4B12 is on an autosome and therefore detects similar intensity signals in all *four lanes.* Probe pERT87 is located on the short arm of the X chromosome within the region deleted in BB. It can be seen that the intensity of the signal in the other *three lanes* is a function of a number of X chromosomes, confirming that this probe is located on X. (From Kunkel LM, Monaco AP, Middlesworth W, et al.: Specific cloning of DNA fragments absent from the DNA of a male patient with an X chromosome deletion. Proc Natl Acad Sci USA 82:4778, 1985.)

of cell lines from individuals who have anywhere from one to four X chromosomes, as shown in Figure 9.6. If the amount of DNA in each *lane* of the Southern blot has been carefully kept constant, a probe located on the X chromosome (pERT87) will be four times more intense in the 49,XXXXY cell line than in the 46,XY line. An autosomal probe (p4B12), on the other hand, will look the same in all of these *lanes.*

Chromosome Aberration

The Duffy blood group mapping described at the beginning of this chapter is an example of this approach. Its attractiveness is that when it works it is very simple and direct, but the disadvantage is that one must depend on a rare event, which may not be found for every possible application. However, such rare events, when identified, can play an extremely critical role in the mapping and eventual cloning of an elusive disease gene.

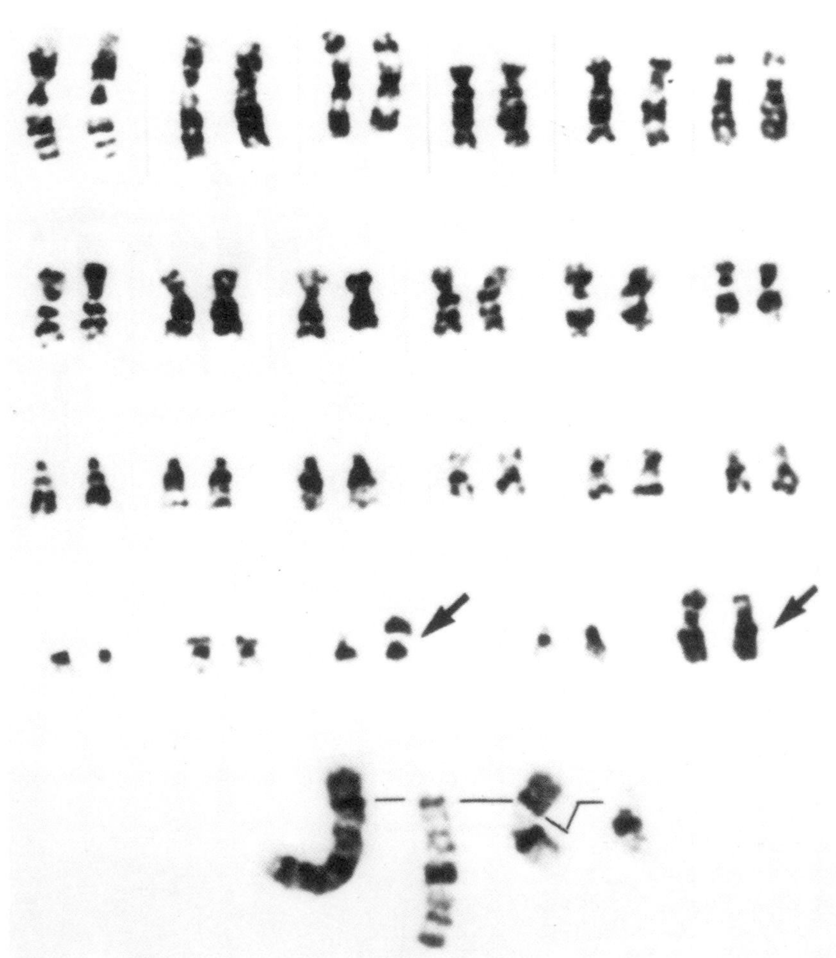

Figure 9.7. Karyotype of a female with muscular dystrophy. As indicated by the *arrows,* there is an apparently balanced translocation between chromosome 21 and one of the X chromosomes in this female. In the *bottom row* are shown high resolution pictures. On the *left* is the normal X chromosome. Next to that is a derivative X that has exchanged the *top half* of the short arm with a small piece of chromosome 21. Next to that is the other counterpart of the translocation, a chromosome 21 that has distal Xp attached to its short arm. On the *right* is the normal chromosome 21. The breakpoint on the X chromosome is at p21, which turns out to be the location of the muscular dystrophy gene. (From Verellen-Dumoulin C, Freund M, DeMeyer R, et al.: Expression of an X-linked muscular dystrophy in a female due to translocation involving Xp21 and non-random inactivation of the normal X chromosome. Hum Genet 67:115, 1984.)

A very important example of this phenomenon is provided by the identification of translocations between the X chromosome and an autosomal chromosome in females who have the phenotype of Duchenne muscular dystrophy. As discussed in Chapter 3, Duchenne muscular dystrophy (DMD) is normally an X-linked recessive disease, so finding a female affected with this disease is very unusual. Possible explanations would include homozygosity for the disease gene or extreme lyonization (see Chapter 8). However, cytogenetic studies on several such affected girls have universally revealed X-autosome translocations; the autosome involved in each case has been different, but the breakpoint on the X chromosome has always been in band p21 (Fig. 9.7). The simplest explanation for this phenomenon is that the translocation has actually broken within the DMD gene in each of these cases. One might wonder, therefore, why these girls would be affected, since they also carry a normal X chromosome. The answer lies in the phenomenon of X-inactivation; in all cases, the normal X chromosome is inactivated and the translocation X remains active, leaving no functioning copy of the normal gene at the DMD locus. (Fig. 9.8). The reason for this selective X-inactivation may well be that in those cells where the translocation X tries to inactivate, the autosomal sequences attached to this region are also suppressed. This

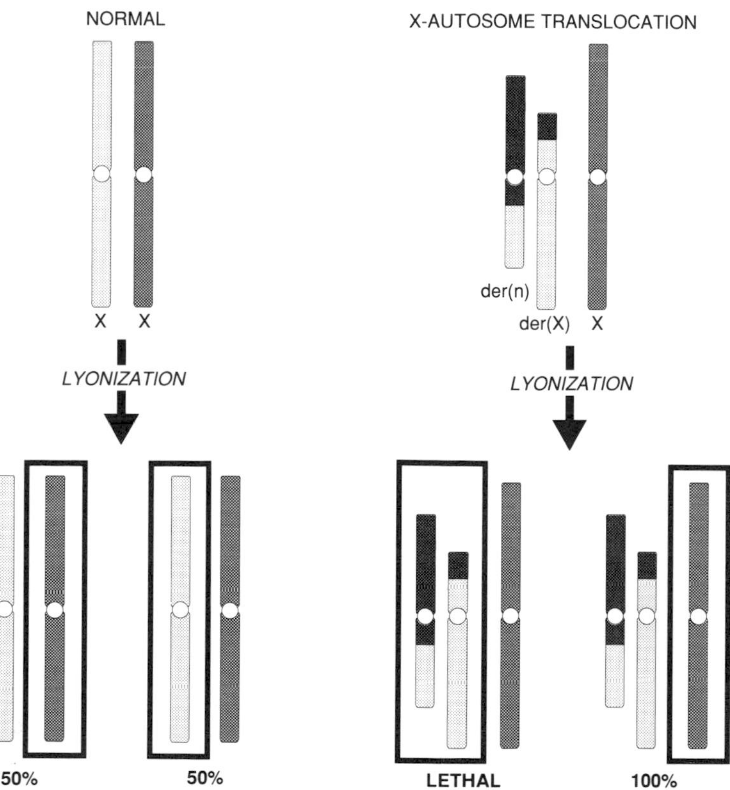

Figure 9.8. The consequences of X-inactivation in the presence of an X-autosome translocation. In the normal situation, about 50% of the cells will have inactivated each X chromosome. (Inactivation is indicated by the *closed box* around a chromosome.) In the presence of an X-autosome translocation, however, cells that inactivate the X chromosome involved in the translocation also inactivate the attached autosomal material, which is presumably lethal to the cell. As a result, virtually 100% of the somatic cells of such an individual are found to have inactivated the normal X. This explains the occurrence of Duchenne muscular dystrophy in a female with an X-autosome translocation interrupting the DMD gene on Xp21, even though such a person carries a normal DMD gene on the normal X. For simplicity, only the X chromosomes and the translocated autosomes are shown in this diagram.

presumably is lethal to that cell, since monosomy for autosomal sequences is not well tolerated. As a result, only those cells that inactivate the normal X chromosome will have normal growth potential.

Thus, the discovery of these rare individuals led to the conclusion that the DMD gene most likely maps to Xp21. As we shall see later in this chapter, the translocation breakpoint from one of these individuals was actually used to assist in the cloning of the gene.

Not only translocations but also deletions can assist in the mapping of a gene for human disease. Again, DMD provides an instructive example. Even small chromosomal deletions are likely to involve a number of genes, so a clue to the possible presence of a chromosomal deletion is the occurrence of more than one genetic defect in a single individual. A boy (BB) with no family history of any genetic disorder was discovered to have DMD, chronic granulomatous disease (a disorder of white cells which seriously impairs the ability to fight off infection), and two other X-linked traits. The simultaneous occurrence of these four X-linked conditions led to a careful cytogenetic analysis, which revealed an extremely small deletion of band Xp21.2 (see Fig. 9.9). Since neither parent carried such a deletion, this appeared to be a de novo occurrence and allowed the mapping of these four X-linked conditions to that part of the X chromosome. As will be described in more detail below, this unique individual also provided a critical clue in the puzzle that led to the cloning of the DMD gene and the beginnings of a molecular understanding of the nature of the disease.

Linkage Analysis

A final method for mapping genes to human chromosomes is called linkage analysis, because using this method one maps the gene by its proximity to another locus on the same chromosome. Such loci are then

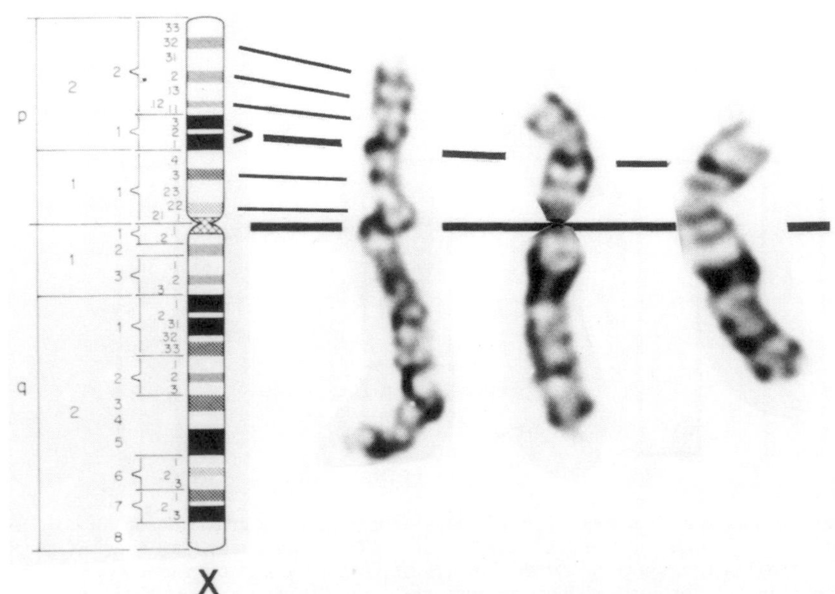

Figure 9.9. Occurrence of a very small interstitial deletion in Xp21.2 in a boy (BB) with Duchenne muscular dystrophy, chronic granulomatous disease, and two other X-linked conditions. On the *left* is shown a diagram of the normal banding pattern, and on the *right* are three representations of the X chromosome from this boy. A very subtle decrease in the size of the Xp21 band is present, and the light band Xp21.2 is never visible. (Photo courtesy of Dr. Uta Francke.)

said to be "linked." This method is extremely powerful, but it is conceptually the most complex of those we have considered.

In order to understand this approach, it is essential to have a firm grasp on the events that occur during meiosis I, especially as regards crossing over. In Figure 9.10, a pair of homologous chromosomes is shown undergoing meiosis. In the *left-hand* part of the figure, the two loci being followed are far apart on the chromosome, which makes it likely that a crossover will occur between these. The result, shown at the *bottom,* will be chromosomes that have undergone a patchwork reassembly of their alleles. In the example, what began as a chromosome with A and B alleles and a chromosome with a and b alleles results in all possible combinations after meiosis.

On the *right-hand side* of the figure, the two loci are shown close together. In that event, a recombination between these two loci will be a less common event, and thus, A and B will tend to stay together, and a and b will also. Thus, recombination between two loci can be used as a rough measure of their distance apart.

The use of this approach to follow the inheritance of a Mendelian disease is illustrated in Figure 9.11. The principle of the approach is simple: if the disease locus is quite close to another polymorphic locus (often called the "marker locus") whose inheritance can be followed in an affected family, it is possible to predict who is going to be affected by following the inheritance of the marker locus. The chance of being mistaken in this analysis is a function of how far apart the marker locus and the disease locus are. In the figure, the father is affected with a dominant disorder; hence, his genotype is DN at the disease locus, whereas his normal wife is NN. At the marker locus, he happens to be Aa, whereas his wife is AA. Looking at his offspring, all but II-4 show perfect linkage of the disease locus and the marker locus, because all of those who have inherited the father's A allele have also inherited the disease gene, and all who inherited the a allele inherited the normal allele at the disease locus. In fact, one would need this sort of information to determine that the disease gene in the father is on the same chromosome as the A allele at the marker locus; this is called "determining the phase" of these two loci.

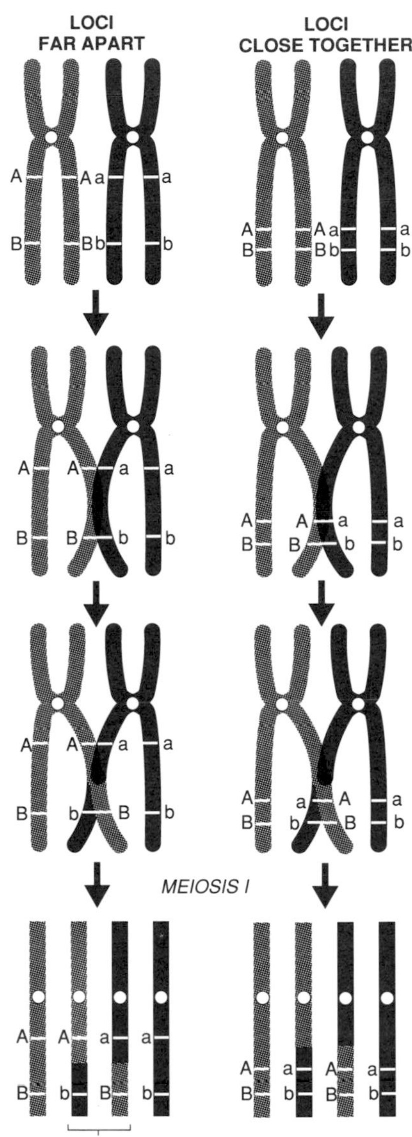

Figure 9.10. Crossing over between homologous chromosomes in meiosis. On the *left* is shown an example where two loci are relatively far apart, in which case recombination is likely to occur between them. On the *right* is shown a situation where they are close together, in which case recombination between them will be a rarer event.

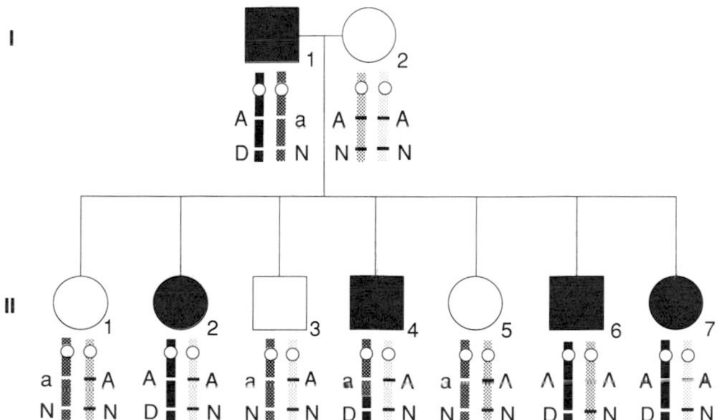

Figure 9.11. Linkage of a disease gene to a marker locus. The individuals shown by *solid symbols* are affected with a dominantly inherited disease and have genotype DN, whereas unaffected individuals are NN. The father (I-1) carries the disease gene on a chromosome that has the A allele at the marker locus, whereas his normal chromosome carries a. The unaffected mother is homozygous AA at the marker locus. The seven offspring are shown below with the paternal chromosome on the *left* and the maternal chromosome on the *right.* Individual II-4 demonstrates recombination between the marker locus and the disease gene, because this person has inherited an a allele from his father at the marker locus, but has inherited the disease allele D. The rest of the siblings are nonrecombinants.

Individual II-4, however, is an exception. This offspring is affected with the disease, but inherited an a allele from his father. This is an example of recombination between these two loci.

It is important to appreciate in this sort of analysis that the allele at the marker locus is not in itself the cause of the disease. Thus, for example, finding an individual with genotype AA at the marker locus in some other family with no history of this disease would not indicate that that individual has the disease (I-2 is an example of this). An important corollary is that linkage analysis to follow the inheritance of a disease gene can in general only be performed when several family members are available, including some who are affected with the disease. Furthermore, the analysis shown in Figure 9.11 would have been impossible if the father were homozygous AA or aa because, in that instance, one could not distinguish his two chromosomes at the marker locus. Hence, in linkage analysis, the most useful marker loci are those that are highly polymorphic.

The distance apart of two loci is defined in genetic terms in units of centiMorgans (cM). If two loci are 1 cM apart, there is a 1% chance of recombination between these loci as the chromosome is passed from parent to child. Thus, one can think of centiMorgans as a rough unit of distance along the chromosome, although the relation to physical distance is not truly linear because regions vary somewhat in recombination potential. The average chromosome contains about 150 cM; there are about 3300 cM in the whole human genome, which corresponds to 3×10^9 bp. Therefore, on the average, 1 cM is about 1 million bp (1000 kb). In order for a marker locus to be tightly linked to a disease gene, therefore, it must in general be not only on the correct chromosome but in the same region of that chromosome. Markers that are a long distance away on the same chromosome may not even appear to be linked because of relatively free recombination between the two loci.

The marker loci can be anything polymorphic. Originally, many were proteins such as red blood cell antigens (ABO, Rh, etc.). An example showing probable linkage of the gene for myotonic dystrophy (an autosomal dominant form of muscular dystrophy associated with frontal baldness, cataracts, and intellectual deterioration) to the secretor locus is shown in Figure 9.12. In *A* of the figure are shown the results of secretor testing of the members of the pedigree, as well as their disease status. In order to interpret the secretor pattern, one must know that there are two alleles at the secretor locus, Se and se. The Se allele is dominant, so that "+" individuals are either Se/Se or Se/se. Individuals marked "−" must be homozygous se/se. In *B,* the genotypes at the secretor locus have been reconstructed based on this information. This reconstruction is aided by the fact that both parents of a "−" individual must carry a se allele, which allows definition of the ambiguous members of the pedigree. Only individual III-1 cannot be fully assigned a genotype. Inspection of the pedigree indicates that the Se allele carried by individual I-1 is traveling with myotonic dystrophy, with no definite examples of crossover.

Unfortunately, the number of polymorphic protein loci is limited, so that many important disease genes cannot be mapped this way, as no protein polymorphism will be close enough to show linkage. More recently, with the appearance of recombinant DNA technology, DNA markers that detect restriction fragment length polymorphisms (RFLPs, see Chapter 5) have added enormously to the number of polymorphic loci. In 1980 it was realized that if a large number of such markers could be generated for each human chromosome, any Mendelian disorder could be mapped to its proper locus, provided sufficient families were

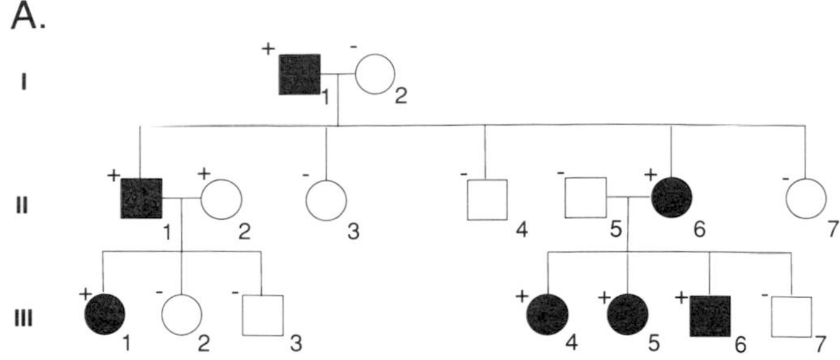

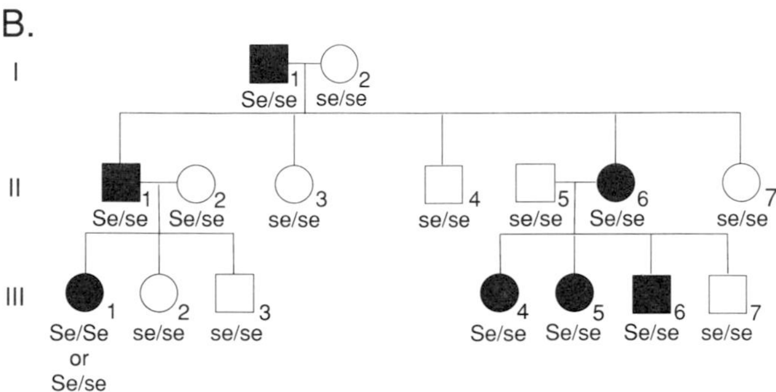

Figure 9.12. Pedigree showing probable linkage of the gene for myotonic dystrophy to the secretor locus. Individuals with *solid symbols* are affected with autosomal dominant myotonic dystrophy. In **A** are shown the secretor phenotypes (+ or −) for each of the individuals in the pedigree. Genotypes are inferred in **B** using the fact that the Se allele is dominant, so that + individuals are either Se/Se or Se/se, and − individuals must be se/se. The genotypes of all of the + individuals except for III-1 can be inferred by the necessity of Mendelian inheritance at the secretor locus. Thus, for example, individual I-1 must be Se/se, not Se/Se, because he has three se/se offspring. Inspection of **B** shows that the myotonic dystrophy gene and the Se allele at the secretor locus are apparently linked in this pedigree.

available. To be fully useful, it would be necessary to have highly polymorphic markers spaced at 5–10 cM intervals over the entire genome. One would then apply a panel of such markers (approximately 200–300 usually would be necessary) to families with the disease and search for evidence of linkage to one or more of the markers. While the cloning of such a panel of RFLPs was a substantial undertaking, that task was essentially accomplished over the next 8 years.

To fully perceive the nature of linkage analysis, it is essential that we delve a bit more into the mathematical facets of this approach. It may have occurred to you that the appearance of linkage in a family like the one shown above for myotonic dystrophy could occasionally occur by chance. Furthermore, if the marker locus and the disease locus are not terribly close together, then recombinants are likely to be seen in the families being analyzed, and there must be some way to account for this in the analysis, and even to use this information to calculate distances. The most common method used to generate this information is the method of lod scores. This is based on a likelihood ratio that a given set of data would have been observed, given that the *true* value for the recombination fraction between two loci was θ. The likelihood ratio is computed as a relative number by comparing it to the possibility that the two loci were completely unlinked.

$$\text{Likelihood ratio } (\theta) = \frac{\text{likelihood (data} \mid \theta)}{\text{likelihood (data} \mid \text{no linkage)}}$$

where likelihood (data | θ) indicates the mathematical likelihood of obtaining a particular linkage data set if the recombination fraction were θ.

In practice, this ratio is computed for several values of θ and the results are expressed as the $\log_{10}$ of the above ratio, which is called the lod score (Z). The most likely recombination fraction ($\hat{\theta}$) is the value of θ which gives the highest positive lod score ($\hat{Z}$). Positive lod scores favor the presence of linkage, whereas negative lod scores indicate linkage is less likely. By convention, a positive lod score of $+3$ or greater is considered definite evidence of linkage; because lod scores are based on a base 10 logarithm, a lod score of $+3$ indicates 1000 to 1 odds that the linkage being observed did not occur by chance. A lod score of ≤ -2 (indicating 100 to 1 or greater odds *against* linkage) is taken as evidence of exclusion of linkage for this value of θ.

This more formal mathematical analysis can be understood best by considering an example. Figure 9.13 diagrams a pedigree of a family in which autosomal dominant neurofibromatosis (NF1) is occurring and shows the results of a Southern blot with an RFLP marker for which the two alleles are 3.0 and 4.7 kb. Inspection of the pedigree shows that the 4.7-kb allele carried by individual I-1 is travelling with the neurofibromatosis gene in this family. Again, note that this RFLP marker does not itself detect the disease gene; individual II-8 is homozygous for the 4.7-kb allele but does not have neurofibromatosis. The one exception to linkage is individual III-7, who has inherited his father's 3.0-kb allele but is affected with neurofibromatosis.

While simple inspection of this pedigree certainly suggests that the marker locus and neurofibromatosis are linked and III-7 is a recombinant, the actual analysis of this requires some mathematics, which in general is carried out using a computer program. The results of such a lod score analysis are shown in Table 9.2. Note that lod scores have been computed for several values of θ. If $\theta = 0$, the lod score is negative infin-

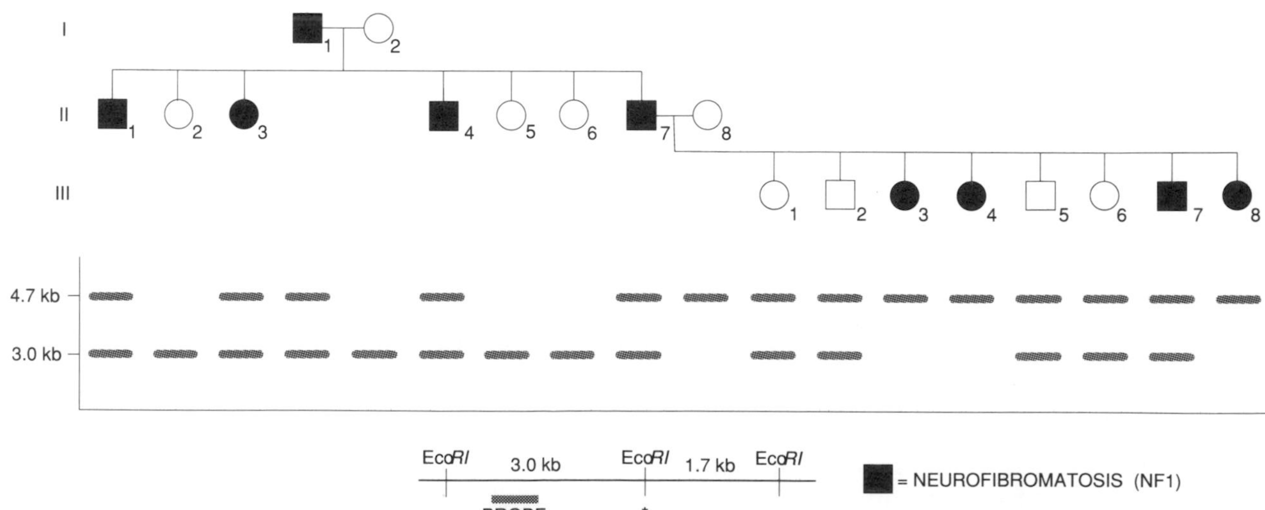

Figure 9.13. Linkage analysis of NF1 with a probe on chromosome 17. The probe, as diagrammed at the *bottom* of the figure, recognizes a 3.0-kb allele in chromosomes that have the *Eco*RI site marked with an *asterisk* present, and a 4.7-kb allele if this site is absent. The Southern blot pattern is shown for each individual in the pedigree below their respective pedigree symbol. The NF1 disease allele carried by individual I-1 can be seen to be traveling on a chromosome carrying the 4.7-kb allele for the marker probe, except for individual III-7, who appears to be a recombinant.

Table 9.2. Lod Score Analysis for Pedigree in Figure 9.13

	Lod (Z) Scores for various θ					
θ =	0.00	0.05	0.10	0.20	$\hat{Z}$	$\hat{\theta}$
NF1 vs. marker	$-\infty$	3.0	3.1	2.2	3.4	0.07

ity. To understand this, keep in mind that the lod score is a logarithm, and the logarithm of 0 is minus infinity. Thus, this finding indicates that there is zero likelihood of observing this set of data if the marker is identical with the neurofibromatosis gene. The likelihood of this is zero because a definite recombinant has occurred in III-7. As θ is allowed to increase from 0, the lod score becomes positive and peaks at $\hat{Z}$ = 3.4 with $\hat{\theta}$ = 0.07, or 7 cM. For larger values of θ the lod score starts to drop off, indicating that for this family the most likely distance between the marker locus and neurofibromatosis is 7 cM. Note that this distance makes some intuitive sense from inspection of the pedigree in Figure 9.13. There are 15 offspring (children and grandchildren) of the original ancestor I-1, and of these, only one shows a recombination. Thus, the percent recombination is approximately $\frac{1}{15} \times 100$, which is very close to the 7% obtained in a more formal calculation. This data would be taken as definitive evidence for linkage between NF1 and the marker, because the lod score at $\hat{\theta}$ exceeds 3.0.

Comparison of Mapping Methods

Table 9.3 summarizes the methods of human gene mapping we have discussed so far, together with the situations in which each method is applicable. Note that for a cloned DNA sequence, the methods of in situ hybridization, somatic cell hybrids, and dosage are useful. Proteins can also be mapped using somatic cell hybrids and dosage. For mapping a human disease gene where the nature of the protein product is unknown, none of these first three methods can be used. It is important to realize that the majority of human Mendelian disorders fall in this category. Diseases like Huntington disease, cystic fibrosis, and neurofibromatosis are known to be due to a single gene because of their inheritance in a classic Mendelian fashion, but the normal function of the gene involved in these disorders is unknown. Only the last two methods in the table can be used for mapping this sort of gene. As noted above, chromosome aberrations are extremely useful for this purpose, but cannot be counted upon to be found for every disease whose map location is being sought. Linkage analysis, on the other hand, is a much more generalizable approach, since any human single gene disorder can be mapped providing a sufficiently large panel of probes and families is available. Note that linkage analysis can be used also to map cloned genes and proteins if they are polymorphic, although other options are available in that situation.

Table 9.3. Comparison of Gene Mapping Methods

Method	Cloned Gene	Protein	Mystery Disease
In situ hybridization	+	−	−
Somatic cell hybrids	+	+	−
Dosage	+	+	−
Chromosome aberration	−	−	+
Linkage	+	+	+

HUMAN DISEASE GENES: LINKAGE ANALYSIS AND "REVERSE GENETICS"

We have already had several occasions to refer to specific uses of linkage analysis, particularly the example of neurofibromatosis mentioned above. In this section three other diseases for which linkage analysis has played a key role will be described in more detail.

Huntington Disease

In Chapter 3, Huntington disease was mentioned as an example of a dominant disorder with delayed onset. The disease affects about 1 in 20,000 individuals and is characterized by onset at an average age of 37 years, with the symptoms consisting of personality changes, memory loss, and a peculiar series of motor problems including chorea, an involuntary movement of the arms and legs. Pathologically, those who have died of the disease are found to have dramatic neuronal loss in parts of the basal ganglia of the brain, especially the caudate nucleus. Despite years of research, no evidence for any specific protein abnormality has ever been obtained in comparing tissues from Huntington patients to normal tissues.

It was appreciated early that with its classic Mendelian inheritance and high penetrance (essentially 100% by age 80), Huntington disease is a prime target for gene mapping by linkage analysis. Initial studies with protein polymorphisms, however, did not indicate the location of the gene. When RFLPs were described, Huntington disease seemed like a natural target, and researchers began the arduous process of collecting family material and developing a series of probes, expecting that 100–300 such probes would have to be tried out before a linkage was found. By good fortune, the 12th probe that was tried, called G8, turned out to be tightly linked to the Huntington disease (HD) locus. This fortunate finding provided immediate impetus for other investigators to enter the field of linkage analysis using DNA polymorphisms. The G8 marker detects two polymorphic *Hin*dIII sites, as diagrammed in Figure 9.14. Because there are two polymorphic sites, there are four possible chromosome patterns, called haplotypes, denoted A, B, C, and D, depending on which sites are present or absent. All possible genotypes have been observed, as shown by Southern blot in Figure 9.14. In Figure 9.15 is shown a portion of a very large Venezuelan pedigree in which Huntington disease is occurring. Because of the large number of affected individuals in this family, it has been of enormous use in carrying out the linkage analysis. Indicated on the pedigree are the genotypes at the G8 locus as determined by RFLP analysis. Inspection reveals that all individuals with Huntington disease have inherited the C allele from their affected parent, except for the shaded individual in generation IV, who must represent a recombinant. Again, note that the RFLP analysis simply helps one track the Huntington chromosome in this family, and having the C allele does not equate with having Huntington disease, as should be obvious from the fact that several unrelated spouses also have a C allele. Lod score calculations from this pedigree and others indicate that the genetic distance between G8 and the Huntington disease locus is about 3 cM. The linkage between G8 and HD is absolutely unquestionable, with odds in favor of linkage currently more than 10^{80} to 1! Such a high lod score could only have been obtained by studying a very large number of affected individuals within families. Using in situ hybridization, the G8 marker has been mapped to the tip of the short arm of chromosome 4, which indicates that HD must also be close to this location. Subsequently,

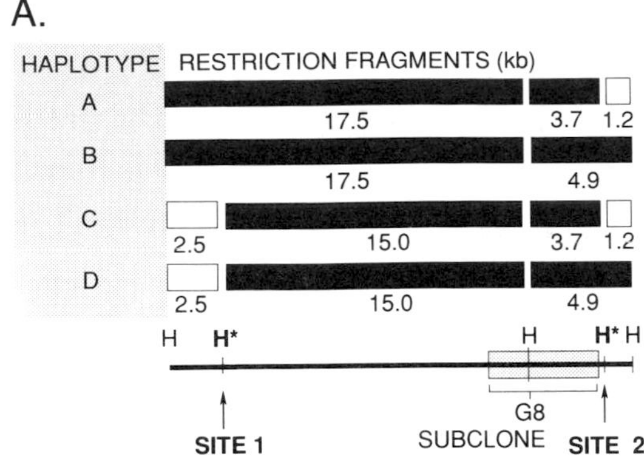

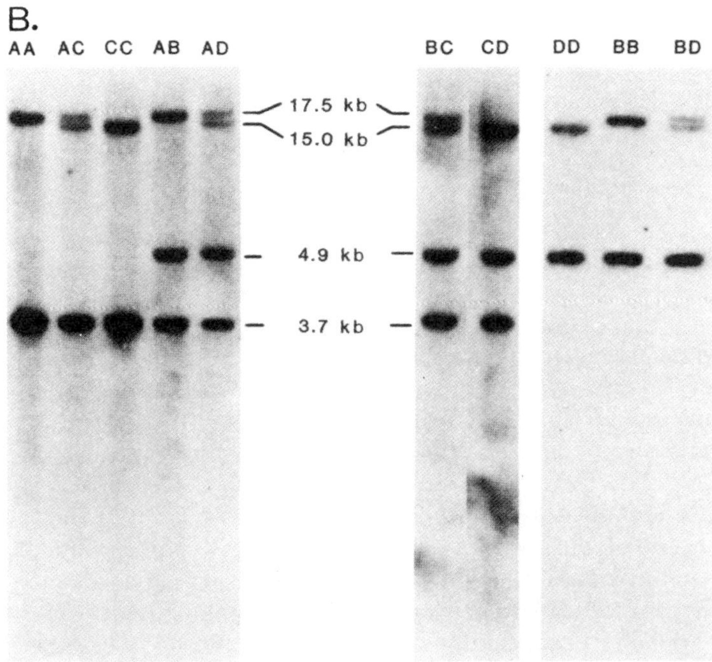

Figure 9.14. A, Diagram of the G8 locus. This RFLP is more complex than others we have described, because it detects two polymorphic *Hin*dIII sites. The polymorphic sites are marked with *asterisks* and invariant sites are also shown. Depending on whether sites 1 or 2 are present or absent, a total of four different patterns can appear from each chromosome. These are designated by "haplotypes" A, B, C, and D. The position of the probe is indicated at the *bottom* of the diagram. Notice that the 2.5-kb band from haplotype C and D and the 1.2-kb fragment from haplotypes A and C will not be visualized on the Southern blot using this probe, because the probe does not overlap these fragments. **B,** Southern blot showing each of the 10 possible genotypes at the G8 locus. Note that the pattern observed for the genotype AD is identical to that for BC, so these can only be distinguished by typing close relatives. (From Gusella JF, et al.: DNA markers for nervous system diseases. Science 225:1320. ©1984 by the AAAS.)

additional markers has been derived from this region of chromosome 4, and some of them are even closer to HD than is G8.

These RFLP markers have already begun to be used clinically. Individuals with a parent affected with Huntington disease face a serious dilemma. On the one hand, it might be advantageous for them to know whether they carry the Huntington disease gene even prior to the onset of symptoms, so that they could plan accordingly, especially as regards their own childbearing. On the other hand, obtaining such information, if the result indicates a high likelihood of developing the disease, presents such a severe psychological burden that many individuals would prefer to remain uncertain about their status. The decision to obtain such infor-

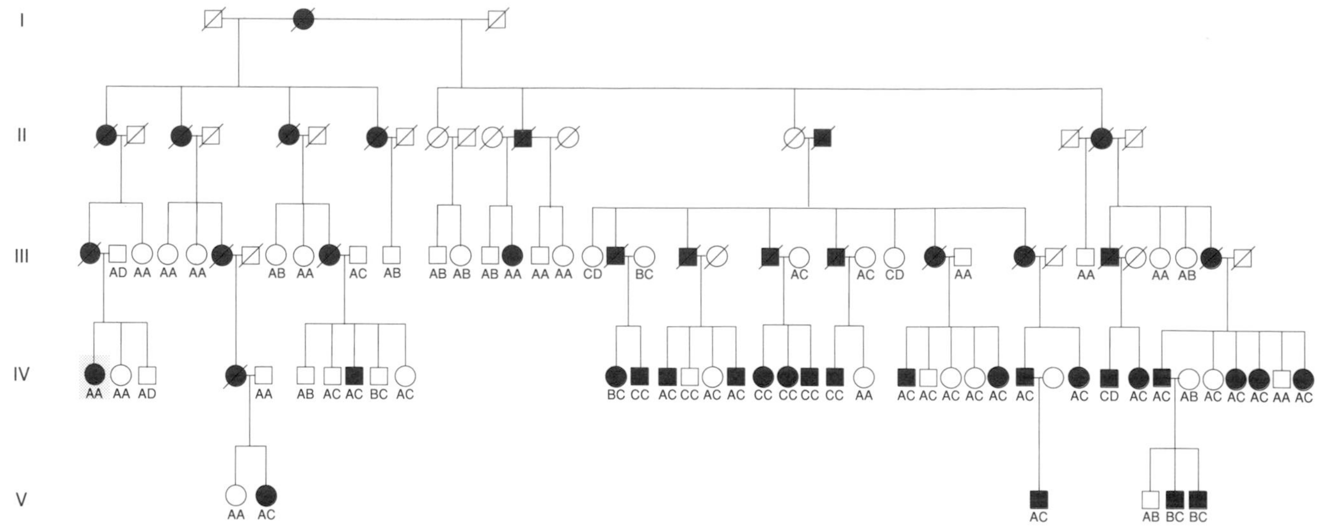

Figure 9.15. A portion of a large Venezuelan pedigree affected with Huntington disease. Note that many individuals in the earlier generations are deceased. It is still possible, however, to carry out linkage analysis by allowing the computer program to consider all possible genotypes for deceased individuals that are consistent with Mendelian inheritance. Note that all affected individuals have a C allele for G8, except for the *shaded* individual in generation IV. (From Gusella JF et al.: DNA markers for nervous system diseases. Science 225:1320. © 1984 by the AAAS.)

mation was in the past a theoretical one. With the advent of these markers it has become feasible to determine the likely status of an individual within a family where Huntington disease is occurring. Again, because the RFLP marker is not detecting the gene itself, such an analysis is possible only if other family members are available, so that the affected chromosome can be identified. An example of this sort of situation is shown in Figure 9.16. Individual II-1, who already has had two children and is considering whether to have more, wishes to know his risk of developing Huntington disease, which affects his mother and brother. After counselling about the possible outcomes, he wishes to pursue RFLP testing, and using the G8 marker the blot results shown in the figure are obtained. As in previous examples, it is important to look at the affected individuals in order to determine which allele is travelling with the disease gene. The patient's mother, I-2, has a 3.7- and a 4.9-kb allele (the rest of the G8 bands on the blots are not shown for the sake of simplicity), whereas her affected son, II-3, is homozygous for the 4.9-kb allele. Therefore, it is the mother's 4.9-kb allele that seems to travel with the Huntington disease gene. Individual II-1 also has inherited this allele from his mother, which indicates that his risk of having the Huntington disease gene is high. However, because of recombination, the risk is not 100%. There are two ways in which a recombination could have occurred in this family in such a way as to change his status. If II-1 himself represents a recombination between G8 and HD, which has a 3% chance, then he would not have inherited the disease gene. Alternatively, if II-3 is a recombinant, then we would have made the wrong conclusion about which G8 allele is travelling with the Huntington disease gene, and it would be the mother's 3.7-kb allele which is on the abnormal chromosome; therefore, II-1 would not be at risk. Each of these recombination events has an approximately 3% chance of occurring. Taking both into consideration, II-1's risk is approximately 94% rather than 100%.

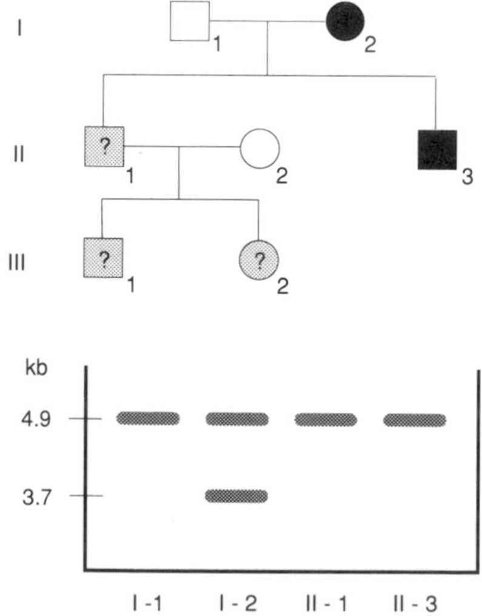

Figure 9.16. Application of RFLP analysis to prediction of risks for developing Huntington disease. Individual II-1 has inherited the same maternal allele at the G8 locus as his affected brother II-3 and therefore has a high likelihood of developing the disease.

Note that RFLP analysis can be carried out only if the marker being used is "informative," that is, it allows a distinction between the two chromosomes of an affected individual. Using only the information given above, for instance, it would not be possible to apply this approach to individuals III-1 and III-2, since their at-risk father is homozygous at the G8 locus. If one wished to pursue this, it would be necessary to find another marker for which he is informative.

Duchenne Muscular Dystrophy and Reverse Genetics

The application of human gene mapping to actually clone the gene responsible for a disease is commonly referred to as reverse genetics. One of the first successful applications of reverse genetics was the cloning of the Duchenne muscular dystrophy gene. As described above, DMD is an X-linked condition with onset of weakness in affected boys in early childhood. These boys are usually wheelchair-bound before the age of 10 years and death usually occurs from complications of muscle degeneration by about age 20 years. As described above, the gene was mapped to Xp21.2 based on the observation of X-autosome translocations in affected females (Fig. 9.7), as well as the occurrence of a small Xp21.2 deletion in a boy who had Duchenne muscular dystrophy and three other X-linked recessive diseases (Fig. 9.9). The gene was also mapped by RFLP analysis, and that mapping agreed with localization to Xp21.

Cloning of the gene itself was accomplished by two groups of researchers using two different approaches. One group was able to clone a portion of the gene by working with the X-autosome translocation shown in Figure 9.7, in which the translocation connects X-chromosome sequences to DNA from the short arm of chromosome 21. This region, like the short arms of chromosomes 13, 14, 15, and 22, contains ribosomal genes, which are repeated sequences coding for the ribosomal RNAs. Because those sequences were known, it was possible with some ingenuity to clone the breakpoint in this affected female, which connected ribosomal sequences to DNA from the X chromosome. As expected, this X-chromosome sequence turned out to lie within the DMD gene.

Another approach was taken by another group of researchers using DNA from the boy with the small Xp21.2 deletion (Figure 9.9). Using a clever subtraction technique, they were able to obtain cloned fragments of DNA that are present on a normal X chromosome but absent in this boy's DNA. One such clone, pERT87, is shown in Figure 9.6; the *46,Y,del(X) lane* is DNA from the boy with the Xp21.2 deletion. When they tested these clones on boys who had DMD with *no* visible cytogenetic deletion, pERT87 was also missing in the DNA from some of these boys (Fig. 9.17). This suggested that this fragment of DNA might include part of the DMD gene itself. These researchers extended the cloned region of DNA to include about 140,000 bp, and tested additional fragments (87–1, 87–8, and 87–18) within this region for deletion in boys with DMD. As shown in Figure 9.18, additional deletions were found in this region. Whereas these seemed to focus around the middle of the pERT87 region, some extended off in both directions. These data could be reconciled only with the notion that the DMD gene is very large and extends to both sides of this cloned region. Several fragments within this region were then tested to see whether any of them might include exons of the DMD gene, and eventually a 16-kb muscle-specific transcript was detected on Northern blots (Fig. 9.19). The cDNA for this gene was subsequently cloned, and it was determined that the genomic DNA sequence encoding the DMD gene is truly mammoth, occupying approximately 2 million bp, or more than 1% of the X chromosome.

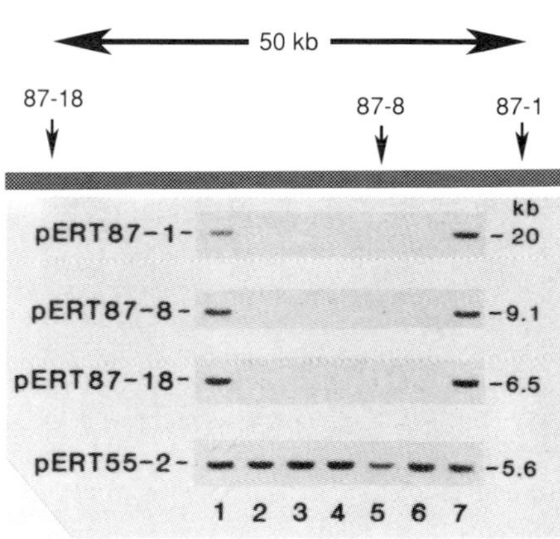

Figure 9.17. Southern blotting of DNA from seven boys with DMD, using clones from the pERT87 region. The relative positions of the 87-18, 87-8, and 87-1 are shown in the diagram at the *top* of the figure. DNA in *lanes 1* and *7* show no evidence of deletion, whereas *lanes 2–6* indicate deletion of the 87-1, 87-8, and 87-18 clones. None of these boys had cytogenetically visible deletions. (From Monaco AP, Bertelson CJ, Middlesworth W, et al.: Detection of deletions spanning the Duchenne muscular dystrophy locus using a tightly linked DNA segment. Nature 316:842, 1985.)

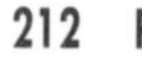

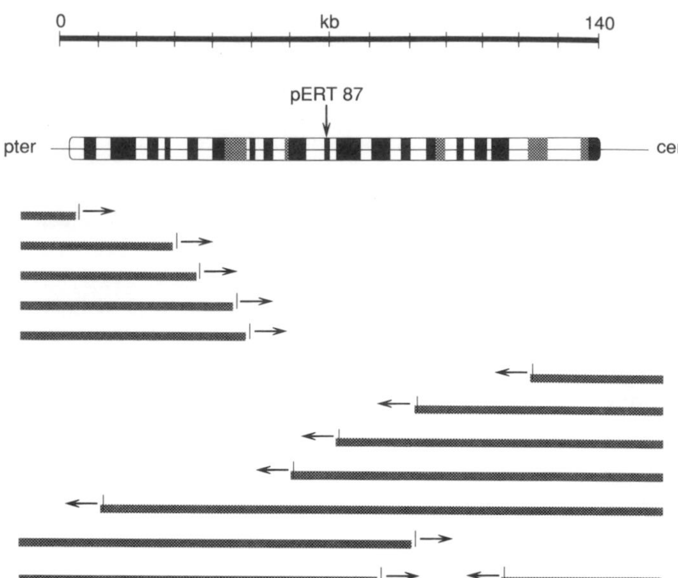

Figure 9.18. Additional deletions found by chromosome walking from the original pERT87 probe. The diagram shows the extent of deletions found in different males with DMD, as determined by Southern blotting using a series of probes spread over 140 kb. *Arrows* indicate the deleted regions; *solid red lines* indicate nondeleted regions. It is apparent that deletions can extend off to both sides of pERT87; in one situation *(last line)*, an interstitial deletion is present. (Reprinted by permission from Kunkel LM, et al.: Analysis of deletions in DNA from patients with Becker and Duchenne muscular dystrophy. Nature 322:73. ©1986, Macmillan Magazines Ltd.)

The protein encoded by this gene, named "dystrophin," has had its sequence completely predicted based on the cDNA sequence and the use of the genetic code. The protein has features that suggest its involvement in the contractile apparatus of striated and cardiac muscle. As expected, this protein is completely missing in boys with DMD. Immunological techniques have demonstrated that the protein is localized to the muscle cell membrane (Fig. 9.20), and its function is under active investigation.

Interesting, a milder form of X-linked muscular dystrophy, called Becker muscular dystrophy (BMD), is distinguished from Duchenne muscular dystrophy by a later age of onset, a later age of requiring wheelchair support, and a longer life span. Linkage analysis indicated that the BMD gene was also located in Xp21. BMD patients have been found to also have DNA abnormalities in the DMD gene, and muscle tissue from BMD patients contains reduced amounts of dystrophin, or sometimes a protein of an abnormal size. Thus, DMD and BMD represent examples of allelic heterogeneity.

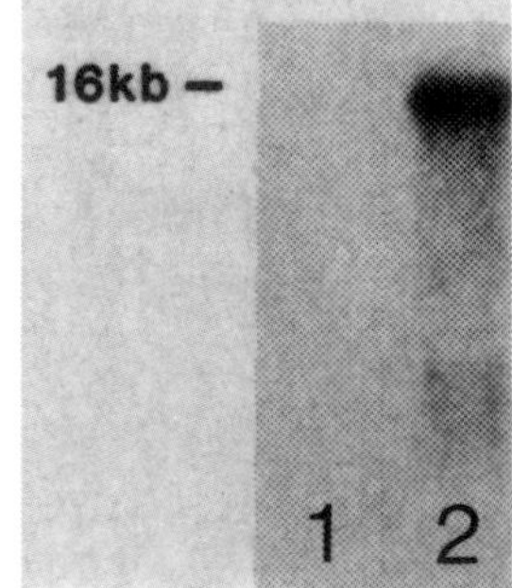

Figure 9.19. Northern blot, demonstrating a 16-kb transcript in RNA obtained from fetal skeletal muscle *(lane 2)* but not in a nonmuscle cell RNA sample *(lane 1)*. The probe is a cDNA clone that was derived by screening a cDNA library with a clone from the pERT87 region. This is a very large mRNA, and represents the normal transcript of the DMD gene. (From Monaco AP, Neve RL, Colletti-Feener C, et al.: Isolation of candidate cDNAs for portions of the Duchenne muscular dystrophy gene. Nature 323:646, 1986.)

Cystic Fibrosis

Cystic fibrosis (CF) is the most common autosomal recessive disease of Caucasians, affecting approximately 1 in 2500 newborns. From Hardy-Weinberg considerations, one can then calculate that the frequency of heterozygous carriers is about 1 in 25 individuals. The disease is characterized clinically by sticky viscous secretions of the pancreas and lungs. It may be recognizable at birth by a condition called "meconium ileus," which is an intestinal obstruction. The diagnosis is commonly made by demonstrating an elevation of chloride in sweat. This is both a highly sensitive and specific finding in CF. Children with this disorder usually develop pancreatic insufficiency, which can be managed with enzyme supplementation. Their chronic pulmonary infec-

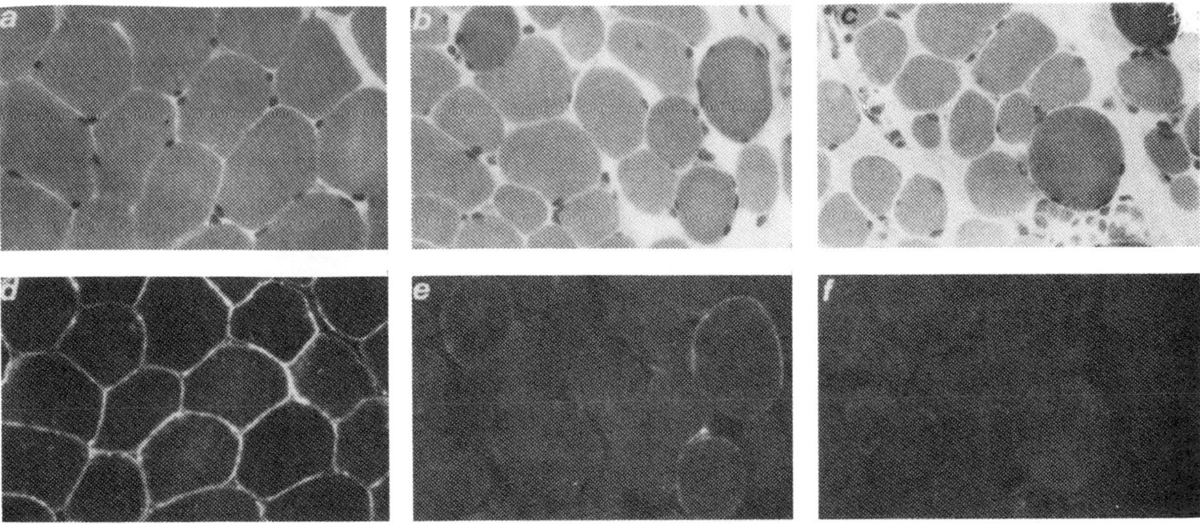

Figure 9.20. Localization of the DMD gene product using immunofluorescence. In **a** is shown a section of normal muscle under light microscopy; **b** shows a section of BMD muscle; **c** shows a similar section of DMD muscle. In **d, e,** and **f** are shown immunofluorescent stains of the normal, BMD, and DMD muscle sections using an antibody that had been produced against a synthetic polypeptide derived from the predicted amino acid sequence of the DMD gene product. The staining is seen to be on the muscle cell membrane in the normal sample. Staining is much reduced in BMD muscle (**e**) and completely absent in DMD (**f**). (Reprinted by permission from Arahata K, Ishiura S, Ishiguro T, et al.: Immunostaining of skeletal and cardiac muscle surface membrane with antibody against Duchenne muscular dystrophy peptide. Nature 333:861. ©1988, Macmillan Magazines Ltd.)

tions are more difficult to manage, however, and in spite of gains in survival based on vigorous treatment of the chest infections with antibiotics and physical therapy, the current average survival is about 25 years. Decades of direct research have failed to identify the specific gene product involved in cystic fibrosis, although considerable indirect evidence has been collected to indicate that an abnormality in ion transport across cell membranes seems to be involved.

Thus, CF also represents a prime target for gene mapping by linkage analysis, and this effort was initiated in the early 1980s by several groups. Here, finding the linked marker was less rapid than for Huntington disease, and several years of searching were required. However, in 1985 linkage was demonstrated to markers on chromosome 7 (Fig. 9.2*C*). Very quickly, several more markers on chromosome 7 were tested, and the CF gene was found to lie quite close to the markers *met* and J3.11, as shown in Figure 9.21. Physical mapping techniques indicated that the distance between these markers was about 1.6 million bp, which is a large enough region to contain approximately 50 genes. Additional markers were sub-

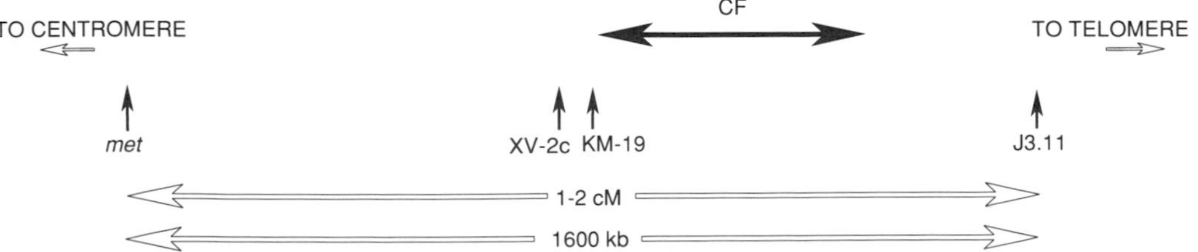

Figure 9.21. Map of the CF region on 7q31. DNA markers in the region include the *met* oncogene, whose mapping to chromosome 7 was shown in Table 9.1. Markers XV-2c, KM-19, and J3.11 are DNA probes that detect RFLPs.

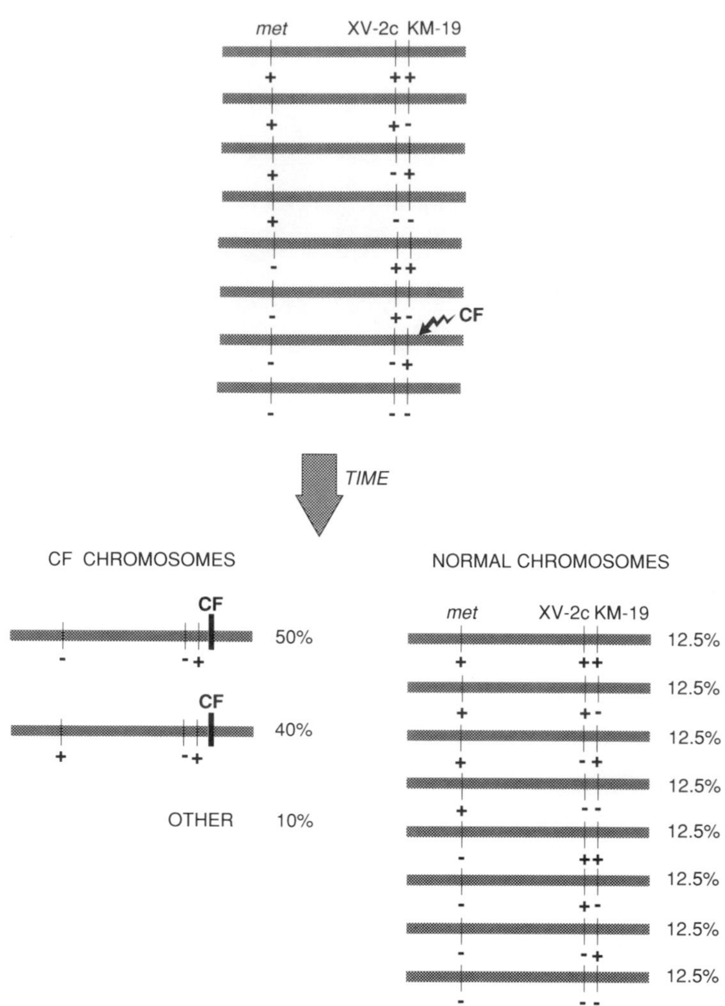

Figure 9.22. Mechanism for the occurrence of linkage disequilibrium. In this example, the CF mutation is shown as having arisen only once on an ancestral chromosome, which had a − allele at the *met* locus, a − allele at XV-2c, and a + at KM-19. In the next few generations after the mutation arose, all CF chromosomes had these alleles at the nearby marker loci. Over time, however, recombination has occurred between CF and the more distant marker *met,* so that there is relatively little linkage disequilibrium between these two loci. However, close linkage disequilibrium still exists between XV-2c, KM-19, and CF, indicating that these loci are very close and relatively little recombination has occurred since the original mutation. The net result is that the distribution of alleles seen in CF chromosomes for closely linked markers is different than for normal chromosomes.

sequently obtained within this interval and allowed the position of the CF gene to be even further narrowed down (Fig. 9.21).

An interesting feature of cystic fibrosis emerged as very closely linked markers were identified. Two such markers, shown in Figure 9.21 as XV-2c and KM-19, are not part of the CF gene itself; both detect polymorphic sites. The surprising finding is that the vast majority of chromosomes carrying the CF mutation also carry particular alleles for XV-2c and KM-19, namely a − allele for XV-2c and a + allele for KM-19. This −/+ haplotype is found in approximately 25% of normal chromosomes, with the rest of the normal chromosomes having other patterns. This preferential occurrence of a disease gene in association with specific alleles of nearby markers is called "linkage disequilibrium." In this setting, linkage disequilibrium indicates that most chromosomes carrying the CF mutation are descended from a common ancestor. The mechanism for the generation of linkage disequilibrium is diagrammed in Figure 9.22. This sort of disequilibrium would only be expected to be seen if: (*a*) most CF chromosomes carry the same mutation, and (*b*) the markers being tested are quite close to the disease gene. In fact, the linkage disequilibrium between CF and the more distant markers *met* and J3.11 is quite weak.

Very recently, the cystic fibrosis gene has been cloned by careful study of the approximately 500,000-bp candidate interval defined by genetic analysis (Fig. 9.21). Without the availability of major rearrangements, which were so helpful in the DMD search, a major problem was to identify the *correct* gene. In fact, three possible genes from this region were studied, which turned out *not* to be responsible for CF, before the correct gene was finally cloned.

Initial suggestions that the fourth candidate gene was correct came from evolutionary conservation and Northern blotting results. As shown in Figure 9.23, a transcript is present in lung, pancreas, sweat glands, intestine, and liver, all of which are affected in CF. This gene,

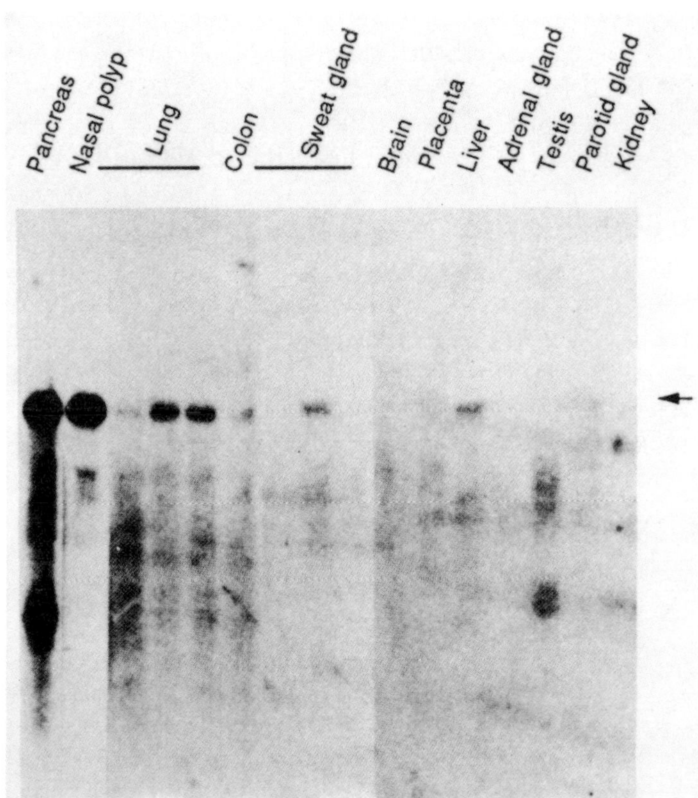

Figure 9.23. Northern blot showing the pattern of expression of the cystic fibrosis gene. The probe for the blot is a fragment of a cDNA prepared from normal human sweat glands. The genomic sequences used to derive this cDNA lie in the 500,000-bp CF candidate region (Fig. 9.21). *Each lane* of the Northern blot contains RNA from a different normal human tissue. A 6.2-kb mRNA is apparent in lung, pancreas, and sweat gland, but not in all tissues (e.g., brain). This is consistent with expectations of the CF gene transcript, which presumably performs an important normal function in these organs; when both copies of the gene are defective, CF is the result. (From Riordan JR, Rommens JM, Kerem B, et al.: Identification of the cystic fibrosis gene: Cloning and characterization of complementary DNA. Science 245:1066, 1989.)

which was discovered to code for a 1480-amino acid protein, is quite large, containing 26 exons and stretching across 250,000 bp of DNA (Fig. 9.24). The mRNA transcript is 6129 bp long. By reference to the genetic code (Table 2.2) the complete sequence of the 1480-amino acid protein could be predicted; careful study of this sequence and comparison to other proteins whose functions are better known makes the strong prediction that the protein product is anchored in the cell membrane, probably binds ATP, and probably functions as a molecular pump, although the nature of its substrate remains unclear.

To prove the correctness of this candidate gene, it was necessary to identify mutations which correlate with disease. This was a formidable

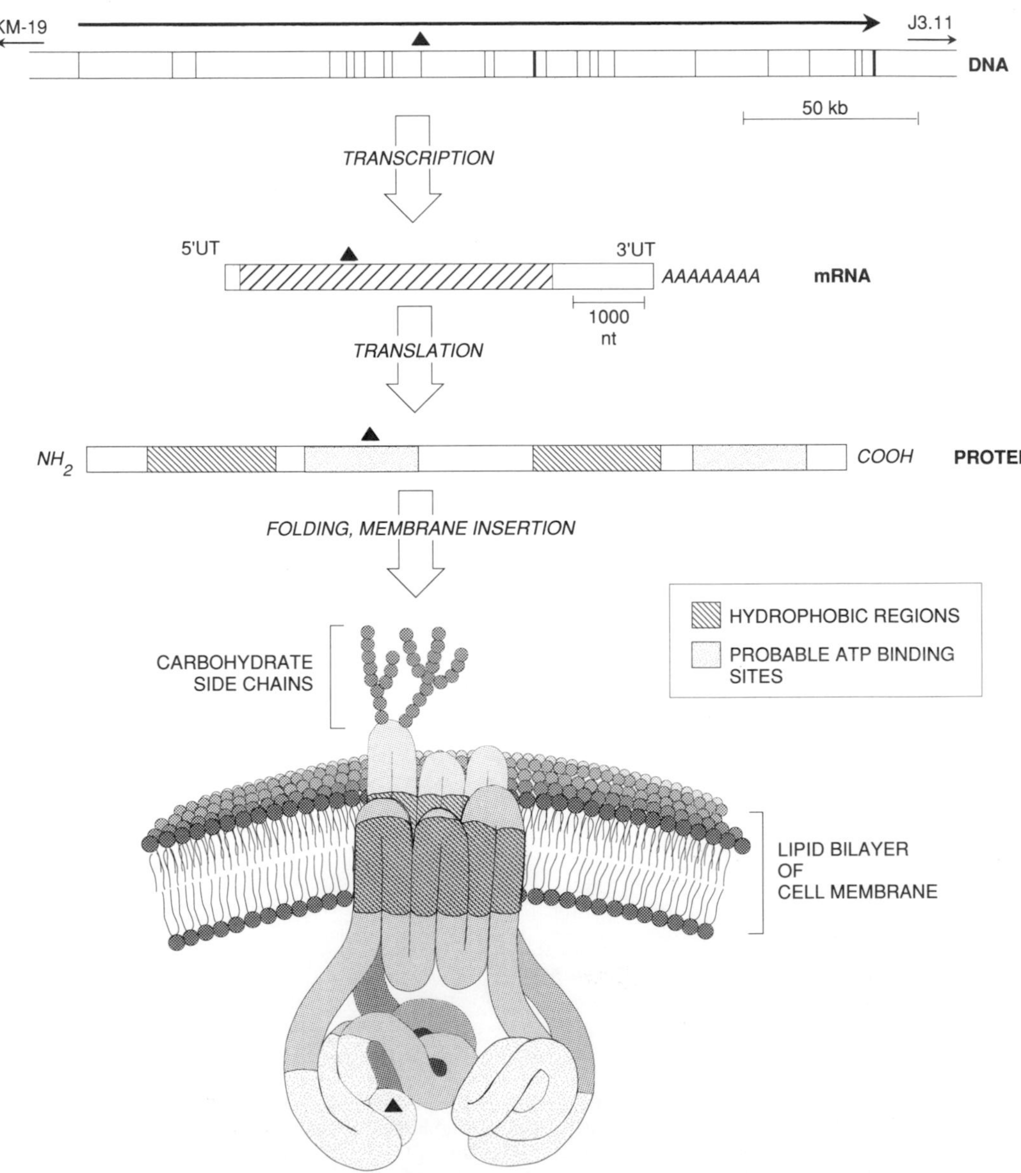

Figure 9.24. Gene, transcript, and protein implicated in cystic fibrosis, as identified by reverse genetics. The folding of the protein and its localization in the cell membrane are thus far hypothetical. ▲ indicates the location of the 3-bp deletion in exon 10, which represents the common mutation in CF. This leads to a loss of a single amino acid in the protein product, also indicated by ▲.

NORMAL								
DNA	*..GAA*	*AAT*	*ATC*	*ATC*	*TTT*	*GGT*	*GTT*	*TCC..*
PROTEIN	Glu	Asn	Ile	Ile	Phe	Gly	Val	Ser
POSITION	504	505	506	507	508	509	510	511

CYSTIC FIBROSIS								
DNA	*..GAA*	*AAT*	*ATC*	*AT-*	*--T*	*GGT*	*GTT*	*TCC..*
PROTEIN	Glu	Asn	Ile	Ile		Gly	Val	Ser

Figure 9.25. The common mutation responsible for cystic fibrosis. A deletion of CTT in exon 10 results in the loss of a phenylalanine at position 508 of the 1480 amino acid protein. The isoleucine at 507 is unaltered because ATC and ATT both code for isoleucine.

task, as such mutations turned out to be quite subtle. Cloning and sequencing a cDNA prepared from sweat glands of a CF patient, however, eventually revealed an unequivocal difference from the normal sequence in exon 10: a 3-bp deletion was found, which would have the effect of deleting a single amino acid (a phenylalanine) at residue 508 (Fig. 9.25). That this represents a mutation *causative* of CF, and not a neutral polymorphism, was subsequently demonstrated by detecting this same mutation in 70–75% of CF chromosomes, and in 0% of more than 600 chromosomes known *not* to harbor a CF mutation.

The cloning of the CF gene has major consequences. Most immediately, it allows the possibility of detecting heterozygotes for this autosomal recessive disease (4% of the Caucasian population) and thus allows couples at risk for having an affected child to obtain this information prior to starting their families (see discussion of genetic screening in Chapter 11). At this writing, only 70–75% of carriers can be identified, but it is expected that the allelic mutations responsible for the other 25–30% will be defined in the near future.

Secondly, the cloning of the CF gene allows a powerful attack on understanding the basic biology of the disease, which was simply not possible before. Such understanding will likely lead to new approaches to treatment, in both the drug therapy and gene therapy (Chapter 12) arenas.

Thirdly, the success in cloning the CF gene by reverse genetics, even in the absence of gross genetic rearrangements to lead the way, has led to much enthusiasm that this approach may succeed in identifying the genes for a large number of human disorders for which no information exists about the normal gene function.

The general strategy of the reverse genetics approach is therefore as follows. Using a large panel of polymorphic markers in a large number of families with the disease in question, the disease gene is first mapped to a particular part of a particular chromosome. Cytogenetic abnormalities are extremely helpful and are used whenever possible. By successive iterations, it is usually possible to obtain markers within 1 to 2 cM of the gene. This region (approximately 1–2 million bp) must then be searched for the actual gene. While there is no one best way to do this, the search includes looking for deletions in patients with the disease, looking for exons that are expressed as mRNA in the affected tissue, and looking for sequences conserved in evolution, which indicate the presence of an expressed gene. While this entire process is arduous, it offers the only available means to identify the gene for a large number of human disorders and provides an approach to understanding human medical genetics that was previously not thought possible.

THE HUMAN MAJOR HISTOCOMPATIBILITY COMPLEX (HLA)

We have considered the general features of polymorphic loci in humans, as well as their usefulness in genetic mapping. A particular cluster of genes on human chromosome 6 is worthy of special attention because of its high degree of polymorphism and relation to disease, especially immunologic disorders. The human major histocompatibility complex (MHC, also frequently called HLA for human leukocyte antigen) was originally defined by reference to a similar complex in mice (called H-2), which appeared to be responsible for the ability of skin grafts to survive after transplantation. Such grafts were successful when the mice were from identical genetic backgrounds, but often were rejected if they were not. Through a complex series of experiments, the genetics of transplant rejection were worked out, and as transplants became clinically applicable in humans, it was clear that similar constraints existed.

The human HLA genes are located on the short arm of chromosome 6, occupying about 3000 kb of DNA. Figure 9. 26 shows a diagram of this gene cluster, which is divided into three groups of genes, called classes I, II, and III. The class I genes are called A, B, and C. A full discussion of the function of the protein products of these genes (the human leukocyte antigens) falls outside of the scope of this book (see Suggested Readings). In general, however, class I antigens are critical for recognition of foreign substances on the surface of a host cell by so-called "killer T cells." In order for killer T cells to recognize a foreign antigen, they must "see" this in association with a class I gene product. The HLA proteins are anchored to the cell membrane, leaving the majority of their structure outside the cell.

Class II genes are represented by the DP, DQ, and DR loci. The protein products of these genes are also anchored in the cell membrane and play a role in antigen recognition; this time, however, the primary role is in recognition by helper T cells.

Finally, the class III gene cluster is located between class I and class II and includes several genes that are part of the complement pathway. This includes C2, C4A, C4B, and properdin factor (Bf).

The class I and class II loci are among the most polymorphic genes ever described, with each locus represented by more than 10 alleles in the population. It is presumed that this degree of polymorphism developed because it has some benefit to the species, but the reasons for this are still not entirely clear. One proposal has been that the degree of polymorphism makes it very unlikely that a mother and her fetus will share all of these antigens, so that, should some fetal cells escape into the mother's circulation, they would be recognized by the mother's immune system as foreign. Alternatively, the presence of so many different alleles may have prevented the possibility of any mimicking foreign agent (such as a virus) being able to evade recognition in all hosts and destroy the species.

The inheritance of HLA alleles precisely follows the expectation for

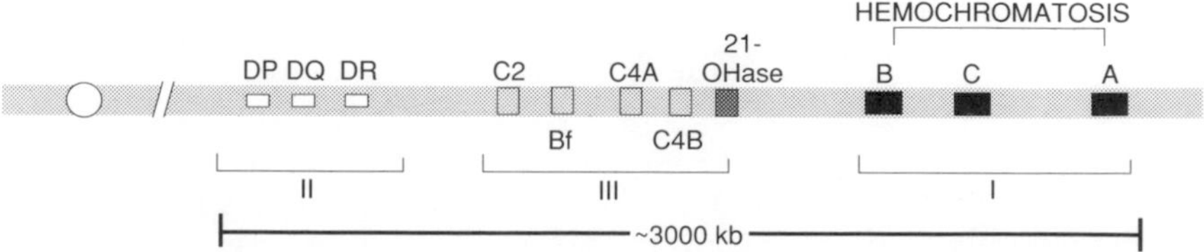

Figure 9.26. Diagram of the human major histocompatibility complex on the short arm of chromosome 6.

A.

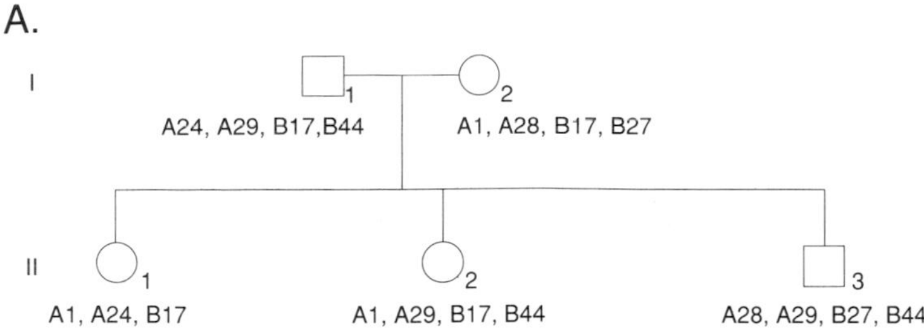

B.

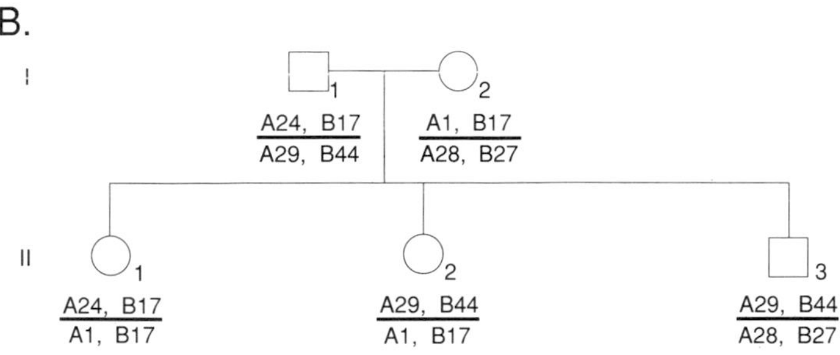

Figure 9.27. Demonstration of Mendelian inheritance of alleles at the HLA-A and HLA-B loci. In **A** is shown the results of HLA typing of two parents and three offspring. The typing itself does not completely establish the genotype, as one must determine which A allele and which B allele are on the same chromosome. This is referred to as "haplotyping," and has been done in **B.** Haplotyping is accomplished by noting that individual II-1 has only the B17 antigen, which means that she must have an A1, B17 chromosome and an A24, B17 chromosome. The A24, B17 chromosome must have come from her father and the A1, B17 chromosome from her mother, which then allows haplotyping of the rest of the family.

a codominant Mendelian system. In Figure 9.27 is shown a nuclear family with a typical inheritance pattern. Crossovers between the loci within the HLA complex do occur, because the total genetic distance within the locus is about 3 cM, but they are unusual.

The major practical application of HLA typing at the present time is for tissue transplantation. For example, the long-term results of renal transplantation, whether the donor is a related individual or an unrelated cadaver, are improved if there is a good match between the HLA alleles of the donor and those of the recipient. The same is true for platelet transfusion. Platelets, like almost all cells in the body except red blood cells, carry class I antigens on their surface. If there is not a good match between donor and recipient, the donor platelets can be rapidly destroyed. Therefore, individuals being given large amounts of platelets (often because of leukemia) need to be HLA typed and have their platelets obtained from a well-matched donor.

Because the HLA complex is so polymorphic, it makes an ideal marker for linkage studies. Furthermore, the various alleles can be detected by a panel of serologic antibodies, so that alleles at this locus were possible to score 30 years before the genes involved were cloned. A large number of genetic analyses have been carried out in the past several decades using HLA as the marker, testing this against a variety of diseases. As expected, most of those disorders did not show linkage, but in three important instances, a specific linkage has been identified. The first of these is a dominant neurological disorder called spinocerebellar ataxia. In at least some of the families with this disorder, characterized by the onset of an unsteady gait in middle life, clear evidence of linkage to HLA has been demonstrated. In other families, however, there has been no evidence at all of linkage, so that there appears to be locus heterogeneity in this disorder.

A second disorder linked to HLA is deficiency of the enzyme 21-hydroxylase. This is an enzyme of steroid metabolism, and its insufficiency leads to a block in the normal synthesis of glucocorticoids. As a result, precursor molecules are shunted down alternate pathways, leading to an overproduction of androgens. Thus, females with 21-hydroxylase deficiency (also called congenital adrenal hyperplasia or the adrenogenital syndrome) are often born with ambiguous or masculinized genitalia. There is also a tendency to lose salt because of a simultaneous deficiency of aldosterone. The gene for 21-hydroxylase is located next to the gene for C4B in the class II region of the HLA complex (Fig. 9.26). Whether there is any significance to this location remains unclear.

A third disorder that maps to the HLA region is idiopathic hemochromatosis. This is an autosomal recessive disease in which excessive iron accumulation occurs in affected adults. Homozygous individuals absorb iron from the gastrointestinal tract at high rates throughout their life. The normal control of iron in the body operates at the level of intestinal absorption, but the mechanism that would normally act to slow absorption in the setting of adequate stores is defective. The excess iron deposits in the heart, liver, pancreas, skin, and endocrine system, leading to a variety of symptoms including heart failure, cirrhosis, pituitary hormone deficiency, and "bronze diabetes" (skin pigmentation and pancreatic endocrine insufficiency). Females often do not show symptoms until after menopause, as menstrual iron loss is protective against the most damaging levels of iron accumulation. Males, however, often show evidence of disease by middle adulthood. The most effective treatment is periodic removal of blood, since this is a simple way to remove iron. As this is usually successful, it is always a tragedy to miss this diagnosis. Because the disease is recessive, it is essential to examine other members in a family at risk, especially siblings, when one individual is diagnosed.

The gene for idiopathic hemochromatosis is located within the MHC, between the B and the A genes of the class I cluster. The gene itself has not yet been cloned. However, once the diagnosis is made in one individual, a very accurate assessment of the risk of siblings can be made by knowing the linkage to HLA. An example is shown in Figure 9.28. HLA typing of this family shows that a younger brother of the affected proband carries the same HLA alleles as does his affected brother, and therefore, will almost certainly develop hemochromatosis. While reliable tests to

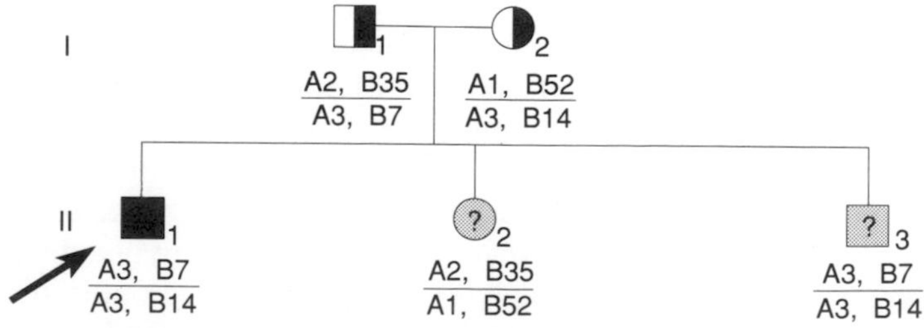

Figure 9.28. Pedigree of a family in which individual II-1 has been found to be affected with idiopathic hemochromatosis. His sister, II-2, has inherited different HLA alleles from both parents, and therefore would be predicted to be homozygous normal. On the other hand, his younger brother, II-3, who so far has no symptoms of iron overload, has identical HLA genotypes to the proband and therefore can be predicted to be homozygous for the hemochromatosis gene. This discovery will allow close follow-up of II-3 and early treatment of increasing iron storage. The A3, B7 and A3, B14 chromosomes carrying the hemochromatosis gene in this family are typical (see text).

indicate the presence of iron overload are available, HLA linkage testing is capable of detecting the presence of the disease even *before* iron overload occurs, which allows ideal management of this potentially curable disease.

Idiopathic hemochromatosis also represents another example of linkage disequilibrium, which was introduced in the discussion of cystic fibrosis. The majority of hemochromatosis mutant alleles travel on a chromosome that is either A3, B7 or A3, B14 for the class I A and B loci. This presumably reflects the fact that most of these mutant chromosomes derive from a common ancestor who had an A3 allele at the A locus.

Another highly interesting feature of the human HLA complex is the association of certain alleles with a group of diseases often referred to as "autoimmune" disorders. These conditions, many of which are characterized by the presence of antibodies directed against self antigens, provide considerable circumstantial evidence for an immune system gone awry, though the actual steps involved in the initiation of this situation are quite obscure. The list of autoimmune diseases is long; many of these are rare, but the list includes common disorders such as juvenile-onset diabetes mellitus, rheumatoid arthritis, and multiple sclerosis. For these disorders an association has been noted between the presence of particular HLA alleles and the risk of getting the disease. Notice that there is a distinction between an association of this sort and a linkage. In genetic terms, an association indicates that the distribution of alleles at a locus seen in affected individuals differs from unaffected individuals. The most obvious interpretation of such a result is that linkage between the disease and the marker locus exists and that there is linkage disequilibrium present. Note that linkage *alone* is not necessarily sufficient to result in an association; for example, although the G8 marker is closely linked to the Huntington disease gene, there is no association between a particular allele at the G8 locus and the presence of Huntington disease. Table 9.4 lists associations that have been reported for a variety of autoimmune diseases with respect to particular HLA antigens. The percent of patients who have a particular allele is compared to controls; when a discrepancy appears, an association is suggested.

Perhaps the most dramatic association is that between ankylosing spondylitis and the B27 allele at the HLA-B locus. Ankylosing spondylitis is a large-joint form of arthritis that affects the sacroiliac joints and the spine and has a genetic component. Ninety percent or more of individuals with ankylosing spondylitis are found to have the HLA-B27 allele, whereas only about 8% of controls have this.

Other associations are not as strong as this, but are highly statistically significant. Juvenile-onset diabetes mellitus is associated with the DR3 and DR4 alleles in the class II cluster of genes. A child who has a DR3 allele on one chromosome 6 and DR4 on the other has an approx-

Table 9.4. Examples of Associations between HLA and Disease

Disease	HLA Allele	Frequency of Allele (%)	
		Patients	Controls
Ankylosing spondylitis	B27	90	8
Diabetes mellitus, juvenile-onset	DR3	50	21
	DR4	38	13
Multiple sclerosis	DR2	55	23
Systemic lupus erythematosus	DR3	70	21
Graves disease	DR3	53	21
Psoriasis	C6	50	23

imately 50-fold increased risk of developing insulin-dependent diabetes. For multiple sclerosis it is the DR2 allele that seems to carry an increased risk.

The meaning of these associations is still not entirely clear, but several hypotheses have been proposed. One is that it is the HLA protein itself that is responsible for the predisposition to disease. This could occur if a particular HLA product in combination with a particular foreign agent such as a virus were incapable of inducing an effective immune response, so that a chronic infection resulted. Alternatively, if the immune response to the foreign agent in the context of a particular HLA allele in some way crossreacted with the host and led to destruction of normal cells, an autoimmune situation would be created. Another proposed mechanism is that the HLA loci themselves are not responsible for the predisposition to disease, but this phenomenon derives from other as yet unidentified loci within this cluster, which are in linkage disequilibrium with HLA. This hypothesis would suggest that autoimmune diseases are similar to idiopathic hemochromatosis, except that they do not follow strict Mendelian inheritance patterns. At the very least, one would have to propose the presence of reduced penetrance, other modifier genes, or an interaction with the environment. At present, it is not possible to distinguish between these various hypotheses.

STATUS OF THE HUMAN GENE MAP

What began on a small scale has now become a major endeavor in multiple laboratories throughout the world. As a result, the number of mapped loci in the human genome has been increasing exponentially over the past several years. With such a large amount of rapidly accumulating information, it is crucial that quality control be exerted over the data, and this function has been carried out by the Human Gene Mapping Workshops, which are held approximately every 2 years. By convention, a map assignment is considered provisional until it is confirmed by a second group, and the Human Gene Mapping Workshops act to keep track of this information and publish an updated map at regular intervals. Table 9.5 shows in tabular form the numbers of genes and arbitrary DNA segments assembled at the last five Human Gene Mapping Workshops. While items in all of these categories of mapped loci have been increasing, the most rapid increase has occurred in cloned arbitrary DNA segments. Many of these are probes that detect restriction fragment length polymorphisms and therefore have contributed greatly to the ability to do linkage analysis of single gene disorders in humans.

Many of the major human single gene disorders have already been mapped by this approach, as shown in Table 9.6. A number of these disorders have already been alluded to in the above discussion. In most of these, prenatal or presymptomatic diagnosis is now possible (Chapter 11)

Table 9.5. Mapped Genes and Markers, as Assembled at the Human Gene Mapping (HGM) Workshops from 1981 to 1989

	HGM6 1981	HGM7 1983	HGM8 1985	HGM9 1987	HGM10 1989
Cloned genes	16	104	249	610	945
Cloned arbitrary DNA segments	35	215	559	2057	3417
Total cloned DNA segments	51	319	808	2667	4362[a]

[a] 1886 of these segments detect RFLPs.

Table 9.6. Representative Autosomal Single Gene Disorders Mapped by Linkage Analysis

Disease	Chromosome Arm
Alzheimer disease (some families)	21q
Cystic fibrosis	7q
Friedreich's ataxia	9q
Hemochromatosis	6p
Huntington disease	4p
Multiple endocrine neoplasia, type I	11q
Multiple endocrine neoplasia, type II	10
Myotonic dystrophy	19q
Nail-patella syndrome	9q
Neurofibromatosis, type 1	17q
Neurofibromatosis, type 2	22q
Polycystic kidney disease	16p
Spinocerebellar ataxia (some families)	6p
von Hippel Lindau disease	3p
Wilson disease	13q

based on linkage analysis with closely linked probes, provided the family is available for analysis and there is no locus heterogeneity. Eventually, all of these disease genes may be specifically identified using the reverse genetics process.

A complete pictorial map of the human genome can be generated from the human gene mapping effort and is rapidly becoming quite complex. Figure 9.29*A* shows as an example the current map of human chro-

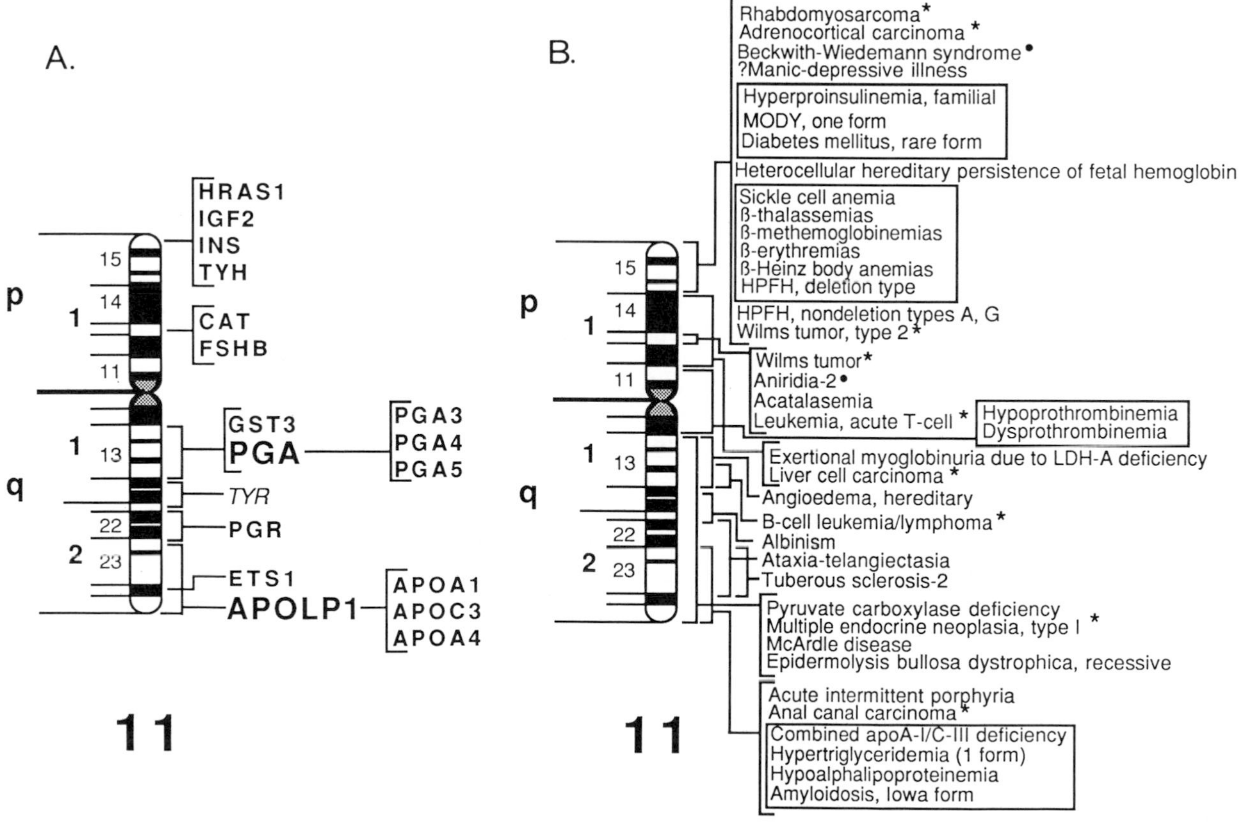

Figure 9.29. **A,** Map of representative loci currently assigned to human chromosome 11. **B,** The "morbid anatomy" of chromosome 11, indicating the location of DNA regions that have been associated with disease.

mosome 11, including known expressed genes, but not including the large number of arbitrary DNA segments which map to this chromosome. Designations of loci follow standardized Human Gene Mapping nomenclature. For example, INS is insulin (see Fig. 9.2), CAT is catalase, and so on. The *brackets* beside the chromosome indicate the interval within which a particular locus has been mapped, using a combination of the approaches discussed above. In Figure 9.29*B* is shown the "morbid anatomy" of chromosome 11, indicating the human diseases that map to this chromosome. Many of these have been placed there based on knowledge of the specific gene involved in their pathogenesis. For example, sickle cell anemia and β-thalassemia are mapped to chromosome 11p, because their structural gene (β-globin) is known to be located there. Other human disorders have been mapped to this chromosome based on linkage analysis. Finally, some disease genes on chromosome 11 have been mapped based on cytogenetic abnormalities. Examples are the Wilms' tumor and aniridia loci, which have been placed in 11p13 based on the occurrence of deletions of this chromosome band in patients with Wilms' tumor of the kidney and absent iris.

CONCLUSION

One of the fastest moving fields in human genetics is gene mapping. Over the past two decades several thousand assignments of cloned DNA segments to specific autosomes have been made. Powerful methods have been developed for mapping cloned DNA segments or proteins. Linkage analysis offers the opportunity to also map human disease genes when the causative gene has not been identified. The ultimate application of this approach, namely the reverse genetic cloning of those previously unapproachable disease loci, is just beginning to be successfully applied, but promises to fill in many of the gaps in our understanding of the molecular basis of human genetic disease.

SUGGESTED READINGS

Auffray C, Strominger JL: Molecular genetics of the human major histocompatibility complex. Adv Hum Genet 15:197–247, 1986.

Gusella JF, et al.: DNA markers for nervous system diseases. Science 225:1320, 1984.

McKusick VA: The morbid anatomy of the human genome: a review of gene mapping in clinical medicine. Medicine (Baltimore) 65:1–33, 1986; 66:1–63, 1987; 66:237–296, 1987; 67:1–19, 1988.

Monaco AP, Kunkel LM: Cloning of the Duchenne/Becker muscular dystrophy locus. Adv Hum Genet 17:61–98, 1988.

Riordan JR, Rommens JM, Kerem B-S, Alon N, Rozmahel R, Grzelczak Z, Zielenski J, Lok S, Plavsic N, Chou J-L, Drumm ML, Iannuzzi MC, Collins FS, Tsui L-C: Identification of the cystic fibrosis gene: cloning and characterization of complementary DNA. Science 245:1066–1080, 1989.

Rommens JM, Iannuzzi MC, Kerem B-S, Drumm ML, Melmer G, Dean M, Rozmahel R, Cole JL, Kennedy D, Hidaka N, Zsiga M, Buchwald M, Riordan JR, Tsui L-C, Collins FS: Identification of the cystic fibrosis gene: chromosome walking and jumping. Science 245:1059–1065, 1989.

White R, Lalouel JM: Chromosome mapping with DNA markers. Sci Am 258:40–48, 1988 (Feb.)

9/ Study Questions

1/ Inspect the somatic cell hybrid panel below. Where does gene H appear to map?

Segregation of Gene H and Human Chromsomes in Human-Hamster Hybrids

Cell	Gene	Human Chromosome																						
Hybrid	H	1	2	3	4	5	6	7	8	9	10	11	12	13	14	15	16	17	18	19	20	21	22	Y	X
1	+	+	−	+	+	+	+	−	+	+	−	+	−	−	−	−	−	−	−	+	+	+	−	−	+
2	−	−	+	−	−	−	−	+	−	+	−	+	−	+	+	+	−	−	−	−	−	−	−	−	+
3	+	−	−	+	+	−	−	−	−	−	−	−	−	−	−	−	+	−	−	+	−	+	−	−	+
4	+	+	−	+	+	−	+	−	+	−	+	+	+	+	+	−	−	−	−	+	+	+	+	+	+
5	+	−	+	+	+	−	−	+	+	−	+	+	+	−	+	+	+	−	−	−	+	−	−	−	+
6	+	−	−	+	−	−	+	+	−	−	+	+	−	+	−	−	−	−	−	−	+	−	+	−	+
7	+	+	+	+	−	−	−	+	−	+	+	+	−	+	−	−	+	−	+	−	−	+	+	−	+
8	−	−	−	−	−	−	−	−	−	−	−	+	−	+	−	−	−	−	+	−	−	−	+	−	+
9	+	−	−	+	+	+	+	−	−	−	−	+	+	−	+	+	+	+	+	−	−	+	+	−	+
10	+	−	+	+	+	+	+	−	−	−	−	+	−	−	−	−	+	−	+	+	−	+	−	+	+

2/ Observe the following lod score table for two markers.

θ	lod
0	$-\infty$
0.05	−10.32
0.10	−1.48
0.15	2.74
0.20	4.45
0.25	4.88
0.30	4.37
0.35	3.73
0.40	2.56
0.50	0

Graph these lod scores. What is the maximum likelihood estimate for θ? What is the lod score at that θ? Are these two markers tightly linked, loosely linked, unlinked? What can you conclude from the data?

3/ Hereditary elliptocytosis is an autosomal dominant disorder in which red blood cells have an abnormal elliptical shape and have a shortened life span, resulting in anemia due to increased destruction of red blood cells in the spleen.

In one large family, you observe the following lod scores in a linkage study between the Rh blood group on chromosome 1 and elliptocytosis:

θ	lod
0	$-\infty$
0.05	4.74
0.10	5.44
0.15	5.35
0.20	4.89
0.25	4.22
0.30	3.39
0.35	2.49
0.40	1.54
0.50	0

What can you conclude about the relative location of elliptocytosis and the Rh locus?

In a second family, the following lod score results are found:

θ	lod
0	$-\infty$
0.05	−2.9
0.10	−1.44
0.15	−0.73
0.20	−0.34
0.25	−0.12
0.30	−0.01
0.35	0.03
0.40	0.02
0.50	0

What can you conclude concerning the elliptocytosis and the Rh blood group loci in this family? Give two explanations for the different results seen with these two families.

4/ Describe the techniques used to map Huntington disease to the tip of the short arm of chromosome 4.

5/ Apply the correct descriptive term to each of the following observations concerning studies of HLA in a hereditary disease:

Linkage
Association
Linkage disequilibrium

a. A particular allele at the HLA B locus is found in 75% of individuals with a hereditary disease and 4% of normal controls.
b. In families with multiple siblings with the disease, affected individuals often inherit the same alleles from their parents while unaffected individuals often have the other parental alleles in common.
c. In a disease known to be linked to HLA, two particular alleles at

the HLA A and B loci are found 15 times more frequently in individuals affected with the disease than in matched controls.

* **6/** Suggest an explanation for why linkage disequilibrium is extremely unlikely between an X-linked disease and a set of RFLP loci, even when the RFLPs are located within the introns of the gene that, when defective, causes the disease.

10

Cancer Genetics

"Another possibility is that in every normal cell there is a specific arrangement for inhibiting, which allows the process of division only when the inhibition has been overcome by a special stimulus. To assume the presence of definite chromosomes which inhibit division, would harmonize best with my fundamental idea . . . cells of tumors with unlimited growth would arise if those "inhibiting chromosomes" were eliminated . . . on the other hand, the assumption of the existence of chromosomes which promote division, might (also) satisfy this postulate. On this assumption, cell division would take place when the action of these chromatin parts, which are as a rule too weak, should be strengthened by a stimulus; and the unlimited tendency to rapid proliferation in malignant tumor cells would be deduced from a permanent predominance of the chromosomes which promote division."

—Theodor Boveri, 1911

The above quotation, which at first glance may seem densely written and difficult to follow, actually represents an uncannily accurate description of the genetics of human cancer, set down by Boveri 60 years before the tools became available to confirm or refute his ideas. Of all the areas of application of human molecular genetics, hardly any could be said to have generated more excitement than the investigation of the mechanism of cancer. This story is still very incompletely understood and will be evolving over the next several decades. Because of its fundamental importance in human disease, however, it seems appropriate to devote an entire chapter to this subject. The story of the effort to understand the molecular basis of cancer is also helpful in underlining principles derived in previous chapters, as it brings together aspects of Mendelian inheritance, cell biology, cytogenetics, virology, and molecular biology.

MOST HUMAN CANCER IS GENETICALLY INFLUENCED, BUT NOT MENDELIAN

With the scourges of malnutrition and infectious disease under relatively good control, cancer has emerged as a leading cause of death in the developed world, with approximately one-third of the population dying of this cause. Of course cancer is not one disease, but a multitude of different diseases, characterized by the site, tissue type, and grade of the malignancy.

The majority of human cancers cannot be easily modeled using single gene inheritance patterns. This is not to say, however, that common cancers are nongenetic. Decades of research indicate that the first degree relatives of a person with a particular type of cancer have a somewhat increased risk of developing the same tumor. A full discussion of the possible models for such relatively weak genetic risks is outside the scope of this book, because such analyses are complicated by the role played by the environment in many cancers (for example, smoking and lung cancer). The multifactorial model (Chapter 4) postulates that contributions from the environment and several genes contribute to risk, but a true understanding of the mechanism of the genetic predisposition to common cancers will await the definition of the actual predisposing genes, as well as an increased understanding of the environmental causes.

Some features of the genetics of common cancers are, however, accurately predicted by the multifactorial model. Thus, for example, in breast cancer the occurrence of bilateral cancer and/or onset before menopause, both of which signify more severe disease, increase the risk of breast cancer in a first degree relative. Table 10.1 shows in tabular form the approximate empiric risks of breast cancer depending on the proband's status. Note that the presence of more than one affected relative also increases the risk as predicted by the multifactorial model (Chapter 4).

For the most part, calculation of genetic risks of cancer based on family history depends upon empirical figures derived from the study of large numbers of families. Counseling about such risks, however, is an extremely important part of preventive medicine and should be an important result of the careful taking of a family history by the physician about to assume the care of a patient (see Chapter 11). The fact that many of the common cancers (colon, breast, cervix, etc.) have a far better prognosis if detected early and appropriately managed adds additional importance to an understanding of cancer genetics.

MENDELIAN FORMS OF CANCER

While rarer than the common forms of cancer, there are about 100 well-described single-gene disorders that have malignancy as a prominent part of their phenotype. The majority of these are inherited in an auto-

Table 10.1 Empirical Lifetime Risk of Breast Cancer Depends on Family History[a]

Family Background	Risk to Proband
	%
Negative for breast cancer	5–6
Sister with postmenopausal breast cancer	10–15
Sister with premenopausal unilateral breast cancer	10–15
Sister with premenopausal bilateral breast cancer	30–50
Sister and mother with premenopausal bilateral breast cancer	40–60

[a]From Ottman R, King M-C, Pike MC, Henderson BE: Practical guide for estimating risk for familial breast cancer. Lancet 2:556, 1983 and Anderson DE: Genetic study of breast cancer: Identification of a high risk group. Cancer 34:1090, 1974. © JB Lippincott.

somal dominant fashion, although a few recessive disorders have also been described (see below). The single-gene disorders often can be distinguished from their multifactorial counterparts by the following features: (*a*) familial pattern of inheritance fitting the predictions of the effects of a single gene (for many of these disorders, however, penetrance may not be 100%, so that the recognition of single gene inheritance may be somewhat difficult unless a relatively large family is available); (*b*) early onset of cancer relative to this cancer type in the general population; and (*c*) the frequent occurrence of multiple primary tumors. The latter is a rare feature of common malignancies, but is present more frequently in single gene disorders.

While it is outside of the scope of this book to consider a catalog of such familial cancer syndromes, it is worth considering a few of these in more detail in order to derive some basic principles.

Familial Polyposis Coli

This is a relatively common (1 in 10,000) autosomal dominant disorder. The colon is normal at birth, but during the first 20 years of life, hundreds of small polyps appear in the colon and occasionally elsewhere in the intestinal tract. While these polyps are asymptomatic, their major significance is the risk of progression to colon cancer, which approaches 100% in a patient with this disease by age 50 years. A total colectomy in early adulthood completely prevents this outcome. Figure 10.1 shows an x-ray film and a pathologic specimen from a patient with this condition, illustrating the innumerable polyps. Because this is an autosomal dominant disorder, making the diagnosis in one individual obligates the physician to investigate the rest of the family, because there may be no other warning signs of the presence of the disease until the appearance of malignancy. Because surgical therapy is so successful, individuals at risk should have investigations carried out by the age of 20 years using radiologic studies and/or colonoscopy.

The gene for familial polyposis coli has recently been mapped to the long arm of chromosome 5, using the sort of linkage analysis described in the preceding chapter. The gene itself has not yet been identified. On reflection, one can perceive that the mechanism of the development of cancer in a patient with familial polyposis coli must be complex. While all of the cells of such an individual contain the polyposis mutation, the entire colon does not become one enormous polyp, but the polyps are separated by regions of relatively normal colonic mucosa. Thus, the development of a polyp must represent an additional event or series of events, in the context of a background of cells that all carry the same germline mutation. Furthermore, the cancers that develop in this condition invariably arise in a polyp, but the vast majority of polyps do not become malignant. This indicates that a further event or events must be responsible for the transition from polyp to carcinoma. This multihit theory of carcinogenesis is very well supported, both epidemiologically and genetically, and we shall return to this theme later on.

Interestingly, there is another autosomal dominant disorder called Gardner syndrome, which is characterized by the same sort of colon polyps but has additional features not seen in the usual familial polyposis, including osteomas of the jaw and dense tumors of the abdominal cavity called desmoids. The relationship between these two disorders has been unclear; however, linkage analysis has demonstrated that the gene for Gardner syndrome maps to the same region of chromosome 5 as does

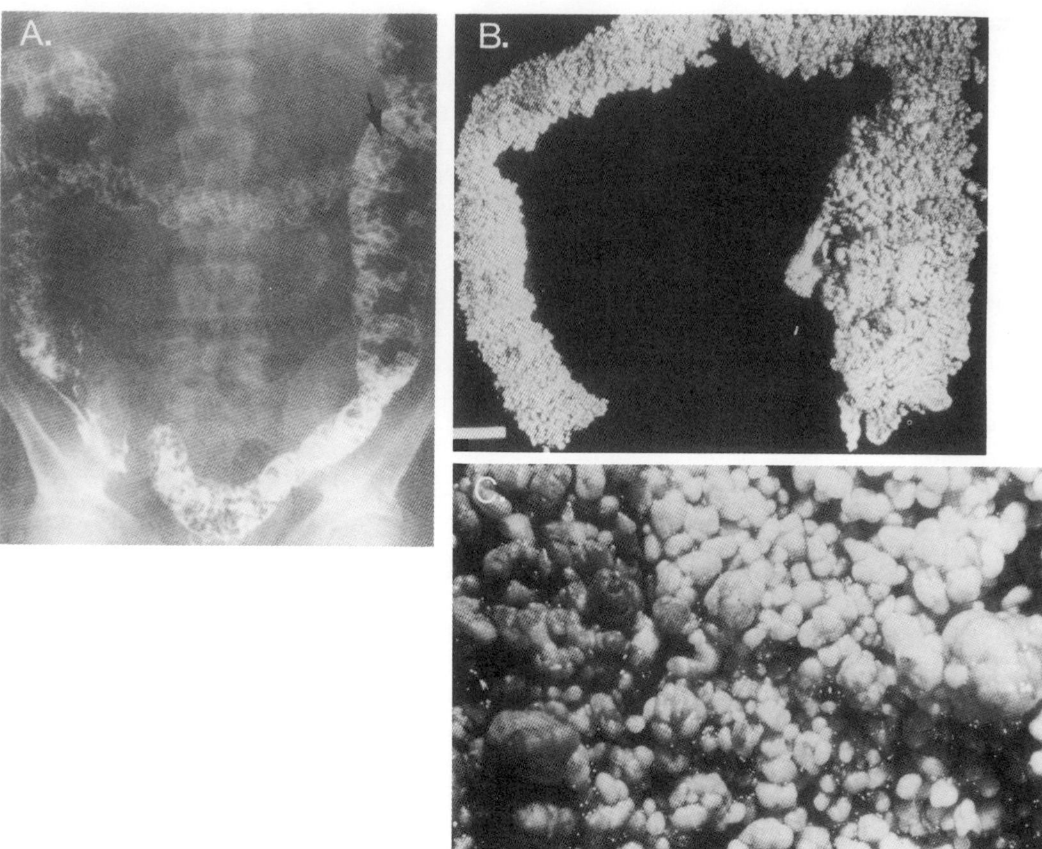

Figure 10.1. Familial polyposis of the colon. A, Barium enema of an affected patient. The colon has been filled with radio-dense barium, and the innumerable polyps in the large bowel appear as filling defects in the lumen. **B**, Excised colon from an affected patient, demonstrating the multiple polyps carpeting the entire length of the large intestine. **C**, Close-up of an excised specimen. Because each polyp has a risk of developing into a carcinoma, it is apparent why a total colectomy is the only successful approach to management. (From Sleisenger MH, Fordtran JS: *Gastrointestinal Disease: Pathophysiology, Diagnosis, Management.* 4th Ed. Philadelphia, WB Saunders, 1989, p. 1502.)

that for familial polyposis, indicating that these are probably allelic disorders.

Neurofibromatosis

This autosomal dominant disorder has already been mentioned in Chapters 3, 5, and 9. There are actually two major forms of neurofibromatosis: von Recklinghausen and bilateral acoustic.

VON RECKLINGHAUSEN NEUROFIBROMATOSIS (NF1)

This disorder, for which photographs are shown in Figure 3.8, is characterized by café au lait spots of the skin, Lisch nodules of the iris, and usually numerous neurofibromas growing from small peripheral nerves, which increase in number and size with age. It is considered a familial cancer syndrome because of the significant (5–10%) risk of malignancy in affected individuals, particularly for optic glioma, a tumor growing from the optic nerve, and for neurofibrosarcoma, a malignant tumor arising from a deeply located "plexiform" neurofibroma.

BILATERAL ACOUSTIC NEUROFIBROMATOSIS (NF2)

This disorder, which is considerably rarer than NF1, bears some superficial similarity due to the occurrence of café au lait spots, although these are usually less frequent in number than in NF1. The major clinical characteristic of the disease is the development of benign neuromas growing from the eighth cranial nerve, which are called acoustic neuromas. These result in hearing loss or dizziness and are frequently bilateral in affected individuals, requiring delicate surgical management. Tumors of brainstem and upper cervical nerve roots are also a frequent occurrence in this disorder. The superficial similarity to NF1 has led to some clinical confusion between the two disorders in the past, but the recent demonstration that NF1 maps to chromosome 17, whereas NF2 maps to chromosome 22, has clarified the issue. Thus, this is an example of locus heterogeneity.

Fanconi Anemia

As an example of an autosomal recessive familial cancer syndrome, Figure 10.2 shows a photograph and pedigree of an individual with this rare disorder. The clinical features include short stature, short or absent thumbs, a triangularly shaped face, learning disability or mental retardation, and darkly pigmented skin. These children characteristically develop anemia in the first few years of life, with eventual reductions in

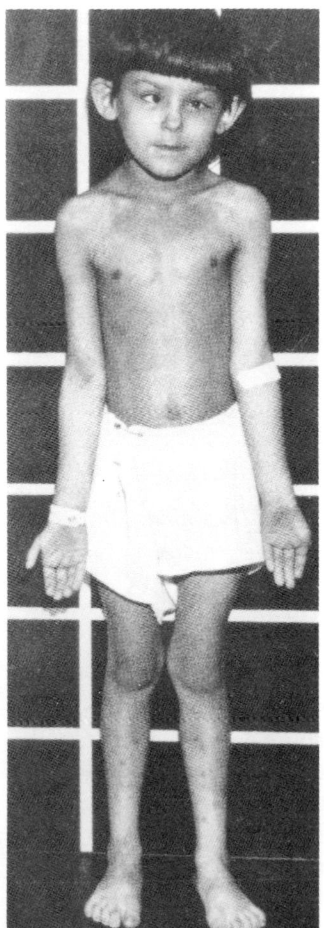

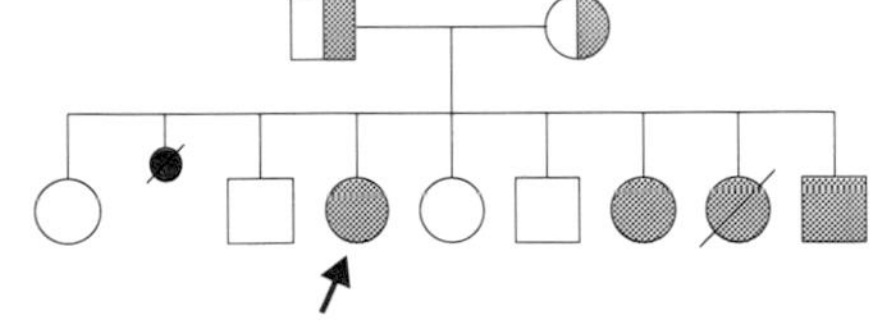

Figure 10.2. A 7-year-old child affected with Fanconi anemia. Note the short stature, darkly pigmented skin, and absence of the left thumb. The pedigree demonstrates the typical autosomal recessive inheritance. (From Smith DW: Fanconi pancytopenia syndrome. J Pediatr 70:479, 1967.)

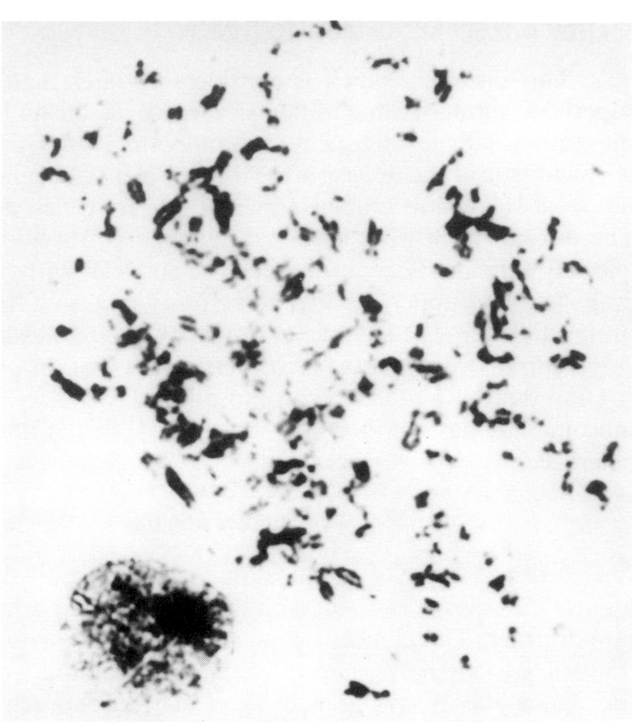

Figure 10.3. Chromosome analysis of a patient with Fanconi anemia. The large number of chromosome breaks is apparent in this metaphase spread after diepoxybutane exposure. (Courtesy of Dr. T. Glover).

red cells, white cells, and platelets. They frequently go on to develop full-blown leukemia. At present the only successful treatment is bone marrow transplantation.

A peculiar characteristic of Fanconi anemia is fragility of the chromosomes in cultured peripheral white cells. When one does a standard karyotype from an individual with this disorder, a high proportion of the chromosomes show spontaneous breaks, and this degree of breakage can be dramatically accentuated by adding chemical agents such as diepoxybutane (Fig. 10.3). This observation suggests that there may be a defect in DNA repair, such that the breaks, which probably occur frequently in normal cells, cannot be effectively reconnected. Presumably this repair problem plays a role in the development of anemia and leukemia. This places Fanconi anemia into a small group of disorders characterized by chromosomal breakage and DNA repair abnormalities, which includes xeroderma pigmentosum, Bloom's syndrome, and ataxia telangiectasia.

THE CLONAL NATURE OF CANCER

A critical question in the understanding of the progression from a normal to a malignant phenotype is whether this reflects a change in the genetic material of a cell or whether cancer is the result of change in the external environment, to which the cell is responding. In the first case, one would expect all of the cells of a tumor to share genetic characteristics of the original transformed cell, that is, to be "monoclonal" (often just designated "clonal"); in the latter case, potentially many cells would be responding simultaneously to the external influence, so the cancer would be polyclonal. The discovery that most cancers are in fact monoclonal, and that therefore cancer is heritable at the cellular level, has been a major factor in reaching the conclusion that changes in DNA sequence of individual cells are responsible for malignant change of those cells.

Several assays have been used for demonstrating this clonality. A very important one was previously described in Chapter 8 and depends upon the inactivation of one X chromosome by the lyonization process in females. Females who have developed various tumors and are heterozygous for the G6PD polymorphism described in Chapter 8 have been investigated. Almost invariably the tumor tissue is found to express one but not both of the G6PD alleles. This is indicative that the tumor arose from a single cell.

In other special situations indications of clonality have been obtained by other means. In certain tumors, characteristic cytogenetic abnormalities are found. An example is the Philadelphia chromosome, which occurs in the malignant cells of the majority of patients with chronic myelogenous leukemia (CML). Figure 10.4 shows an example of the typical balanced translocation between chromosomes 9 and 22 seen in CML; the small shortened chromosome 22 is referred to as the Philadelphia chromosome. The fact that this translocation appears in all of the malignant cells of an individual with CML supports the notion of clonality of the tumor. As we shall see shortly, this conclusion is further strengthened by the demonstration that the translocation activates a growth-promoting gene.

Another example that has allowed the demonstration of clonality in tumors has been provided by leukemias and lymphomas that arise from B cells. As described in Chapter 5, the immunoglobulin genes that code for antibody production undergo rearrangement in B cells, and the specific rearrangement in a particular cell is quite unique, allowing the wide range of antibodies that can be produced. It is possible to use the uniqueness of a particular immunoglobulin gene rearrangement as a marker for clonality, because precisely the same rearrangement is extremely unlikely to occur in two different cells. Figure 10.5 shows how this phenomenon can be used to demonstrate the clonality of a B-cell lymphoma. The analysis depends on the use of the Southern blot to detect a specific rearrangement of immunoglobulin genes. Were the tumor *(lane 2)* not clonal, the

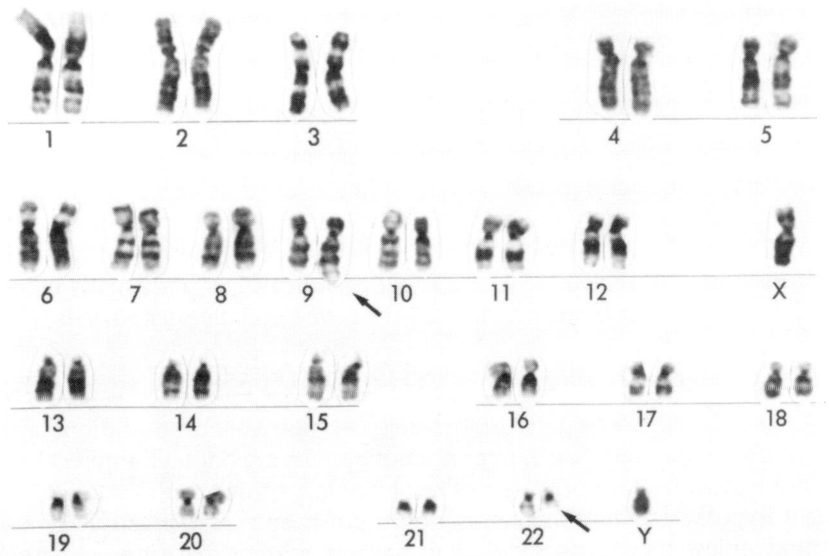

Figure 10.4. Karyotype demonstrating the typical t(9;22) translocation seen in chronic myelogenous leukemia (CML). The shortened chromosome 22 is called the Philadelphia (Ph[1]) chromosome. (Courtesy of Dr. T. Glover.)

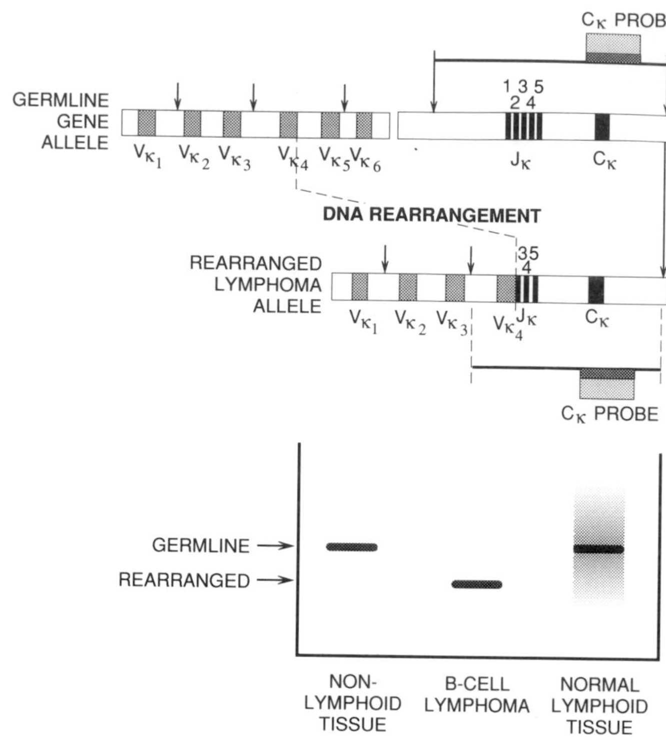

Figure 10.5. Clonality in a B-cell lymphoma. At the *top* is a schematic diagram of the κ light chain gene. As described in Chapter 2, in the germline this gene is unrearranged, but in B cells a DNA rearrangement occurs to generate an expressible gene sequence. Each B cell undergoes an essentially unique rearrangement, thus generating the necessary antibody diversity. *Vertical arrows* indicate the location of restriction sites for the enzyme *Bam*HI. The Southern blot at the *bottom* diagrams the result when nonlymphoid tissue *(lane 1),* a clonal B-cell lymphoma *(lane 2),* or nonclonal lymphoid tissue *(lane 3)* is digested with *Bam*HI and probed with Cκ, which is derived from the constant region of the κ light chain. Nonlymphoid tissue generates a single band whose length is defined by the *Bam*HI sites on either side of Cκ. In a lymphoma derived from a single original B cell, however, the specific signature of that cell will be present in all of the DNA in the tumor, because one particular rearrangement of the κ gene was present in this original transformed cell. Thus, a band different than that in the germline appears. The exact size depends on which Vκ region was used in the particular rearrangement present in the cell responsible for the malignancy. Finding a rearranged band in this situation is an indication of clonality. On the other hand, *lane 3* shows the results of analyzing normal lymphoid tissue; because this is made up of a large number of different rearranged κ genes, as well as some unrearranged alleles, no predominant rearranged band will appear.

blot would have been expected to show a heterogeneous smear of different DNA fragments corresponding to different possible rearrangements, as is seen in *lane 3* for a normal lymph node. However, the lymphoma tissue demonstrates one specific rearranged band, indicating that virtually all of the cells in the lymphoma are derived from one specific precursor B cell.

DOMINANT TRANSFORMING GENES: "ONCOGENES"

The clonality of most tumors suggests that genetic mutations are capable of conferring a malignant phenotype. An area of high interest has been the identification of the genes responsible for this phenomenon. One might hypothesize that organisms would not keep such dangerous genes around unless they performed an important normal function, and one might further hypothesize that their function might involve control of cellular growth. Both of these suppositions turn out to be true. A molecular understanding of these genes has only recently begun to emerge and represents an extremely exciting and promising advance. Pieces of this puzzle have been provided by diverse and unexpected areas of research and require us to take a brief detour into the world of RNA tumor viruses. While such viruses are a rare cause of cancer in humans, it turns out that the study of their biology in other organisms provided a critical clue to an understanding of cancer genetics.

Transforming Retroviruses

Beginning with Peyton Rous' pioneering studies in chickens, a variety of transmissible agents that were capable of inducing cancer were identified in avian and mammalian species. These studies eventually demonstrated that many transmissible agents fell into a class of RNA viruses called retroviruses. The genome of such a virus is composed of single-stranded RNA. Upon entering a cell, as shown in Figure 10.6*A*, a retrovirus is uncoated and the RNA is copied into DNA, using a unique enzyme called reverse transcriptase. This enzyme is carried along with the retrovirus and encoded by it. The DNA copy is then inserted into the host genome. There it may lie quiescent or may be transcribed to generate multiple RNA copies of itself, which can then be packaged, leading to further rounds of infection. A simple diagram of the usual retrovirus genome is shown in Figure 10.6*B* and indicates the presence of three genes: the *gag* gene encodes a core protein of the virus, the *pol* gene encodes reverse transcriptase, and the *env* gene encodes a capsule or envelope protein. The packaging sequence (ψ) is necessary for the transcribed RNA molecule to be assembled into a viral particle.

Characterization of the transforming retroviruses revealed that these carried additional DNA sequences of unclear origin, which appeared to confer their ability to transform infected cells to a malignant phenotype. Using molecular hybridization, a wide variety of independent transforming retroviruses was eventually identified. Their transforming genes were by convention named using a three-letter abbreviation for the virus from which they were originally identified. Thus, for example, the Simian sarcoma virus transforming gene was called *sis*, the avian myelocytomatosis virus was called *myc*, and so on.

Cloning Human Cancer Genes by a Transformation Assay

Retrovirus researchers continued to identify interesting RNA tumor viruses, but because such viruses were not found in human tumors, their relevance to human cancer was open to question. Other researchers began to apply the techniques of molecular biology to a more direct assault on human cancer. If specific mutations in specific genes are capable of causing a malignant phenotype in human cancers, and if those mutations operate dominantly at the cellular level, then the transfer of DNA sequences from a malignant cell to a normal cell might be expected to result in the transformation to a malignant phenotype. A major advance was accomplished in 1981 when three laboratories simultaneously achieved success in this experiment. The basic principle of the experiment is shown in Figure 10.7. The DNA is prepared from a human tumor cell line; for the initial experiments this was a bladder carcinoma called EJ. This DNA was transfected into a nonmalignant mouse fibroblast cell line called 3T3, using the calcium phosphate precipitate method to cause the DNA to enter the cell.

To interpret the results of the experiment, it is essential to have reliable indicators of benign versus malignant cellular phenotype. Previous

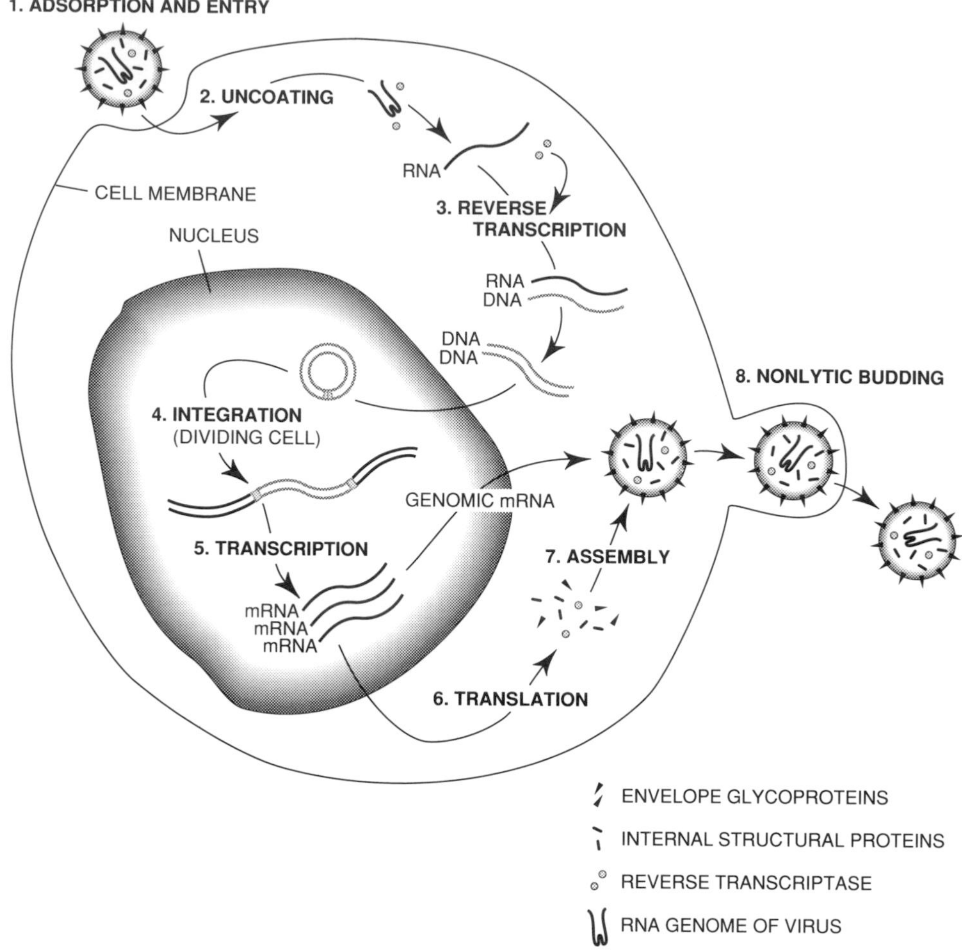

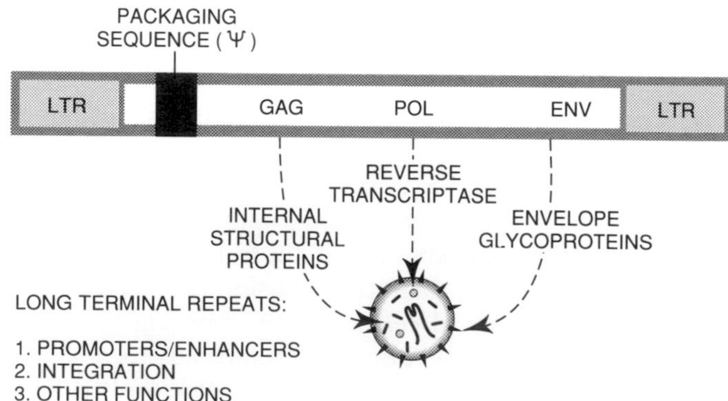

Figure 10.6. **A,** Life cycle of a retrovirus. **B**, Diagram of the genome of a typical retrovirus.

analyses had indicated that normal cells when grown in a culture dish will stop growing when they touch each other (referred to as "contact inhibition"), whereas malignant cells tend to continue to grow in this situation and will pile up on top of each other, forming foci of transformation. A second useful assay is the ability of cells to grow as implants placed into immunologically deficient mice called "nude" mice. Normal cells

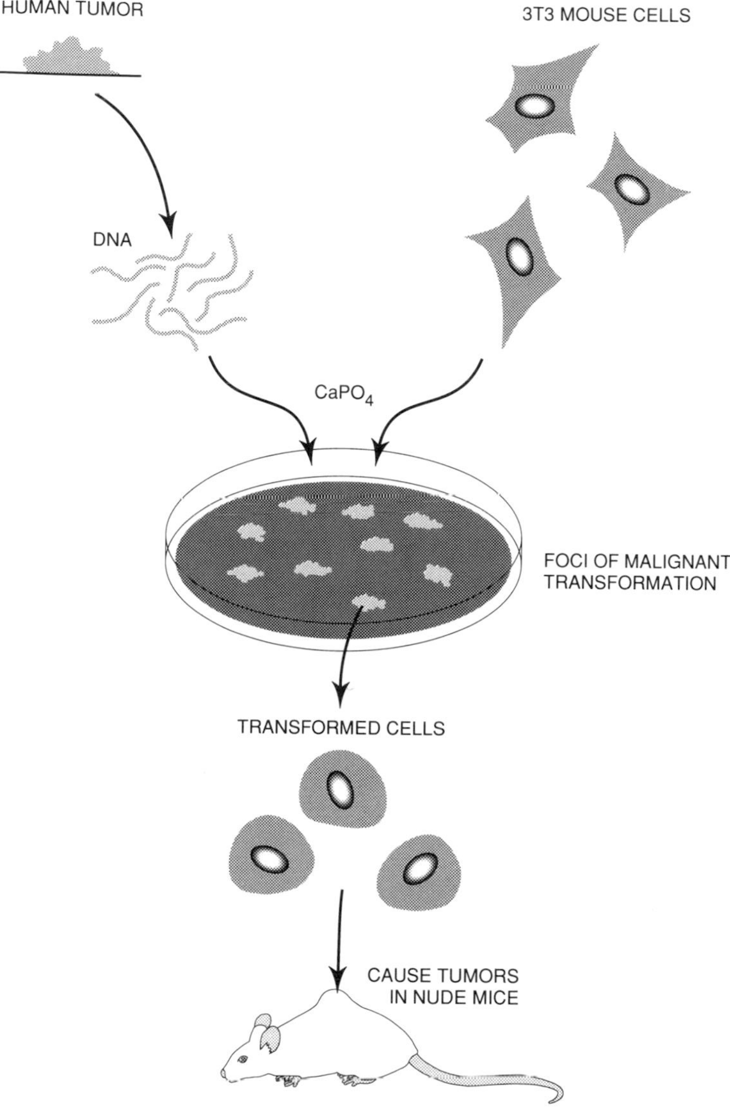

Figure 10.7. Transfection assay of human tumor DNA demonstrating its ability to confer malignant transformation on mouse 3T3 cells. DNA was prepared from the human tumor and transfected into 3T3 cells using calcium phosphate. Cells that received the human cancer gene became transformed and piled up on the plate, forming foci. These transformed cells also created tumors in nude mice when injected subcutaneously, whereas the untransfected 3T3 cells did not.

will not form tumor nodules in this assay, whereas malignant cells will.

When the DNA from the human EJ bladder cancer cell line was introduced into mouse 3T3 cells and the cultures observed, foci of transformed mouse cells appeared. No such foci appeared when DNA from a nonmalignant source was used. This strongly supported the notion that the bladder cancer DNA did contain a dominantly acting cancer gene, which was promptly named an oncogene.

To rescue and molecularly clone this oncogene, a clever strategy diagrammed in Figure 10.8 was used. This approach depends upon the presence of interspersed repetitive *Alu* sequences in human DNA (Chapter 2), which allow its discrimination from mouse DNA. Specifically, those steps were as follows. (*a*) DNA was prepared from a transformed focus, and a Southern blot was carried out. This so-called primary transformant contained many different fragments of human DNA, so that when the Southern blot was probed with human-specific *Alu* sequences, many bands were seen. (*b*) This DNA was used to transform 3T3 cells in a second round. At this point, the majority of the DNA in the transformed foci was mouse in origin, with only a small proportion of human

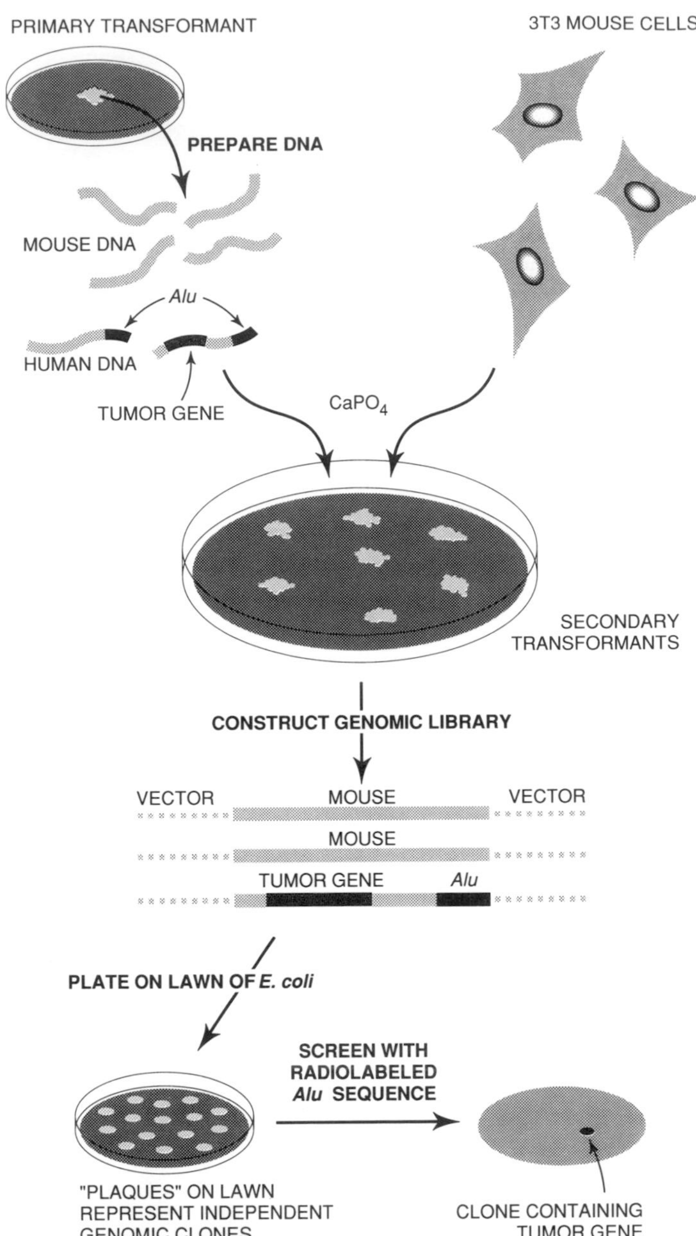

Figure 10.8. Cloning of a dominant oncogene. DNA from a transformed focus (Fig. 10.7) was prepared and mouse 3T3 cells were retransformed with this DNA (a "second round" of transfection, used to limit the amount of human DNA still present in the transformed mouse cells). DNA was then prepared from the resulting foci and cloned into a λ genomic library, as described in Chapter 5. The human sequence then was identified by screening the library with a radioactively labeled sequence corresponding to the human-specific *Alu* repeat element.

DNA still present, containing the oncogene. (*c*) The secondary transformants (foci that appeared after the second round of DNA transfection) also had DNA prepared and were probed with human *Alu* DNA. This time, only one or two hybridizing bands were observed, and a *Bam*HI fragment of 6.6 kb was common to all of the transformants. (*d*) This segment of DNA was molecularly cloned, using the human *Alu* sequence as a probe. The purified DNA, when transfected back into mouse 3T3 cells, yielded foci at extremely high efficiency, indicating that the responsible oncogene had been cloned.

When the sequence of this transforming gene was determined, the research groups found to their surprise that it was extremely similar to the sequence of a retroviral transforming gene called H-*ras*.

How then can these two disparate fields be connected? The answer seems to be that retroviruses, whose life cycle is shown in Figure 10.6*A*, can occasionally do something unusual. After integration into the host genome, a recombination event can occur, such that the retrovirus is excised, carrying along with it a segment of host DNA. If this segment of DNA happens to contain a growth-promoting gene, and if the retrovirus "activates" this gene by use of the strong promoters in the retroviral flanking sequences (called LTRs, see Fig. 10.6*A*), the subsequent infection of other cells by this retrovirus will transform them. Such a virus will provide a growth advantage to cells it infects, and thus will be selected for. Endogenous oncogenes found in human tumors like the EJ bladder cancer, on the other hand, apparently represent activation of a normal growth-promoting gene by a somatic event not involving a virus, but with the same outcome, namely, the development of the malignant phenotype. Normal cellular genes that have this potential are referred to as proto-oncogenes.

Subsequent experiments showed that even the activated *ras* gene, cloned from the bladder cancer cell line, was not able to transform all cell types. Specifically, cultures of human or rodent fibroblasts derived directly from biopsies, without allowing time for "immortalization" to occur in culture (as with 3T3 cells), were not transformed by this gene alone; a combination of two oncogenes, such as *ras* plus *myc*, was able to induce transformation. This apparently indicates that the mouse 3T3 cell line used for the initial experiments is itself not entirely normal. These observations are consistent with the hypothesis that the development of malignancy is an event involving two or more steps. We will return to this theme later.

Cellular Proto-Oncogenes and Their Functions

More than 20 proto-oncogenes have been identified, mostly by their presence in transforming retroviruses. The prediction that these would be genes involved in growth promotion has now been borne out in several specific examples. The *sis* oncogene turns out to be identical to the gene for a subunit of platelet-derived growth factor (PDGF), an important substance produced by platelets and other cells that acts as a strong stimulus to cell growth and division and is involved in normal wound healing. Another class of oncogenes turns out to represent the genes for growth factor receptors, structures that are present on the cell membrane and are activated by the presence of a specific growth factor. Binding of the growth factor to its receptor leads to a chain of events that results in the delivery of a mitogenic signal to the nucleus. The *erb*B1 proto-oncogene is the gene for epidermal growth factor receptor, and the *fms* oncogene encodes the receptor for colony-stimulating factor 1, a growth factor that promotes cell division of a variety of cells in the bone marrow.

Other oncogenes, such as *ras*, seem to play their role by acting in the signal transmission pathway between receptors and the nucleus. A particularly interesting example is *erb*A, which has turned out to be the gene for thyroid hormone receptor. Finally, a number of oncogenes code for proteins that are located in the nucleus and are likely to be involved directly in the regulation of DNA transcription and/or replication. This includes the *myc* and *fos* oncogenes. A summary of these localizations is shown in Figure 10.9.

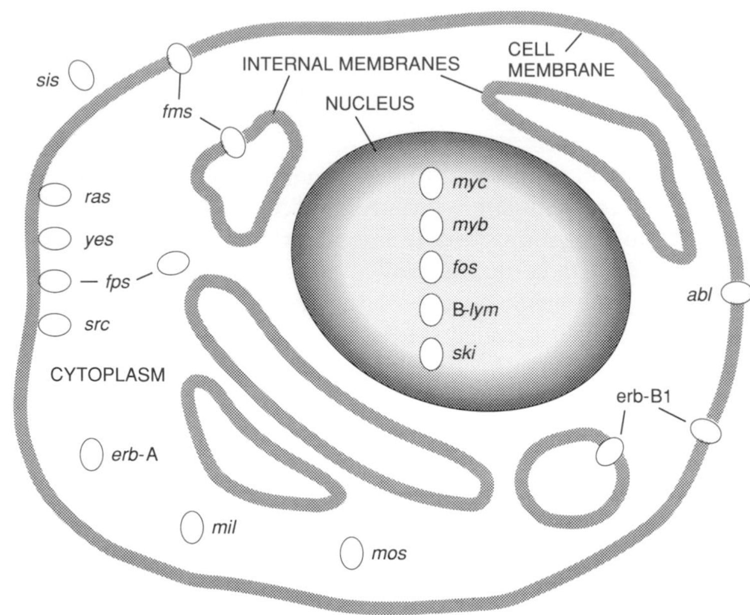

Figure 10.9. Cellular localization of various oncogene protein products. Some, like *sis*, are secreted growth factors; others, like *erb*B1, are growth factor receptors residing in the cellular membrane; others, such as *ras*, are involved in transmission of signals from the membrane to the nucleus, and still others, like *fos* and *myc*, are located in the nucleus itself.

How Are Oncogenes Activated?

If proto-oncogenes represent sequences necessary for normal cell growth, what events are responsible for their activation and subsequent loss of control? Several different mechanisms are possible.

POINT MUTATION

The *ras* gene cloned from human bladder carcinoma cells was initially a puzzle. No major rearrangement of this gene was apparent when comparing it to its normal counterpart in nonmalignant cells. Sequencing the gene revealed a surprisingly subtle abnormality, namely a point mutation in codon 12 of the gene, converting a glycine at that position to a valine.

Analysis of a large number of additional lung and colon tumors using the mouse 3T3 cell transformation assay (Figs. 10.7 and 10.8) also resulted in the cloning of activated H-*ras* genes, as well as activated K-*ras* and N-*ras* genes, which are related members of the same gene family. Remarkably, all of these activated genes contained point mutations in either codon 12 or codon 61 of the *ras* gene, indicating that these positions must be critically important for the normal control of cell proliferation. Recent studies indicate that the *ras* protein product can exist in an active form, which binds to GTP, and an inactive form, which binds GDP. Apparently, these point mutations block the self-conversion of *ras* from the active to the inactive form, and thus allow unregulated cell growth (Fig. 10.10).

AMPLIFICATION

Another plausible mechanism for activation of a proto-oncogene is marked overexpression of its protein product. In some instances this occurs in a cancer cell by actual duplication and manyfold amplification of the DNA sequence encoding such an oncogene. In some instances, a block of DNA as large as several hundred kilobases is tandemly duplicated, with consequent overexpression of the gene within the region. This has occurred, for example, for the N-*myc* gene in some neuroblastomas.

Interestingly, the amplification of the N-*myc* gene in a neuroblastoma is associated with a poorer prognosis.

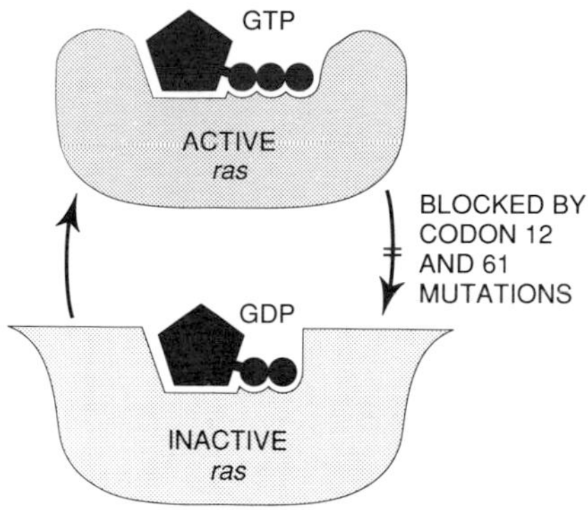

Figure 10.10. Proposed regulation of activation of the *ras* protein. The active form binds GTP, whereas the inactive form binds GDP. Apparently the point mutations in codons 12 and 61, which convert *ras* to a transforming gene, prevent the conversion from the active to the inactive form, so the protein is left in a "locked-on" position.

CHROMOSOME TRANSLOCATION

In some dramatic instances, chromosome translocations occurring at or near a proto-oncogene locus have resulted in activation of the gene. The first such example was found in Burkitt lymphoma, a B-cell tumor, which is rare in the United States but common in parts of Africa. Previous cytogenetic analyses had shown that a high proportion of Burkitt lymphomas are characterized by the appearance of an apparently balanced translocation between chromosomes 8 and 14. Gene mapping efforts carried out in the early 1980s yielded an interesting finding: the *myc* oncogene maps to 8q24, and the immunoglobulin heavy-chain locus maps to 14q32. These are the bands involved in the Burkitt lymphoma translocation (see Fig. 10.11). Subsequent molecular analysis of multiple Burkitt lymphomas has demonstrated that the breakpoints do occur within or near the *myc* locus, and within the immunoglobulin locus. As a result, the *myc* locus is placed close to a gene that is being actively transcribed in a B cell, namely the heavy-chain immunoglobulin gene. Although the exact mechanism of *myc* activation is not clear, and the role of the immunoglobulin enhancer in the event is not consistent, it appears that the *myc* gene is deregulated in an important way by this event, allowing this nuclear oncogene to run amok, resulting in the lymphomatous transformation.

Another example of oncogene activation by chromosome translocation is the Philadelphia chromosome, for which a karyotype is shown in Figure 10.4. Mapping of various cloned oncogenes revealed that the

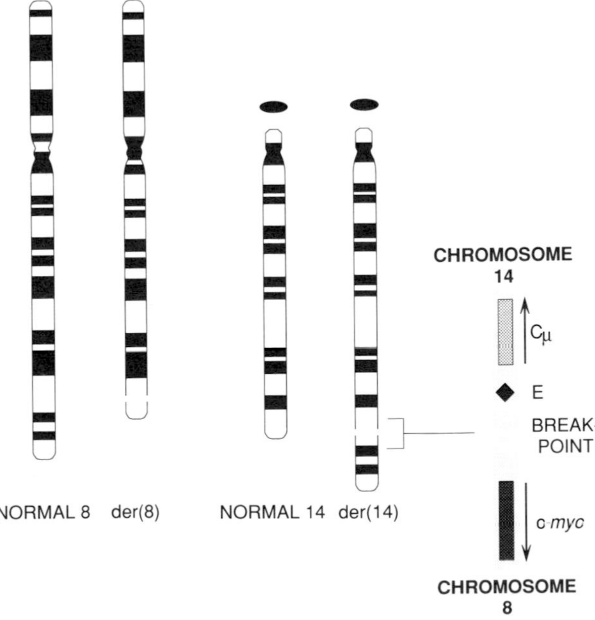

Figure 10.11. Specific translocation seen in Burkitt lymphoma. Most tumors of this sort show a translocation with breakpoints at 8q24 and 14q32. Molecular analysis of these translocations shows that the breakpoint on chromosome 8 is adjacent to or within the *myc* oncogene, whereas the breakpoint on chromosome 14 is in the heavy chain immunoglobulin locus. The exact nature of the rearrangment varies from tumor to tumor, but a typical example is shown in the *right-hand* part of the figure. In some instances, it appears that the enhancer (*E*) of the heavy chain gene (C_μ) may play a role in activating overexpression of the *myc* gene.

abl oncogene maps to the same region of chromosome 9 as the CML breakpoint. Cloning of this region from a CML patient revealed that the *abl* gene is disrupted, placing it under the control of a promoter sequence derived from chromosome 22. The normal function of the chromosome 22 gene, denoted the *bcr* (for breakpoint cluster region) gene, remains to be defined.

In addition to the mechanisms described above, other means of activating proto-oncogenes are also beginning to emerge. A particularly important one involves the truncation of a gene that codes for a cell surface receptor. Some such truncations lead to a receptor that behaves as though it were being continually stimulated by its appropriate growth factor, leading to unrestrained growth.

Do Activated Oncogenes Cause Familial Cancer?

All of the mutations described above, which lead to activation of cellular proto-oncogenes, are somatically acquired events. That is, when the constitutional DNA from patients with these cancers is examined, these mutations are not found, indicating that they were acquired during the process of the development of malignancy. However, as noted above, it seems very likely that more than one such mutational event is required before a transformation to true malignancy occurs. This raises the question as to whether some familial cancer syndromes are due to the germline inheritance of an activated oncogene. Such individuals would be highly predisposed to the development of malignancy should an additional somatic mutation occur.

At the time of this writing, no such mutations have been implicated in the occurrence of human dominant cancer syndromes; however, some evidence has been provided by experiments using transgenic mice. Specifically, in one experiment the *myc* oncogene was placed under the control of the mouse mammary tumor virus promoter, which is known to be induced by steroids in the mouse mammary gland at the time of pregnancy. Transgenic mice were generated with this construct and allowed to breed. While the animals initially appeared normal, females who had experienced one or two pregnancies developed carcinoma of the mammary glands, as shown in Figure 10.12. This pattern was heritable in a dominant fashion, in a manner not too dissimilar from some pedigrees of human breast cancer. Notably, histological examination of breast tissue from transgenic female mice indicated that the vast majority of the breast tissue was normal, with isolated foci of malignant transformation. This provided additional confirmation that an activated *myc* gene alone is not sufficient for the development of malignancy, or all of the breast tissue would have been uniformly transformed. It may well be that a human counterpart of this transgenic mouse model will eventually be uncovered and that germline mutations in cellular proto-oncogenes will be found to play a role in familial cancer. However, the Mendelian familial cancers that have begun to yield to molecular investigation have their mechanism on a somewhat different basis, which we are now ready to address.

TUMOR SUPPRESSOR GENES

As indicated in the opening quotation from Boveri, it is reasonable to hypothesize that there may be genes that normally restrain growth. Inactivation of such genes would be predicted to contribute to the progression toward malignancy. This is an extremely important pathway.

Retinoblastoma and the Knudson Hypothesis

The tumor suppressor gene model has been most thoroughly worked out for hereditary retinoblastoma. Retinoblastoma is a tumor of retinal cells, which develops in children between birth and about age 4 years. It has been known for some time that about half of cases of retinoblastoma are sporadic; these usually involve only one tumor in one eye. The other half of cases, however, occur in an autosomal dominant fashion, usually involve both eyes, and often include more than one tumor in each eye. Treatment is surgical and often involves removal of the affected eye or eyes. Interestingly, those affected with familial retinoblastoma have a high incidence of later developing other malignancies, especially osteosarcoma, a malignant tumor of bone. Figure 10.13 shows typical pedigrees contrasting the familial and sporadic forms.

In Figure 10.14 is shown a section of an eye of an individual affected with the familial form of retinoblastoma. There are two sites of tumor formation visible. However, the entire globe is lined with a layer of retinal cells, and inspection reveals that the vast majority of these retinal cells are behaving in a normal fashion. Nonetheless, all of these cells must carry the retinoblastoma mutation, because this was inherited through the germline from an affected parent. Those cells that have developed into tumors, therefore, must have acquired at least one additional genetic abnormality, which led to their clonal expansion. Because a large number of cells of the retina are at risk, an additional mutation ("second hit") of low frequency would still be sufficient to convert a few of these cells to tumorous behavior.

Nearly 20 years ago Alfred Knudson carried this observation one step further by proposing a specific hypothesis. He proposed that the germline event in familial retinoblastoma is inactivation of one allele of an autosomal tumor suppressor gene. Because the other allele would remain active, only a 50% reduction in the amount of the protein product would occur, which would be expected to have negligible effects. He then proposed that the somatic second hit in retinoblastoma is the loss of the other allele. In a cell in which this had occurred, production of this tumor suppressor protein would be completely abolished, and the result would be unregulated growth. This model leads to a paradoxical conclusion: while inheritance of the tendency to retinoblastoma is dominant, the actual mechanism of tumor development in a specific cell is recessive,

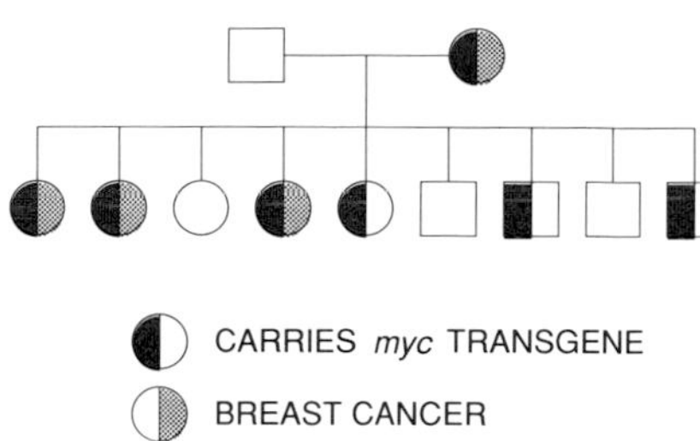

Figure 10.12. Pedigree of a line of transgenic mice carrying an activated *myc* gene. The original founder animal was generated by microinjecting an embryo with a *myc* gene under the control of a steroid inducible promoter that is turned on in mammary tissue during pregnancy. Females carrying the *myc* transgene have a high likelihood of developing breast cancer after pregnancy, whereas males carry the gene but show no phenotype. The resulting mouse pedigree reveals some similarities to the most severe form of human breast cancer (see Table 10.1) and to other familial cancer syndromes.

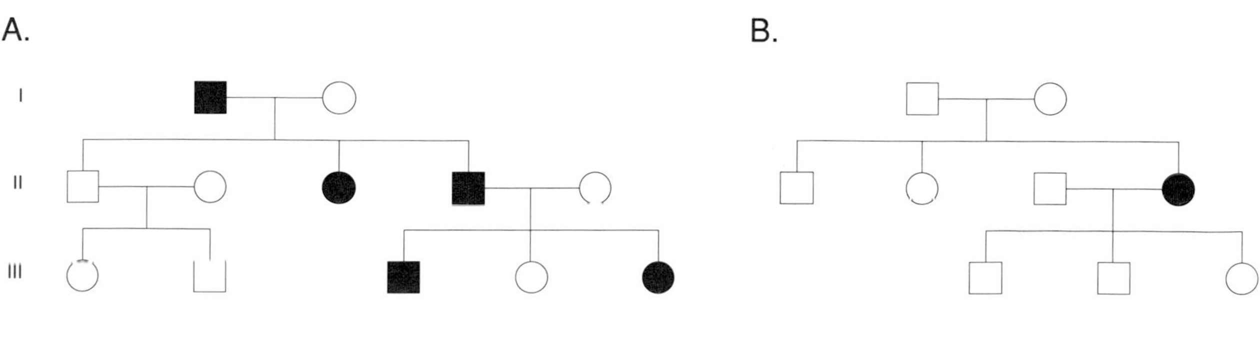

Figure 10.13. Typical pedigrees of retinoblastoma. A, Familial dominantly inherited pattern. In this situation, tumors are usually bilateral and occur at an early age. **B**, Sporadic retinoblastoma. In this situation only one individual in a family is affected, and the tumor is somewhat later in onset and usually unilateral.

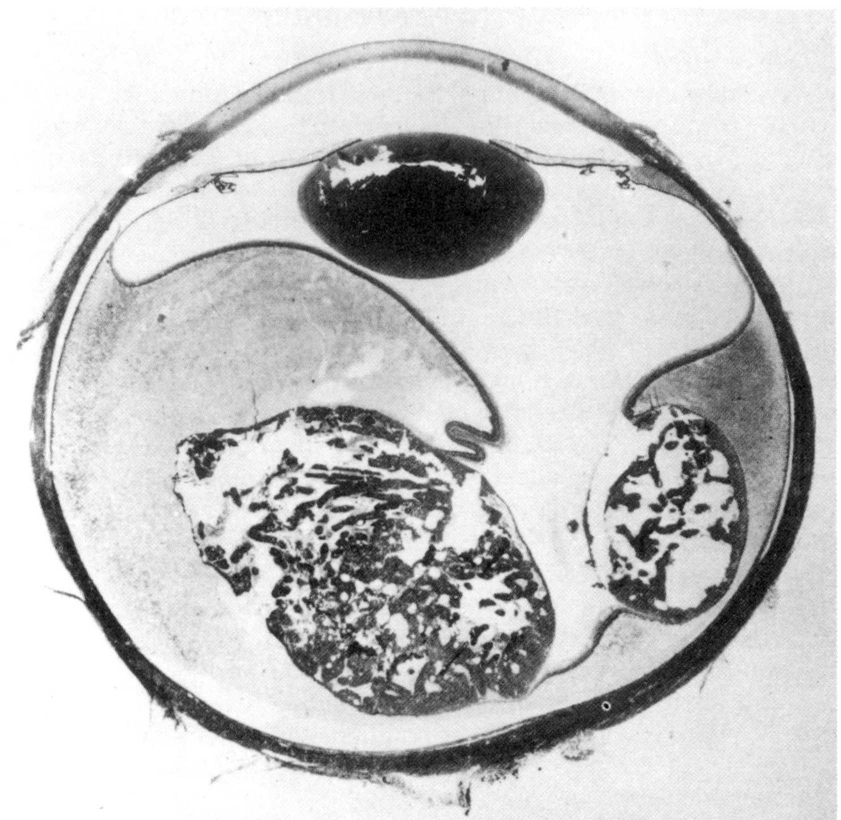

Figure 10.14. **Section of an eye of an individual with familial retinoblastoma.** Note that, although two independent tumors are apparent, the majority of the thin layer of retina (here artifactually separated from the back of the eye in the preparation) is normal. This suggests that tumor formation requires an additional somatic event on top of the germline mutation. (Willis RA (ed): Pathology of Tumours. 3rd Ed. Butterworth, 1960, p 894.)

because tumors appear only when *both* copies of the retinoblastoma gene are inactivated. Thus, tumor suppressor genes are also sometimes called recessive tumor genes. The sporadic cases in this model are proposed to be due to somatic inactivation of *both* alleles in a single retinal cell, without the presence of a germline mutation.

Evidence for the Tumor Suppressor Gene Hypothesis

CYTOGENETIC ANALYSIS

One of the observations that supported Knudson's hypothesis was the identification of rare children with retinoblastoma who also had a variety of birth defects and mental retardation. These were sporadic cases of retinoblastoma, but tumors occurred bilaterally. Careful cytogenetic analysis of most of these patients revealed an interstitial deletion of the long arm of chromosome 13. Figure 10.15 shows some of the deletions identified. Whereas the precise portion of chromosome 13, which is absent, varies from patient to patient, a region of 13q14 is common to all of them. This region, commonly referred to as an SRO (smallest region of overlap), thus seems to be a likely candidate for the location of the retinoblastoma gene. Thus, these unusual patients with cytogenetic deletions had obliterated one copy of the retinoblastoma gene by chromosomal deletion; the deletion was large enough to involve many other genes as well, presumably explaining the other birth defects and mental retardation of these patients.

LINKAGE ANALYSIS OF RETINOBLASTOMA FAMILIES

If the retinoblastoma gene is on 13q14, then one would expect to find linkage to this region in the dominant familial form. A gene in this region of 13q codes for the enzyme esterase D, which is polymorphic at the protein level and therefore usable for linkage. Analyses of a large number of families with retinoblastoma revealed that esterase D and the retinoblastoma gene are extremely closely linked. This evidence supported the notion that the same gene (called RB) is mutated in familial retinoblastoma and is completely deleted in the rarer patients with 13q14 deletions.

GENETIC ANALYSIS OF RETINOBLASTOMA TUMORS

While the above data supported the localization of the retinoblastoma gene to chromosome 13, analysis of tumor tissue itself was necessary to demonstrate that the mechanism of tumor formation involves loss of the normal allele of this gene. There are several mechanisms by which this loss might occur, as shown in Figure 10.16. The simplest would be the loss of the normal chromosome 13 in its entirety. Alternatively, the normal chromosome 13 might be lost, and then the abnormal chromosome 13 duplicated. A more complex mechanism involves mitotic recombination, in which an exchange occurs between homologous chromosomes during mitosis. (Note that, although this is an essential event in meiosis, its occurrence in mitosis was not clearly shown until the investigation of this tumor type.) Finally, the normal chromosome could independently acquire a different mutation in the retinoblastoma gene. The outcome of these events, as well as the effect on a polymorphic DNA marker located close to RB, is diagrammed in Figure 10.16. Note that all of these occurrences except independent mutation would lead to loss of one allele for a closely linked DNA marker in the tumor tissue. Specifically, the allele located on the chromosome carrying the *normal* RB gene

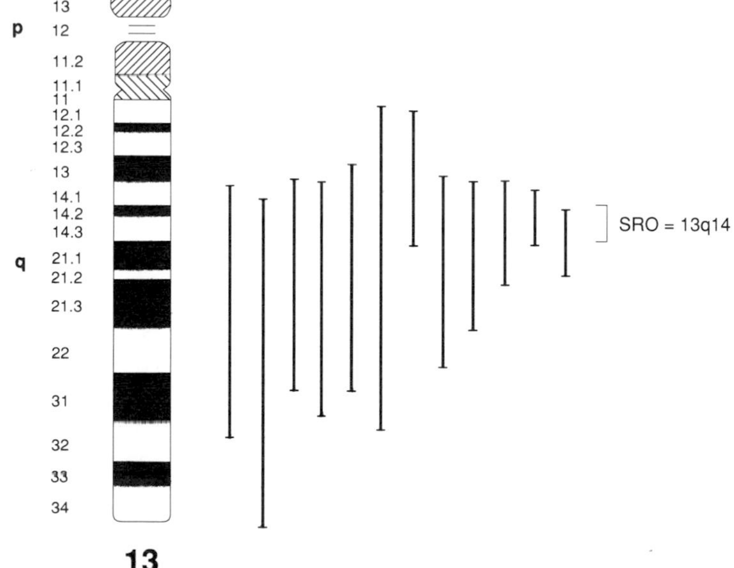

Figure 10.15. Representative examples of chromosome 13 deletions identified in patients with retinoblastoma, birth defects, and mental retardation. While the exact region of chromosome 13 that is deleted varies from patient to patient, all of these have in common a deletion of 13q14 (called the "smallest region of overlap" (*SRO*)), which is therefore likely to contain the retinoblastoma gene.

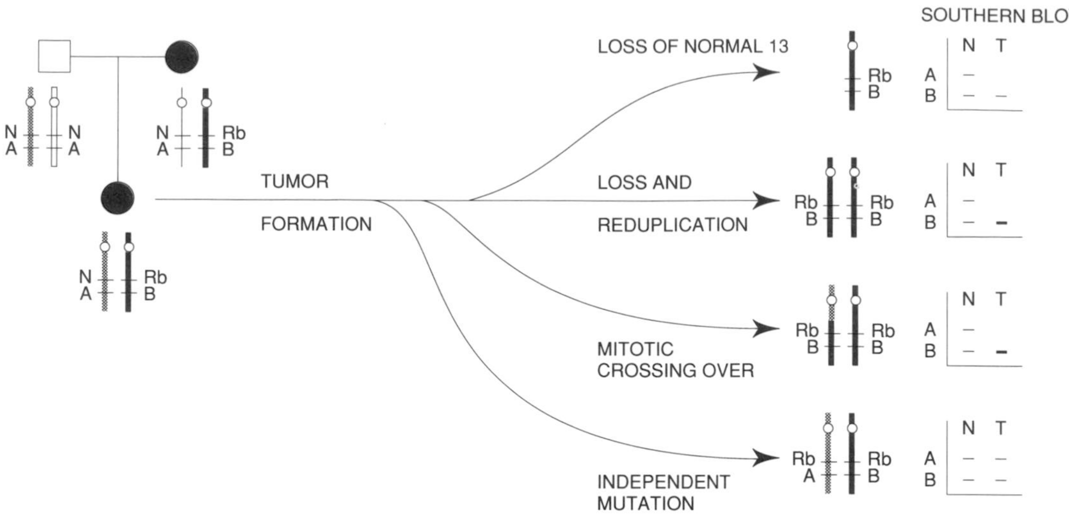

Figure 10.16. Diagram of possible mechanisms for tumor formation in an individual with familial retinoblastoma. On the *left* is shown the pedigree of an affected individual, who has inherited the abnormal (Rb) gene from her affected mother. The four chromosomes of her two parents are drawn to indicate their origin. Just below the retinoblastoma locus a polymorphic marker is also analyzed in this family. The patient is AB at this locus, like her mother, whereas her father is AA. Thus the B allele must be on the chromosome carrying the retinoblastoma disease gene. Tumor formation results when the normal allele (*N*), which this patient inherited from her father, is inactivated. On the *right* are shown four possible ways in which this could occur. In each case, the resulting chromosome 13 arrangement is shown, as well as the results of a Southern blot comparing normal tissue with tumor tissue. Note that in the first three situations the normal allele (A) has been lost in the tumor tissue, which is referred to as reduction to homozygosity for allele B.

would be predicted to disappear in the tumor if one of these mechanisms were operative. This is called "reduction to homozygosity" and can be detected by the use of a Southern blot, comparing constitutional DNA from a retinoblastoma patient to DNA derived from the tumor.

For complete loss of the normal chromosome, with or without duplication of the abnormal chromosome, note that all DNA markers on that chromosome will be reduced to homozygosity. A mitotic recombination, however, will lead to reduction to homozygosity for all markers distal to the site of recombination. If several such events can be detected in independent tumors, it is even possible to obtain a rough idea of where the tumor gene is located, because it must always be reduced to homozygosity in the recombination event.

Careful analysis of retinoblastoma tumors revealed the occurrence of all of these possibilities. By studying families, it was possible to prove that it was always the *normal* chromosome 13 that was lost in tumor formation. Thus, the data agree precisely with the predictions of the Knudson hypothesis and therefore strongly support the presence of a tumor suppressor gene on chromosome 13q14.

Cloning of the Retinoblastoma Gene

All of the above evidence supported the localization of the retinoblastoma (RB) gene in 13q14, close to the esterase D gene. Several researchers proceeded to obtain multiple DNA clones from this region, and eventually a fragment was identified that appeared to have at least one copy deleted in retinoblastoma tumors derived from patients with no cytogenetic abnormality. This piece of genomic DNA was used to obtain a cDNA, following the reverse genetics strategy outlined in Chapter 9. As

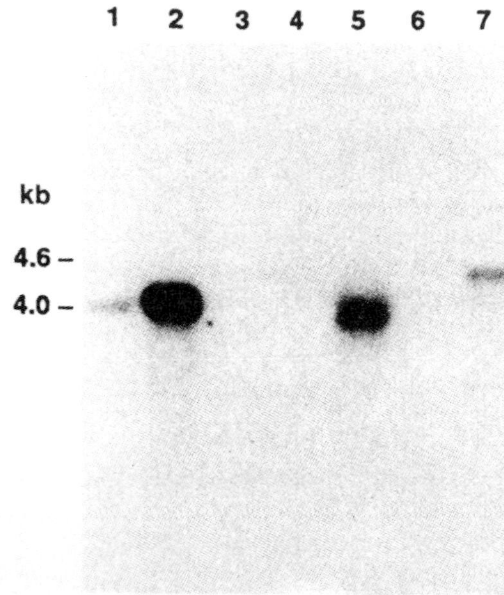

Figure 10.17. Northern blot of RNA from a variety of retinal tumors. The probe used on the Northern blot is a cDNA clone representing the RB gene transcript. *Lanes 1–6* represent RNA samples from six different retinoblastoma tumors, whereas *lane 7* is RNA derived from normal fetal retina. Notice that the normal transcript of this gene is 4.6 kb in length, whereas RNA from the retinoblastoma tumors either completely lacks this transcript (*lanes 3, 4,* and *6*) or contains a shortened abnormal transcript (*lanes 1, 2,* and *5*). Thus, none of the retinoblastoma tumors contain a normal transcript. This indicates that *both* of the alleles of the RB locus are abnormal in these tumors, in accordance with the predictions of the Knudson model. (From Lee WH et al.: Human retinoblastoma susceptibility gene: Cloning, identification, and sequence. Science 235:1394, 1987.)

predicted by the Knudson hypothesis, analysis of retinoblastoma tumors using this cDNA as a probe on Northern blots indicated that in some tumors the message was completely absent, whereas in others an abnormal sized message was seen (Fig. 10.17). In some tumors the messenger RNA appeared normal by Northern blot, but by sequence analysis, point mutations were found. In no instance where careful analysis was carried out was a normal transcript of the gene found in retinoblastoma tumors.

The normal function of the retinoblastoma gene is under active investigation. The protein product of the gene appears to be localized in the nucleus and may well play an important role in regulating the expression of other genes. Somewhat surprisingly, the gene is expressed in a wide variety of tissues, not just the retina. As mentioned above, patients with retinoblastoma who are cured by surgery have a risk of developing other tumors, particularly of bone. Analysis of these bone sarcomas has revealed that a similar mechanism underlies them. There is also growing evidence that this gene may be involved in the genesis of common tumors such as breast cancer and lung cancer, although the lack of apparent increased risk for these tumors in families with dominantly inherited retinoblastoma remains a paradox. The study of this gene now appears to be a good example of the paradigm that the study of rare genetic diseases often sheds light on common diseases as well.

Other Familial Cancer Syndromes

Although the tumor suppressor gene mechanism is best worked out for retinoblastoma, the same mechanism of tumor development has been suggested in several other disorders, using the reduction to homozygosity analysis described above. Familial polyposis coli, described earlier in this chapter, appears to be a case in point, as at least some of the tumors occurring in patients with this disorder appear to have lost the normal allele of this gene on the long arm of chromosome 5. The situation is not simple, however, as other genetic events also seem to be occurring in these colon cancers, as will be described below. Bilateral acoustic neurofibromatosis (NF2) is perhaps a closer situation to retinoblastoma. Here the acoustic neuromas frequently are found to have lost the normal allele of the NF2 gene on chromosome 22, and studies are under way to identify the gene itself. The mechanism of tumor formation in NF1 remains unclear.

A GENERAL MECHANISM FOR CANCER

Several principles can be derived from the information presented in this chapter. There appear to be two major mechanisms for genetically altering a cell in such a way that its growth is increased. These are, in fact, the two mechansims proposed by Boveri in the opening quotation. In fact, if the word "gene" is substituted for "chromosome" in his usage, then that paragraph accurately describes both oncogenes and tumor suppressor genes. We have seen that the activation of proto-oncogenes is a common somatic event in the progression from normal cell to malignant cell. As described above, tumor suppressor genes can also be responsible for dominant familial predisposition to cancer, with loss of the second allele occurring as a somatic event. It is also quite possible, however, for an individual with both alleles normal in the germline to end up losing both of these through somatic mutations. Such is the case, for example, in sporadic retinoblastoma (Fig. 10.13*B*), and also for the instances of breast cancer mentioned above where both alleles of the RB gene appear to be nonfunctional. A recurring theme in these discussions is the fact that more than one mutational event is required to convert a normal cell to a malignant cell. Recently, careful analysis of colon cancer specimens has added stronger evidence to this conclusion. Noted earlier in this chapter is the presence of a putative tumor suppressor gene on chromosome 5,

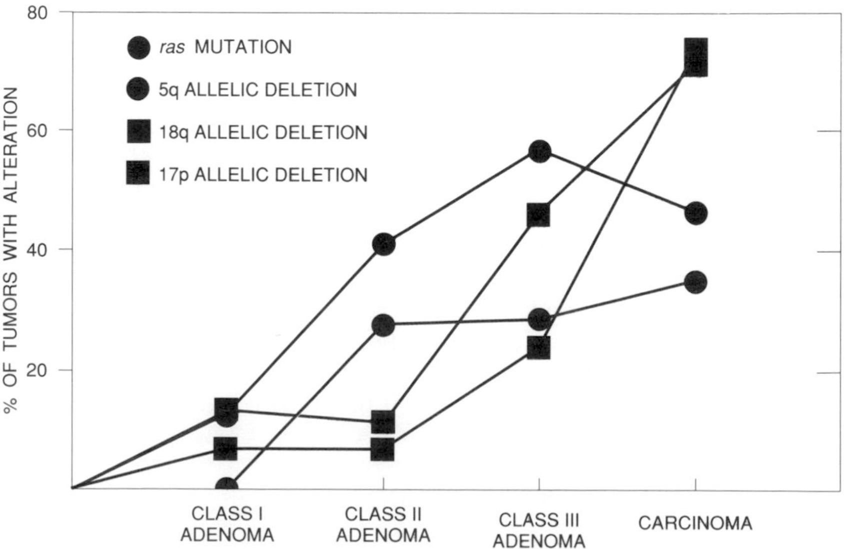

Figure 10.18. Frequency of various mutational events in colon cancer. The percent of tumors with four different genetic abnormalities is shown as a function of the tumor type. Class I adenomas, being the most benign, also have the lowest incidence of genetic abnormalities. As the grade of malignancy increases, so does the number of mutational events. This includes activation of a dominant oncogene *(ras)* as well as inactivation of putative tumor supressor genes on 5q, 18q, and 17p, as deduced by reduction to homozygosity at these loci. (Reprinted with permission from Vogelstein B, Fearon ER, Hamilton SR, et al.: Genetic alterations during colorectal tumor development. The New England Journal of Medicine. 319:525, 1988.)

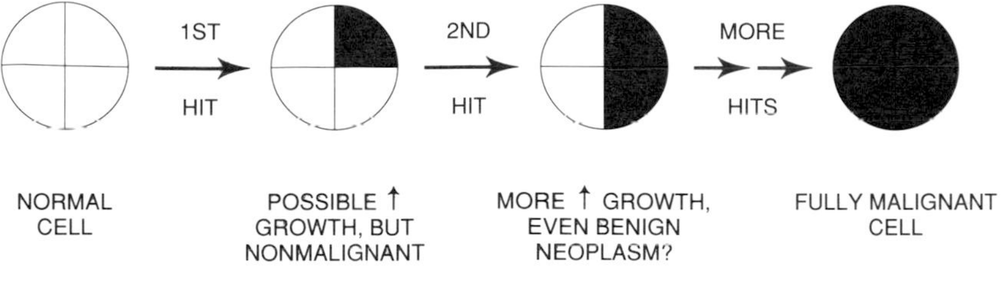

"HITS" MAY BE:

1. ACTIVATION OF DOMINANTLY ACTING ONCOGENES
2. LOSS OF AN ALLELE OF RECESSIVELY ACTING TUMOR SUPPRESSOR GENES
3. ENVIRONMENTAL INFLUENCES
4. OTHER

Figure 10.19. Diagram of the multistep origin of cancer. At least two genetic events appear to be necessary to convert a cell to a neoplastic phenotype, and for some tissues more than two events may be required. A germline predisposition to cancer can be thought of as shifting this diagram one step to the right.

which seems to be involved in colon cancer, at least in familial cases. The activation of the H-*ras* and K-*ras* proto-oncogenes was also described as a relatively frequent event in colon tumors. By careful survey of polymorphic markers from other chromosomes, it also has been discovered that reduction to homozygosity is frequently seen in colon cancers using probes from chromosomes 17p and 18q. Figure 10.18 shows a summary of the abnormalities found in a number of colon tumors ranging from the most benign histological pattern (class I adenoma) to a full-blown carcinoma. Note that the more benign categories have fewer genetic lesions, but the specific genetic lesion varies from tumor to tumor. In general, the more malignant tumors have acquired a larger number of mutational events. In some instances, it is even possible histologically to see that a carcinoma is arising out of an area of epithelium with a lower grade neoplasm, and to show that the more malignant area has acquired an additional genetic event.

This evidence then supports a multistep hypothesis for the origins of cancer, as shown in Figure 10.19. Beginning on the *left* is a normal cell, which possesses the appropriate mechanism to inhibit its own growth when that is appropriate. A single mutation may somewhat increase the ability of that cell to proliferate, but appears insufficient to completely escape the normal control mechanisms. There are, in fact, compelling reasons why this must be so. Given the fact that there are an estimated 10^{14} cells in the body, and during replication a mutation rate of 10^{-6} per gene is estimated to occur, clearly, cancer would be an everyday event if a single mutation were sufficient. The single mutated cell may have a completely normal phenotype or may possess a slight growth advantage allowing it to survive, propagate, and eventually acquire another mutation. With each step along the way, the cell acquires somewhat more autonomy and is therefore able to propagate better than its neighbors. Eventually a point is reached at which the cell is able to grow in spite of signals that would normally arrest its proliferation, and it can then go on to destroy neighboring tissues and spread to other parts of the body.

Familial cancer syndromes, representing germline predisposition to cancer, can be thought of as shifting this diagram one step to the right. The individual with such a germline mutation still is made up of cells that behave essentially normally. However, they are one step closer to malignancy than in the normal situation, and hence a higher risk applies. Two great challenges of the coming years are to understand how this process applies to the genesis of common cancers, and to take the rapidly increasing understanding of the nature of oncogenes and tumor suppressor genes and use them to develop effective therapies against cancer.

SUGGESTED READINGS

Bishop JM: The molecular genetics of cancer. Science 235:305, 1987.

Friend SH, Dryja TP, Weinberg RA: Oncogenes and tumor-suppressing genes. N Engl J Med 318:618, 1988.

Knudson AG: Genetics of human cancer. Annu Rev Genet 20:231, 1986.

Varmus HE: The molecular genetics of cellular oncogenes. Annu Rev Genet 18:553, 1984.

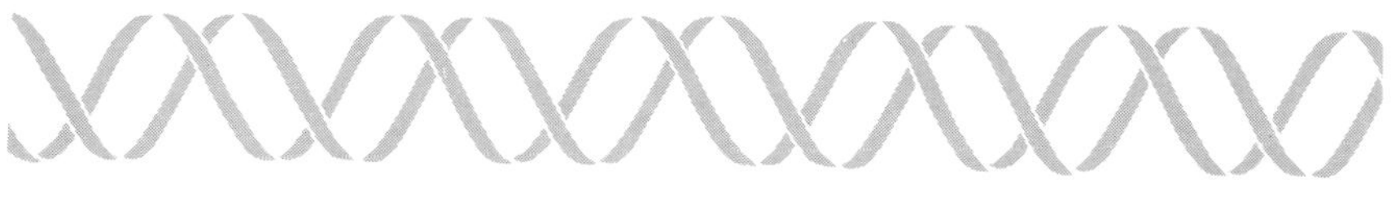

10/ Study Questions

1/ Name four mechanisms implicated in the activation of a proto-oncogene.

2/ Explain why a patient with sporadic retinoblastoma usually has a single focus of tumor growing in one eye, while hereditary retinoblastoma often occurs in both eyes or at multiple sites in one eye.

3/ Why do genetic disorders of DNA repair seem to predispose to malignancy?

4/ What is the risk of breast cancer to a woman whose older sister had cancer of both breasts at age 25 years?

11

Clinical Genetics

"Previously the geneticist was like a 'bookie,' offering odds for any given event to happen. Now that the geneticist is involved in the 'action,' i.e., diagnosis and therapy, he has changed from a bookie to a fixer."

—Roy D. Schmickel
(From Genetic counseling as a form of medical counseling. Univ Michigan Med Ctr J 40:38–43, 1974)

The clinical management of patients with genetic diseases involves many of the same techniques of diagnosis and treatment that are used in other medical specialties. Unique to medical genetics, however, is its focus on the prevention and/or avoidance of disease. Central to this approach are the concept of presymptomatic diagnosis, the provision of genetic counseling, the use of genetic screening programs, and prenatal diagnosis. Each of these topics will be covered in this chapter.

HOW TO TAKE A FAMILY HISTORY—AND WHY

The family history plays a central role in clinical genetics. Properly obtained and interpreted, it is one of the most useful and accessible tools available to physicians caring for patients with genetic diseases.

Before considering how to take a family history, it is worth considering why. First, the family history provides an aid to reaching a correct *diagnosis.* W. H., discussed in Chapter 3 (Fig. 3.3), began to develop chest pain typical of angina pectoris at the age of 25 years, but the diagnosis of coronary artery disease was dismissed because of his age. At age 30 when W. H. experienced his first heart attack, the diagnosis was again missed because it was felt he was too young to have a heart attack. Had his physician obtained the family history of early coronary artery disease in his father and paternal uncle, it should have led to the correct diagnosis of familial hypercholesterolemia and to the early institution of appropriate therapy.

Another illustrative case is that of a 26-year-old woman who sought medical attention because of a breast lump. Her physician recommended that she return in 6 months for a follow-up examination;

the physician did not seriously consider breast cancer because of her young age. Four months later, she again sought medical attention because of severe back pain which proved to be the result of bone metastases from her breast cancer. Family history, subsequently obtained, revealed that one sister had died at age 26 years of metastatic breast cancer and another sister had undergone bilateral mastectomy for breast cancer at age 28 years. Obtaining this simple family history would have alerted the physician to consider seriously the diagnosis of breast cancer and to pursue appropriate studies.

The second reason for obtaining the family history is to determine an accurate *prognosis.* The case of R. B. illustrates the usefulness of the family history in both making a correct diagnosis and providing appropriate prognosis, or information about the future course of the disease. She was referred to the Medical Genetics Clinic at the age of 52 years because of a 5-year history of involuntary movements (chorea) thought to represent Huntington disease. Her movement disorder did indeed resemble Huntington disease, but she did not show any signs of dementia or mental deterioration. A family history, shown in Figure 11.1, revealed that several relatives on her mother's side of the family suffered from a similar illness, suggesting that her disorder was inherited in an autosomal dominant fashion. Strikingly, however, none of these affected individuals developed any signs of dementia, nor did they have a shortened life span. Both of these latter observations are incompatible with the diagnosis of Huntington disease and would suggest that in this family there is a benign form of chorea quite different from Huntington disease in its clinical severity and prognosis. Although many autosomal dominant diseases show a great deal of variability, family history suggested that in this family this particular neurologic movement disorder was fairly constant in its expression in various affected family members. Therefore, it provided useful information upon which to base accurate diagnosis and prognosis.

The third and most important use of the family history is for the *presymptomatic diagnosis of genetic disease and the prevention or avoidance of clinical disease.* Correct interpretation of family history information allows one to offer genetic counseling to individuals or families at risk, and it allows the early diagnosis and therapy of genetic diseases. Specifically, it allows the physician to concentrate intervention in a

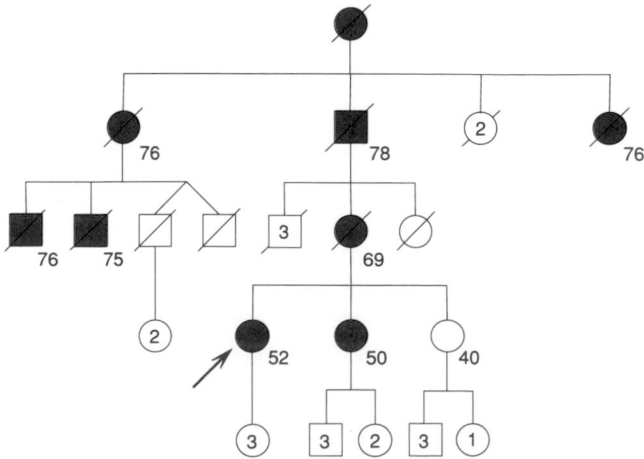

Figure 11.1. Pedigree of a family with benign autosomal dominant chorea. Affected individuals are indicated by the *red symbols.* See text for discussion.

small defined population at high risk. It should be clear that this opportunity also involves a responsibility to extend medical services beyond the individual patient to other family members at risk of disease. Several examples will illustrate these principles.

Once the diagnosis of familial hypercholesterolemia was made in W. H., all of his living first degree relatives could be identified as being at high (50%) risk of this same disease. Although the disease is common (1/500), the risk among W. H.'s first degree relatives is 250 times higher than in the general population. Because early intervention may retard the progress of atherosclerosis, children of affected individuals are the ones in whom we should focus preventive measures. All three of W. H.'s children, although entirely healthy, were affected with familial hypercholesterolemia on the basis of blood lipid measurements. Dietary and subsequently drug therapy was instituted at ages 2, 6, and 9 years with normalization of serum cholesterol levels in all three children. Hopefully, such early intervention should slow the progress of their disease.

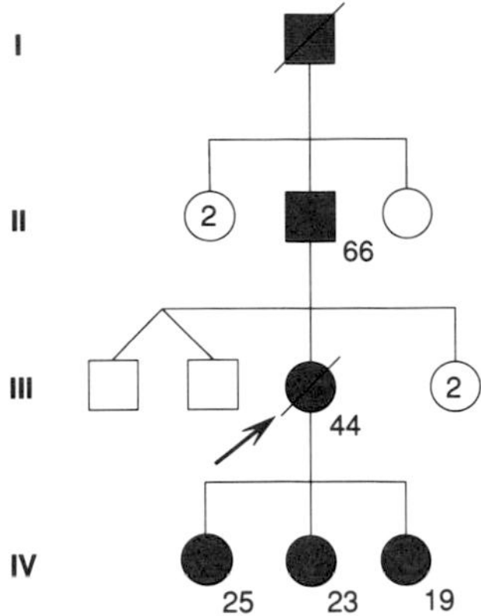

Figure 11.2. Pedigree of a family with familial polyposis of the colon. See text for discussion.

Familial polyposis of the colon provides another unique opportunity to apply the results of the family history to early intervention (Fig. 11.2). The proband had a massive hemorrhage from her large bowel at age 42 years and was discovered to have multiple polyps and cancer of the colon; she died 18 months later of metastases. Her father had undergone removal of the colon for colon cancer and was alive at age 66 years; his father had died of colon cancer. The surgeon caring for this family obtained radiographic and endoscopic studies on the three daughters of the proband. The eldest underwent colectomy at age 18 upon the discovery of multiple polyps in her colon. The middle daughter appeared to be normal when examined at age 16, but was found to have multiple polyps when reexamined at age 18 and underwent total colectomy. The youngest daughter was found to be affected at the age of 16 and underwent colectomy. Although the removal of the colon is a fairly drastic surgical procedure in an adolescent, it prevented the virtual certainty of colon cancer in these young women at risk. With the mapping of the gene for familial polyposis to chromosome 5, DNA markers may now be available for early diagnosis in family members at risk.

Familial polyposis is usually diagnosed in the second decade of life and cancer of the colon usually develops in the third and fourth decades, approximately 30 years earlier than this cancer develops in the general population (Fig. 11.3). However, some families show an earlier age of onset and, once again, a careful family history may prove very useful in prevention of disease. F. H. was diagnosed as having multiple polyposis at the age of 17 years, was found to have cancer of the colon at age 23 and died shortly thereafter of metastatic disease. Among his three children, two had rectal bleeding before the age of 10 years and were shown to have multiple polyps in their colon. Their primary physician was planning to evaluate them further in their late teens. However, because of the very early age of onset of multiple polyposis in this family and of colon cancer in the proband, it was felt that these two children were at high risk of developing colon cancer in their teens as did their father. Therefore, both underwent total colectomy at age 10 years; fortunately, no cancers were found in the colon at the time of surgery. Applying information obtained from the family history led to more aggressive therapy and earlier intervention in this particular family than would be true in the average family with familial polyposis.

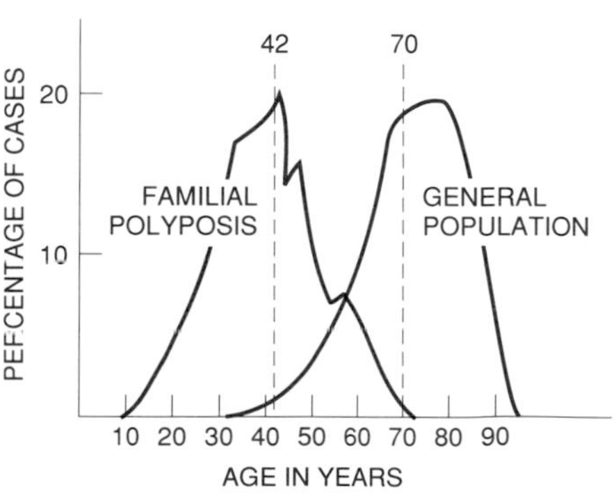

Figure 11.3. Age distribution of cancer of the colon in individuals with familial polyposis of the colon and in the general population. (From Bussey HJR: *Familial Polyposis Coli.* Baltimore, Johns Hopkins University Press, 1975.)

The pedigree shown in Figure 11.4 illustrates the application of family history information to the prevention of a common cancer. C.

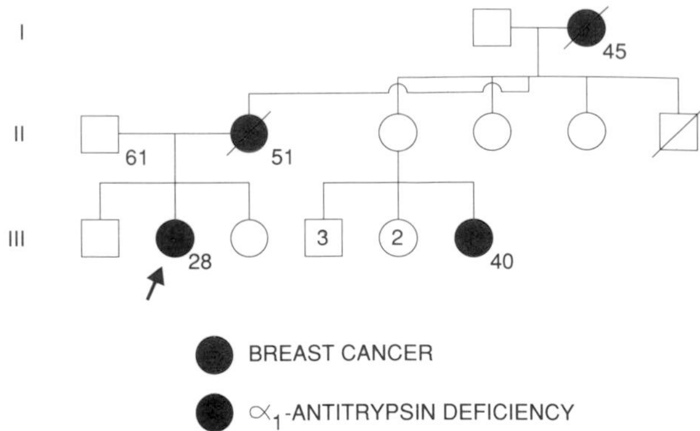

Figure 11.4. Pedigree of a woman with α_1-antitrypsin deficiency. Note, however, that the probands' mother, maternal grandmother, and a maternal first cousin (indicated by the *red circles*) had early-onset breast cancer.

R. was referred to the Medical Genetics Clinic for genetic counseling regarding α_1-antitrypsin deficiency. However, family history also revealed that her mother had died of breast cancer at the age of 51 years, 11 years after the cancer had been diagnosed. Her maternal grandmother developed breast cancer at age 41 and a maternal cousin had recently been discovered to have breast cancer at the age of 40. These three close relatives with premenopausal onset of breast cancer suggest that in this family the risk of developing breast cancer is at least three times higher than in the general population. Therefore, it would be appropriate for C. R. to obtain a mammogram immediately and to have more frequent and more thorough follow-up for the detection of breast cancer than would be advised for a young woman without this family history. Approximately half of all breast cancers have metastasized by the time they are diagnosed by physical examination, but only about 10% of those detected by mammography have metastasized at the time of diagnosis. Therefore, a more aggressive screening program to detect this condition at an early stage when it is treatable is highly recommended based on the information obtained from a simple family history.

Finally, the family history may also provide information that helps in understanding the nature of a given disease. For example, R. B., discussed above, has a movement disorder that is clearly familial. Without having obtained the family history, one would not have known whether this disorder was an acquired illness or a genetic one.

How to Take a Family History

The salient points of the family history are listed in Table 11.1. The family history need not be lengthy, but it must be thoughtful. Most importantly, it must be relevant to the clinical problem at hand.

Table 11.1. Taking the Family History

1. Make it relevant to the "Present Illness."
2. Ask about early-onset preventable diseases.
3. Specifically ask about all first degree relatives.
4. Ask about informative relatives.
5. Record racial and ethnic background.
6. Inquire about consanguinity.
7. Keep it up-to-date.

Although the family history is usually included among that miscellany of items including "Past Medical History," "Social History," and "Review of Systems," it is most relevant and most useful when it is a part of the "Present Illness." Thus, in obtaining the family history one should ask about the same or related diseases found in the index case or patient, rather than about a list of diseases of "familial tendency." If the patient has suspected heart disease, then one should ask whether any other family members have heart disease or have related conditions known to be associated with heart disease such as diabetes mellitus and hypertension. The rote inquiry about any family history of diseases ranging from allergy and asthma to tuberculosis may impress the patient with the physician's memory for a list of diseases, or worse, lull the physician into thinking he or she has obtained a family history, but it rarely yields useful information. An exception to the above dictum is asking about preventable or treatable diseases. Therefore, in addition to asking about diseases related to the patient's current problem, it is worthwhile asking about hypertension, early coronary artery disease, early onset of cancer, or death early in life from any cause. In this way one can detect individuals at greater-than-average risk for common diseases such as hypertension, coronary artery disease, and cancer.

One must ask specifically about first degree relatives (parents, siblings, and children) who share 50% of their genes with the index case. One should ask about their age and state of health, and if they have died, the age and cause of death. One must ask specifically about infant deaths because these are sometimes not reported. In many cases, information that certain relatives are unaffected can be helpful, as will be discussed below. When one is dealing with a known genetic disease, it is essential to ask about informative relatives. For example, one should inquire about male relatives on the mother's side of the family when dealing with an X-linked recessive disease. In contrast, one should specifically focus on siblings when one is dealing with an autosomal recessive disease, and on all first degree relatives on the affected side of the family in the case of an autosomal dominant disease. In the course of obtaining such information, the physician is demonstrating his or her responsibility beyond the individual patient. Information obtained on these other relatives may be used to provide them early intervention or prevention of disease.

Because some genetic diseases show striking differences in their frequency in different racial and ethnic groups (e.g., Tay-Sachs disease, sickle cell anemia, thalassemias, cystic fibrosis), it is useful to record the racial and ethnic background of the family. Although there is strong pressure to eliminate references to race when it is inappropriate, it does not appear that the cause of social justice is served by omitting such potentially important medical information. Finally, although consanguinity is uncommon in the United States, one should also ask about this possibility among parents of an individual suspected of having a rare, autosomal recessive disease.

The family history is frequently deferred in an emergency situation. However, when such information could be helpful in diagnosis, it should be remembered that it takes only a minute to ask whether or not the patient has a family history of related illness. The family history is not static. As individuals get older, the chances increase that they will manifest genetic diseases of late onset. As families at risk of having children with genetic diseases have more children, more information can be obtained. Thus, family history information must be updated.

The pedigree shown in Figure 11.5 indicates the importance of reliable negative information. A young physician and his wife (indicated by the *arrows*) sought genetic counseling because the wife's sister (II-1) had a son with Duchenne muscular dystrophy. The *top half* of the figure (*A*) shows the family history information available at the time of their initial contact with our clinic. On the basis of this information, it is impossible to determine whether the affected boy's disease is the result of a new mutation or has been inherited from a carrier mother. If the latter were the case, the physician's wife would be at increased risk of also being a carrier and of having a child with Duchenne muscular dystrophy. The *bottom half* of the figure (*B*) shows the information obtained at the time the couple actually came for counseling and had had an opportunity to obtain more detailed family history. It is intuitive from the larger pedigree that it is unlikely that the wife's mother (I-2) is a carrier of Duchenne muscular dystrophy because she has five sons who are unaffected. Thus, it is unlikely that either of her two daughters are carriers and much more likely that the affected child's disease is the result of a new mutation. Using Bayes' theorem (discussed below), such "intuitions" can be translated mathematically into more accurate assessment of risk for couples seeking counseling.

As discussed above, the obligations of the physician should extend beyond the individual patient at least to the patient's relatives who might be at risk of a genetic disease and in whom genetic counseling or early intervention might be applicable. This is well illustrated in the cases of familial hypercholesterolemia and familial polyposis of the colon, discussed above, and is shown in Figure 11.6, for a family with Duchenne muscular dystrophy. The man who sought genetic counseling is not at risk of transmitting the disease to his children because he is a healthy 27-year-old and therefore cannot be carrying the mutant allele.

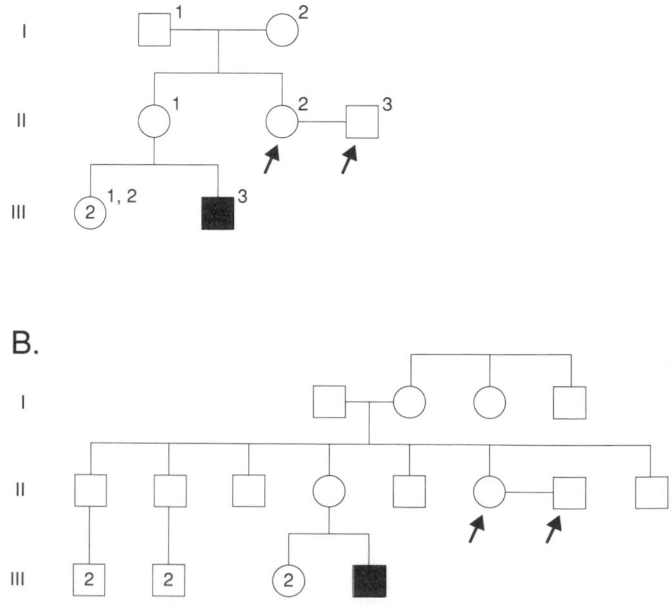

Figure 11.5. Pedigree of a family with a sporadic case of Duchenne muscular dystrophy. The *top half* of the figure (**A**) indicates the information available at the time of initial contact with the clinic and the *bottom half* of the figure (**B**) indicates the family history obtained at the time of the actual genetic counseling. Note the five unaffected males in generation II. The consultands are indicated by the *arrows*.

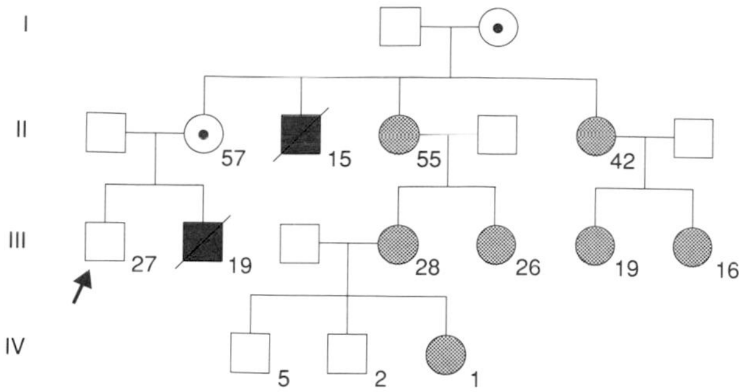

Figure 11.6. Pedigree of a family with Duchenne muscular dystrophy. Note the female relatives (indicated by the *shaded symbols*) who are at risk of being carriers of this X-linked disease.

However, from the family history it is clear that he has several maternal relatives, aunts, cousins, and nieces, who are at risk and should be informed that genetic counseling and carrier detection tests are available. With the cloning of the dystrophin gene (see Chapter 9) and the availability of DNA probes, highly accurate carrier detection and prenatal diagnosis for this disease are now available.

Family histories have also been obtained for a variety of nonmedical purposes and have been recorded in unusual ways. Figure 11.7 shows the first of six paintings from William Hogarth's famous series, "Marriage a la Mode." The fathers of the bride and groom are negotiating the financial aspects of the marriage contract. One father has a scroll in which the family tree arises from the umbilicus of a knightly ancestor. Presumably, the quality of this pedigree is worth money. Figure 11.8 shows a portion of the pedigree of Queen Elizabeth I of England. This 33-foot-long parchment scroll modestly traces the queen's ancestry back to Adam and Eve. The pedigree, exhibited at Hatfield House, north of London, where Elizabeth spent her childhood and adolescence, is depicted in artistic heraldic symbols. Finally, genetics, like any other aspect of science and medicine, can be abused for evil ends.

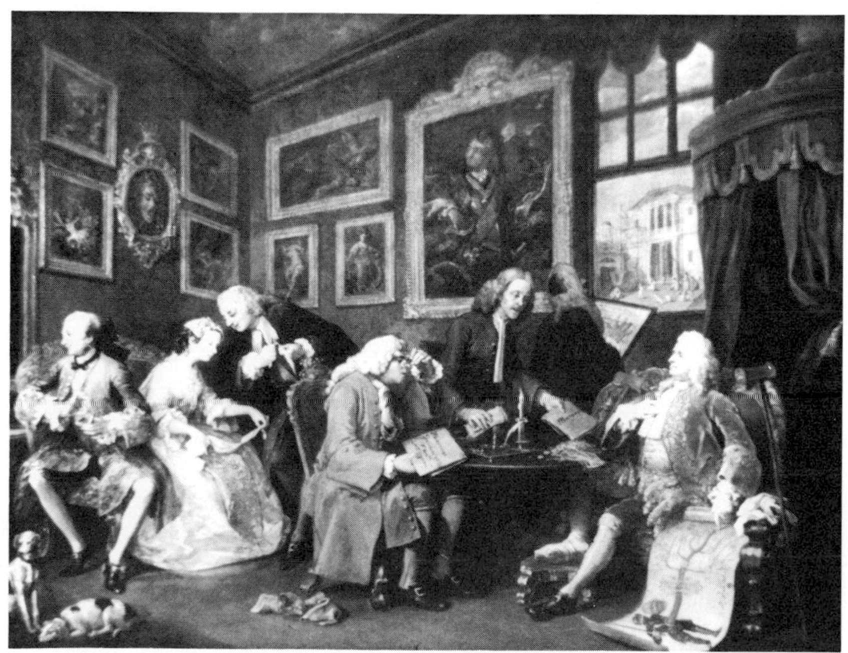

Figure 11.7. "Marriage a la Mode" by William Hogarth. Note the pedigree on the scroll in the *lower right-hand corner* of the painting. This is the first of a series of six paintings that hang in the National Gallery in London.

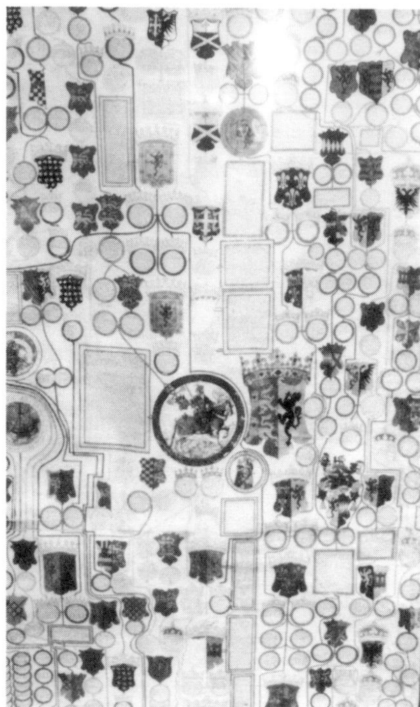

Figure 11.8. Portions of a pedigree of Queen Elizabeth I of England. The large heraldic symbol in the center indicates William the Conqueror. The scroll is displayed at Hatfield House, north of London. (Reproduced with permission of the curator of Hatfield House.)

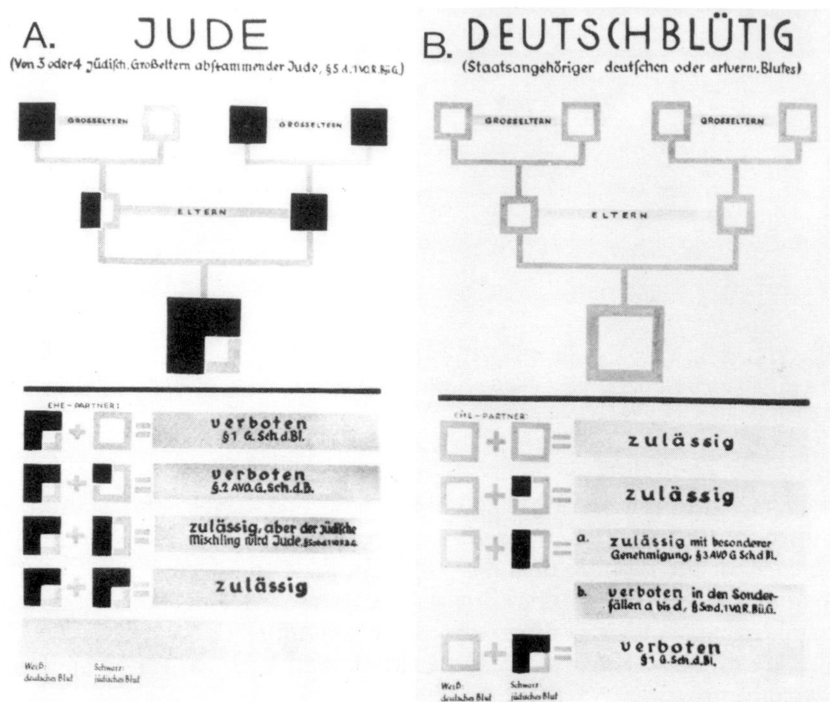

Figure 11.9. Schematic pedigrees from the Nuremberg Racial Laws of 1935 defining Jewishness (A) or German (B) background. (Reprinted with permission from the archives of Yad Vashem in Jerusalem.)

Figure 11.9 shows two schematic pedigrees taken from the notorious Nuremberg Racial Laws of 1935 illustrating the Nazis' view of what determined Jewishness or Aryan background and what kind of marriages were allowed, allowed only under special circumstances, or strictly forbidden.

GENETIC COUNSELING

Genetic counseling is a process of communication, the intent of which is to provide individuals and families having a genetic disease or at risk of such a disease with information about their condition and to provide information that would allow couples at risk to make informed reproductive decisions. The following definition of genetic counseling was adopted by the American Society of Human Genetics in 1975 (From Ad hoc Committee on Genetic Counseling (Epstein CJ, Chairman): Genetic counseling. Am J Hum Genet 27:240–242, 1975. Published by The University of Chicago.)

> Genetic counseling is a communication process which deals with the human problems associated with the occurrence, or the risk of occurrence, of a genetic disorder in a family. This process involves an attempt by one or more appropriately trained persons to help the individual or family to (1) comprehend the medical facts, including the diagnosis, probable course of the disorder, and the available management; (2) appreciate the way heredity contributes to the disorder, and the risk of recurrence in specified relatives; (3) understand the alternatives for dealing with the risk of recurrence; (4) choose the course of action which seems to them appropriate in view of their risk, their family goals, and their ethical and religious standards, and to act in accordance with that

decision; and (5) to make the best possible adjustment to the disorder in an affected family member and/or to the risk of recurrence of that disorder.

Indications for Genetic Counseling

The indications for genetic counseling are listed in Table 11.2. Although the value of genetic counseling for patients and families with known or suspected hereditary diseases is widely recognized by the medical community, the role of genetic counseling in other settings can be equally important. Birth defects and/or mental retardation can occur as part of single gene syndromes or chromosomal disorders, or may result from the interplay of genetic and environmental factors. In every case, accurate diagnostic evaluation and genetic counseling are important parts of patient management and may prevent recurrence in other family members. Pregnancy in women over 35 years of age is associated with an increased risk of Down syndrome (see Fig. 8.16) and other trisomies, and genetic counseling and prenatal diagnosis should be offered to such women. Certain viral infections, such as rubella (German measles), and drugs, such as retinoic acid derivatives used for treating cystic acne and anticonvulsants used for treating epilepsies, are known to be teratogenic. Although not strictly genetic, counseling should be provided for women exposed to potential teratogens during their pregnancy. Finally, as described in Chapter 4, the offspring of consanguineous matings are at increased risk of being homozygous for rare mutant alleles and thus being affected with rare autosomal recessive diseases. The magnitude of this risk varies considerably among different ethnic, religious, and racial groups. There is also a theoretical increased risk for polygenic disorders. It should be noted that for all pregnancies there is a risk of approximately 3% that the child will be born with a serious genetic disease or birth defect. Empirically, the risk to offspring of first cousin matings has been found to be two to three times as great.

Information Conveyed in Genetic Counseling

Table 11.3 lists the major kinds of information we feel are necessary to provide in genetic counseling. Each will be discussed below.

THE MAGNITUDE OF THE RECURRENCE RISK

In order to provide accurate genetic counseling, it is usually necessary to make a correct diagnosis of the condition for which the couple

Table 11.2. Indications for Genetic Counseling

1. Known or suspected hereditary disease in a patient or family
2. Birth defects
3. Unexplained mental retardation
4. Advanced maternal age
5. Teratogen exposure
6. Consanguinity

Table 11.3. Information Conveyed in Genetic Counseling

1. The **magnitude** of the **recurrence risk**
2. The **burden** of the **disease** on the patient and the family
3. The possibility of **modification** of either the burden or the risk
4. Anticipated **future developments**

or family is at risk. Therefore, it is essential to examine the affected patient whenever possible, to obtain appropriate laboratory analysis where it is helpful, and to obtain all relevant medical records. Genetic heterogeneity, discussed in Chapter 3, can create significant problems in reaching an accurate genetic diagnosis. Figure 11.10 shows two infants with rather similar appearing forms of short-limbed dwarfism. The child on the *left* has achondroplasia, which is inherited as an autosomal dominant trait and is often the result of a new mutation, both parents being entirely normal. In this situation, the recurrence risk to these parents is virtually zero. In contrast, the child on the *right* has diastrophic dwarfism, which is inherited as an autosomal recessive trait. Therefore, the phenotypically normal parents of this child face a 25% risk that each subsequent child will be affected with this form of dwarfism. An inaccurate diagnosis in such a case could result in disastrously inaccurate counseling.

Variable expressivity also creates problems in diagnosis. In the case of neurofibromatosis, manifestations may be so mild in some individuals that they may appear to be normal and an affected child may be thought to represent a new mutation. In neurofibromatosis, approximately half of probands have phenotypically normal parents; their disease is thought to result from new mutations. However, a thorough examination of both parents is necessary to ensure that one or the other is not mildly affected. If a parent were affected, then each subsequent child would face a 50% chance of being affected rather than the extremely low risk of a second new mutation.

The inheritance pattern of a condition is often established by careful analysis of the pedigree. When the family history is not informative, but a definite diagnosis can be made, McKusick's *Mendelian Inheritance in Man* is extremely helpful. This catalog provides information on the inheritance patterns of about 4000 Mendelian traits.

Bayes' Theorem. In order to provide optimal assessment of recurrence risk, it is important to use all available information, especially when the genotype of the individual being counseled (the consultand) is unknown. This is commonly accomplished by applying Bayes' theorem,

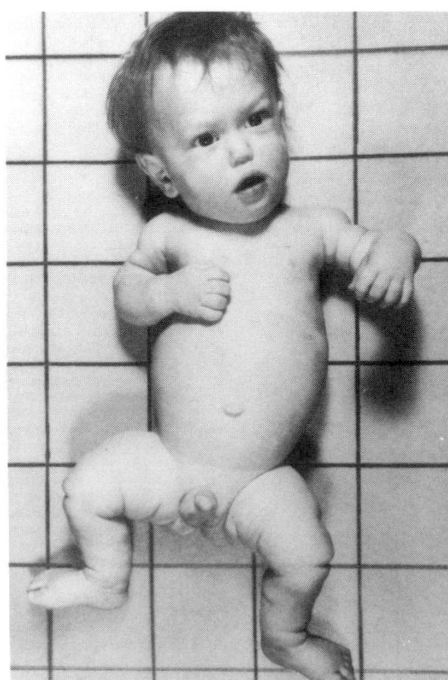

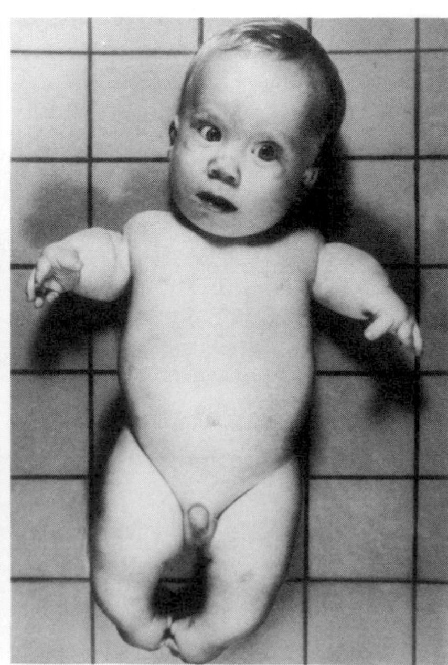

Figure 11.10. Two infants with short-limbed dwarfism. The child on the *left* has achondroplasia. Note the large head, scooped out bridge of the nose, and shortening of the proximal portion of the limbs. The infant on the *right* has diastrophic dwarfism. Note the abnormal thumbs and clubbed feet. The head size is not enlarged. (From McKusick VA: The nosology of genetic disease. In McKusick VA, Claiborne R (eds): *Medical Genetics.* New York, HP Publishing Co., 1973.)

named after an 18th century English scientist-cleric. Bayes' theorem states that, given some event (E) that has already occurred and a set of all causes (C_i) that might have caused that event, then the probability of a particular cause C_i, given E (written as $Pr(C_i | E)$), is equal to the probability of that cause, $Pr(C_i)$, multiplied by the probability of the event given that cause, $Pr(E | C_i)$, all divided by the total probability of event E. The probability of event E is equal to the sum of the probabilities of the potential causes multiplied by the probability of event E given each cause. This can be written as an equation:

$$Pr(C_i | E) = \frac{Pr(C_i)Pr(E | C_i)}{Pr(E)}$$

where

$$Pr(E) = \sum_i Pr(C_i)Pr(E | C_i)$$

As Bayes' theorem is commonly used in medical genetics, E usually refers to an individual who is affected or unaffected with a given disease or who has a certain test result, and C_i refers to a specific genotype. The application of Bayes' theorem can be appreciated by looking first at a simple example (Table 11.4). What is the probability that a clinically unaffected brother of a child with an autosomal recessive disorder, such as cystic fibrosis, is a carrier for that disorder? In this case, the event E is that the brother is clinically unaffected and the cause C_i is that he is heterozygous for the cystic fibrosis allele. At conception, prior to any knowledge of his phenotype, the probability that the brother is a carrier is ½, as shown in the mating diagram for autosomal recessive traits (Fig. 3.12). This is called the **prior probability.** The probability that he would be clinically normal, *given* that he is a carrier, is equal to 1; this is called the **conditional probability.** The **joint probability** that he is a carrier *and* that he is clinically normal, given that he is a carrier, is the product of the prior and conditional probabilities, or ½ × 1 = ½. This is the numerator of the equation shown above. The denominator of the equation is the sum of the probabilities of the different ways in which he could be clinically normal, basically the sum of the different joint probabilities. The first of these ways is that defined in the numerator, i.e., he is a carrier. The second possibility is that he is homozygous normal, which has a prior probability of ¼. If he is homozygous normal, then the conditional probability that he will be clinically normal is of course 1. The joint probability that he would be genotypically homozygous normal *and* clinically normal is ¼ × 1 = ¼. Therefore, the sum of the joint probabilities by which he could be clinically normal is ½ + ¼ or ¾. Now the **posterior probability,** or relative likelihood, that he is a carrier, given that he is clinically normal, $Pr(C_i | E)$, is ½ ÷ ¾ or ⅔.

Table 11.4. Bayesian Calculation of Carrier Status for an Autosomal Recessive Trait

	Unaffected Sibling Is a Heterozygous Carrier	Unaffected Sibling Is Homozygous Normal
Prior probability	½	¼
Conditional probability	1	1
Joint probability	½ × 1 = ½	¼ × 1 = ¼
Posterior probability	$\frac{½}{½ + ¼} = ⅔$	$\frac{¼}{¼ + ½} = ⅓$

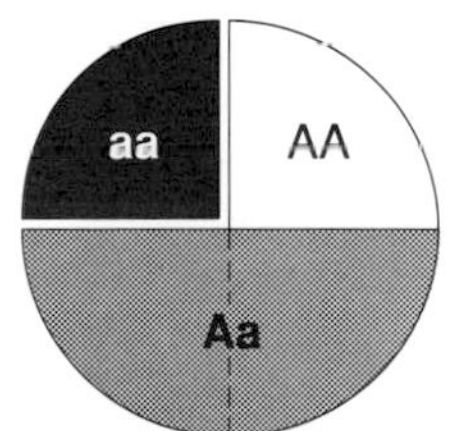

Figure 11.11. Pie diagram showing that the probability that a clinically normal sibling is a carrier (Aa) of an autosomal recessive trait is ¾ ÷ ¾ or ⅔.

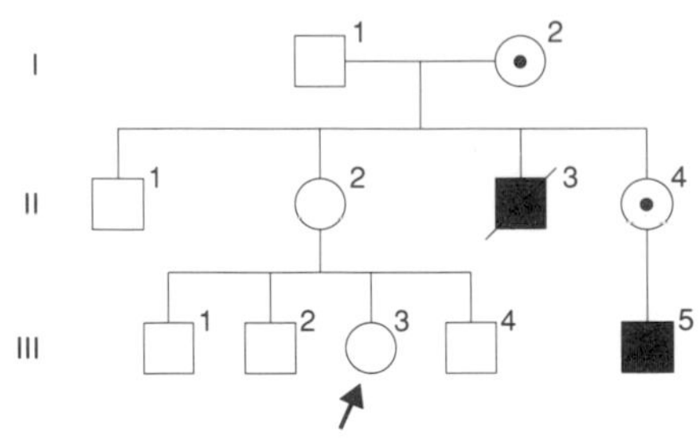

Figure 11.12. Pedigree of a family with Duchenne muscular dystrophy. See text for discussion.

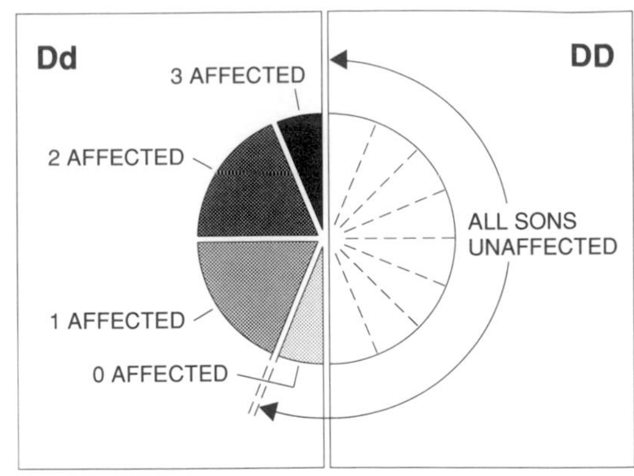

Figure 11.13. Pie diagram showing the probability that II-2 in the pedigree shown in Figure 11.12 is a carrier of Duchenne muscular dystrophy (Dd) given that she has three normal sons. The prior probability of being homozygous normal (DD) is indicated by the *unfilled half* of the *circle.* The prior probability of being a carrier (Dd) is indicated by the *red portion* of the *circle.* From the binomial expansion, it can be calculated that the probability that II-2 would have three affected sons, given that she is a carrier, is ⅛, the probability of having two affected sons is ⅜, the probability of having one affected son is ⅜, and the probability of having no affected sons is ⅛ (*light red* segment). Among the nine segments representing all unaffected sons, the *light red* segment represents one of nine. The probability that II-2 is a carrier (Dd) given that she has three unaffected sons is ⅑.

This conclusion can also be seen graphically by examining the "pie diagram" shown in Figure 11.11. There are three slices of pie corresponding to a clinically normal phenotype, two of these represent the heterozygous carrier genotype Aa. In summary, the unaffected brother had an a priori probability of being a carrier of ½. However, by using the additional information that he is clinically normal, the estimate of the probability that he is a carrier can be refined and given as ⅔. In this simple example this refinement does not make much of a difference; however, in the next example (Figs. 11.12 and 11.13, and Table 11.5) the importance of the application of Bayes' theorem will become clearer.

The pedigree shown in Figure 11.12 is a family with Duchenne muscular dystrophy. The consultand, III-3, whose genotype is unknown, seeks counseling as to whether she is a carrier of the gene for Duchenne muscular dystrophy. In order to be a carrier, she must have inherited the mutant allele from her mother. Therefore, the first question to be answered is whether her mother, II-2, is a carrier. On the basis of the pedigree information one can conclude that I-2 and II-4 are obligate carriers of Duchenne muscular dystrophy. I-2 has an affected son and affected grandson and II-4 has an affected brother and an affected son. Thus, the a priori risk (prior probability) that II-2 is a carrier is ½. However, additional information is available (an event E has occurred); namely, she has had three unaffected sons. If II-2 is a carrier, the conditional probability that any son she has will be affected (or unaffected)

Table 11.5. Bayesian Calculation of Carrier Status for an X-linked Recessive Trait[a]

	II-2 Is a Heterozygous Carrier	II-2 Is Homozygous Normal
Prior probability	$\frac{1}{2}$	$\frac{1}{2}$
Conditional probability	$(\frac{1}{2})^3 = \frac{1}{8}$	$(1)^3 = 1$
Joint probability	$\frac{1}{2} \times \frac{1}{8} = \frac{1}{16}$	$\frac{1}{2} \times 1 = \frac{1}{2}$
Posterior probability	$\frac{\frac{1}{16}}{\frac{1}{16} + \frac{1}{2}} = \frac{1}{9}$	$\frac{\frac{1}{2}}{\frac{1}{2} + \frac{1}{16}} = \frac{8}{9}$

[a]See pedigree in Figure 11.13.

with Duchenne muscular dystrophy is ½ and the probability that all three sons will be unaffected is the product of the probabilities of these independent events, $(\frac{1}{2})^3$ or ⅛. The joint probability that she is a carrier *and* all three sons will be unaffected is ½ × ⅛ or 1/16. The conditional probability that she would have three normal sons if she were not a carrier, i.e., were homozygous normal, would of course be 1, and the joint probability of being homozygous normal and having three normal sons is ½ × 1^3 = ½. Therefore, the posterior probability that II-2 is a carrier given that she has three normal sons is:

$$\frac{(\frac{1}{2})(\frac{1}{8})}{(\frac{1}{2})(\frac{1}{8}) + (\frac{1}{2})(1)} = \frac{\frac{1}{16}}{\frac{1}{16} + \frac{8}{16}} = \frac{1}{9}.$$

By taking into account the three normal sons, the probability that II-2 is a carrier of Duchenne muscular dystrophy is decreased from ½ to 1/9. The probability that the consultand III-3 is a carrier of Duchenne muscular dystrophy is ½ the risk that her mother is a carrier or 1/18, approximately 5%. Without using the additional information about her three unaffected brothers her risk would have been given as ¼ or 25%.

Bayes' theorem is used in various settings in clinical genetics. In the examples discussed above, it allows refinement of recurrence risk estimates in genetic counseling. Bayes' theorem is also used in the interpretation of genetic screening test results and, consciously or unconsciously, in virtually all medical diagnostic decisions. Thus, an effort to understand the principle of Bayes' theorem and to use it in appropriate settings is an important part of medical practice.

THE BURDEN OF DISEASE ON THE PATIENT AND THE FAMILY

It is a common misunderstanding that conveying the magnitude of recurrence risk of a genetic disease is the sum total of genetic counseling, but this is only the first step. Without an understanding of the burden of the disease in question the magnitude of risk may be almost meaningless. The burden of the disease refers to the clinical, financial, social, and emotional burden imposed upon the patient and/or the family. For example, brachydactyly (Fig. 11.14) includes a group of conditions characterized by short fingers and toes. These disorders are inherited in an autosomal dominant fashion so that each offspring of an affected individual has a high recurrence risk, namely 50%. The burden of this disease, however, is primarily cosmetic and causes little functional difficulty for affected individuals. In contrast, the recurrence risk to a woman who has borne a child with trisomy 21 Down syndrome is 1%, that is, a low magnitude of recurrence. However, the burden of Down syndrome, in terms of mental retardation and serious birth defects, is heavy indeed. Thus, the magnitude of recurrence risk must be interpreted in light of the burden of the disease.

At this point, it is important to stress that the burden of any given disease may vary with the severity of the disease itself, but will always vary with the individual and family affected. Down syndrome is a good example. In some families, raising a child with Down syndrome becomes a strengthening and enriching experience; in others, it is quite devastating. The genetic counselor must always keep in mind that the assessment of the burden of a disease is a highly individual one for each family.

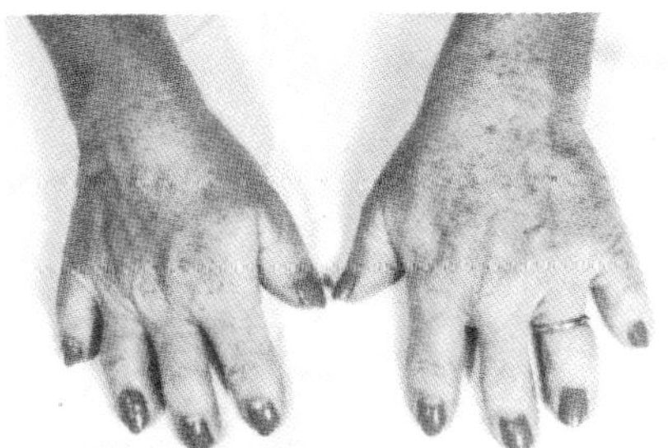

Figure 11.14. The hands of an individual with brachydactyly. (From McKusick VA: *Human Genetics.* 2nd Ed. Englewood Cliffs, NJ, Prentice-Hall, 1969, p. 49.)

THE POSSIBILITY OF MODIFICATION OF BURDEN AND/OR RISK

For a number of genetic diseases, it is possible to modify either the burden or the risk. If the disease is treatable or preventable, as in the case of cancer of the colon secondary to familial polyposis of the colon, or mental retardation secondary to phenylketonuria (discussed below), then the burden of the disease, although still significant, is quite different from what it would be if treatment and prevention were not available. When a condition can be diagnosed prenatally, such as Down syndrome or sickle cell anemia, the geneticist can change a probability statement about recurrence risk to a certainty as to whether the fetus is affected or not. Obviously this information affects the way families view the burden or recurrence risk of a given disease and affects their reproductive decisions.

ANTICIPATED FUTURE DEVELOPMENTS

Because medical genetics is a rapidly progressing field, diseases that were neither amenable to prenatal diagnosis nor treatable just a few years ago may be so today. Thus, the genetic counselor should also offer the best estimate about what might be available in the near future. Individuals often come for genetic counseling early in their reproductive years. Thus, if they have a 20-year span during which they may decide to have children, it is important to know whether the situation is likely to change dramatically during that time. As discussed later in this chapter, there have been rapid advances in the prenatal diagnosis of a number of genetic diseases.

All of these issues are poignantly and clearly raised in the following letter received from a young woman at risk for Huntington disease.

December 5, 1969

Dear Sir:

I am writing to you concerning the hereditary disease Huntington's chorea. I am an 18-year-old college freshman. My mother is now afflicted with Huntington's chorea as were my grandfather and great-grandfather on her side of the family.

I am considering marriage within the next three years. My boyfriend is aware of my mother's disease but I haven't explained all of the hereditary considerations to him as yet. I was wondering if sterilization through ligation and adoption is the only answer, or whether there have been any new developments. Has a process been developed yet in which a donor's egg might be placed artificially in the sterile female?

I know that my mother's condition has affected by parents' marriage, so should I even discard the prospect of marriage all [sic] *together? On the other hand, would it be wrong for me to presume that a cure for Huntington's disease would be developed by the time my children would be grown?*

Please tell me the facts frankly, for I am strong enough to face the truth and follow the best course of action. Thank you for your time and consideration.

This remarkable woman has raised several of the important issues in genetic counseling. She understands the pattern of inheritance from her own family pedigree and has read about the magnitude of recurrence risk. Because she has lived with a mother afflicted with this disease and has seen its effect not only on her mother but on her parents' marriage, she is well aware of the burden of disease on both the patient and family. She has asked whether foregoing having her own children and hoping to adopt children is her only reproductive option or whether there are other possibilities (in vitro fertilization and implantation of a donor egg). She is also asking directly about whether future developments might change this picture over the course of another generation. Her questions are remarkably insightful and prescient. Her letter was written in 1969, at which time the placement of a donor egg in a sterile female was a fantasy. By 1989, in vitro fertilization is an established reproductive option, including the placement of a donor egg into a sterile female. Drug therapy for the movement disorder in Huntington disease has been developed although it is not entirely effective; but no cure or effective treatment is available for the dementia. However, remarkable advances in the molecular genetics of Huntington disease have resulted in presymptomatic and prenatal diagnostic tests for this disease. Therefore, the reproductive options available to this young woman are quite different now than they were at the time she wrote her letter.

The Process of Genetic Counseling

The first step in genetic counseling is to ascertain what question the consultand (the individual(s) seeking counseling) is *really* asking. The major kinds of information that we feel are necessary to provide in genetic counseling have been discussed above, but the consultand may in fact be seeking very specific advice, including counseling to deal with guilt and anxiety. To best help individuals seeking genetic conseling one must carefully determine what is being sought.

Because genetic counseling is a process of communication, several aspects of information transfer must be considered. One must assess the receptivity, both emotional and intellectual, of the individuals seeking genetic counseling. Couples frequently point out that they do better at understanding and accepting counseling when they can receive it together and when they have supportive relatives or friends with them. How much information should be conveyed to those seeking genetic counseling and at what level? Obviously, the information must be conveyed in language that can be understood by the consultands. We believe that candor and honesty are the best way to present such information. Difficulties arise when one must balance raising anxieties against providing unrealistically optimistic prognoses. Again, neurofibromatosis provides an excellent example. One cannot predict which of the various complications of neurofibromatosis will occur in an affected individual nor successfully treat many of them; therefore, is it reasonable to tell consultands about the various complications that can occur with this disease? On the other hand, failure to do so could lead to an unrealistically optimistic expectation and this would be unwarranted because reproductive decisions may be made on the basis of this information.

The information communicated is heavy with emotional content and often contains medical or scientific information that is difficult for individuals to comprehend. It is important that the verbal counseling be followed up by a letter, written in language the consultands can understand, which enables them to read and reread the counseling and to share it with physicians, family members, clergy, or other supportive individuals and allows them time to come to grips with the information.

It is our view that genetic counseling should not be directive. Reproductive decisions are highly personal ones and should be left to individual couples rather than being made by their physicians and counselors. Genetic counseling contains a major component of counseling. One must deal with the anxiety and guilt that often accompanies having a child with a congenital defect and/or genetic disease. The genetic counselor must be attuned to these issues and able to be supportive. He or she should also be able to provide information about social and other support services, which may be very helpful to such families. In many genetic clinics counseling is performed by a team of health professionals including the physician medical geneticist and specifically trained genetic counselors.

GENETIC SCREENING

Screening tests are an essential part of standard medical care and are generally directed at early diagnosis of treatable diseases. Familiar examples include Papanicolaou smears for detection of cervical carcinoma, mammography for early detection of breast cancer, blood pressure screening for detecting hypertension, and skin testing for tuberculosis. Sometimes screening tests and diagnostic tests are the same; more frequently, however, the screening test is aimed at identifying a subset of the population in whom more specific diagnostic tests should be performed. Effective screening tests should be inexpensive, useful for large populations, and capable of selecting efficiently a subset of the population for whom specific diagnostic tests are indicated.

Because any screening test may be positive or negative and a screened individual may be either affected (or a carrier) or unaffected with the trait being screened, there are four possible outcomes of the test (Table 11.6).

The **sensitivity** of a test is defined as the frequency with which the test yields a positive result when the disease is present (A/A + C). The **specificity,** on the other hand, is the frequency with which the test is negative when the disease is absent (D/B + D). The **false-positive rate** (B/A + B) is the proportion of all positive tests occurring in individuals who are not affected, and the **false-negative rate** (C/C + D) is the proportion of all negative results in individuals affected with the trait or disease. Thus, the sensitivity of the test reflects the ability of the test to detect affected individuals, while the specificity indicates the ability of the test to exclude unaffected individuals. The *usefulness* of the screening test, the ability to discriminate between affected and unaffected individuals, is dependent, however, on both the ability to distinguish a positive from a negative test and by the relative sizes of the affected and unaffected populations. This can best be illustrated by a hypothetical example.

Table 11.6. Outcomes of Screening Tests[a]

	Affected	Not Affected
Positive tests	A	B
Negative tests	C	D

[a]False-positive tests are shown in the red-shaded box, false-negatives in the grey-shaded box.

Table 11.7. Screening for Heterozygous Carriers among Unaffected Siblings[a]

	Carrier (Dd)	Normal (DD)
Positive	64	2
Negative	3	31
Total	67	33

[a]False-positive tests are shown in the red-shaded box, false-negatives in the grey-shaded box. See text for discussion.

Let us assume that a test is developed to detect heterozygous carriers of a rare autosomal recessive disease and that this carrier test has a sensitivity of 95% and a specificity of 95%. When this test is applied to 100 clinically unaffected siblings of patients diagnosed with disease D, the following test results are obtained (Table 11.7). Recall that unaffected siblings have a 2/3 chance of being carriers and, therefore, one would expect 67 carriers (Dd) and 33 homozygous normal individuals

(DD). The false-positive rate is 2/66 or 3% while the false-negative rate is 3/34 or 9%. Thus this test appears to discriminate between carriers and homozygous normal siblings with high efficiency.

But now consider the application of this same test to the population of Ann Arbor, Michigan with approximately 100,000 individuals tested. Let us assume that disease D has a frequency of 1/40,000 or 0.000025. The carrier frequency, assuming Hardy-Weinberg equilibrium, is given by 2pq = 0.01. The results of the same screening test applied to the Ann Arbor population are shown in Table 11.8. Under these conditions the false-negative rate is 50/94,050 or 0.05%. However, the false-positive rate is 4,950/5,900 or 84%. In other words, false-positive tests outnumber true-positive tests by more than 5 to 1 and the majority of "carriers" detected by this test are misclassified. Thus, a test that discriminates carriers from homozygous normal individuals with high efficiency in families (in which the sizes of the two groups are similar), seriously misidentifies individuals in the general population in which homozygous normal individuals vastly outnumber carriers. Nevertheless, this test can be useful because positive tests identify a subset of the total population (5,900 of 100,000 individuals) with a significantly higher probability of being carriers (950/5,900 or 16%) than their frequency in the general population (only 1/100 or 1%). If the false-positive tests are a random event, one can simply repeat the same screening test and the false-positive rate will fall to 248/1150 or 22%, and nearly 80% of those with positive tests will indeed be carriers of the disease. In any case, however, a specific diagnostic test must then be applied to those with positive screening tests to identify carriers with a high degree of accuracy.

Table 11.8. Screening for Heterozygous Carriers in the General Population[a]

	Carrier (Dd)	Normal (DD)
Positive	950	4,950
Negative	50	94,050
Total	1,000	99,000

[a]False-positives are shown in the red-shaded box, false-negatives in the grey-shaded box. See text for discussion.

There are two major types of genetic screening tests. The first is aimed at the early recognition of affected individuals in whom medical intervention will have a beneficial effect for the affected individual and/or the patient's family. Within this group are fetal screening, which includes prenatal diagnostic tests for such conditions as Down syndrome, and newborn screening, of which the classical example is screening for phenylketonuria (PKU). A specialized form of prenatal screening is maternal α-fetoprotein screening for pregnant women carrying a fetus with a neural tube defect. The second major form of genetic screening is the identification of individuals at risk of transmitting a genetic disease. Classic examples of this form of screening are carrier detection tests for diseases such as Tay-Sachs disease, sickle cell anemia, and the thalassemias.

Prenatal diagnosis of genetic diseases is discussed later in this chapter. An indirect type of fetal screening is the measurement of maternal blood α-fetoprotein. It has been shown that women carrying a fetus with an open neural tube defect (meningomyelocele or anencephaly) have elevated levels of serum α-fetoprotein. Because serum α-fetoprotein levels vary considerably during pregnancy, it is important to determine accurately the stage of gestation by ultrasound examination of the fetus. It is now known that two consecutive elevated α-fetoprotein levels (3 multiples of the median level) indicate a risk of approximately 1 in 20 that the woman is carrying a fetus with an open neural tube defect. This compares with the frequency of 1 in 1000 in the general population. Therefore, the screening test identifies a group of women at 50-fold higher risk, in whom amniocentesis for measurement of amniotic fluid α-fetoprotein may be offered for prenatal diagnosis of neural tube defects. During the course of such screening programs, it was found that low levels of maternal serum α-fetoprotein may be associated with an increased risk of Down syndrome and other chromosomal trisomies. These latter observations will require extensive confirmatory studies before they should be applied as routine screening procedures.

Newborn Screening for Treatable and/or Preventable Disease: Phenylketonuria

The best example of a newborn screening test is the Guthrie test for the detection of phenylketonuria. PKU is an autosomal recessive disorder occurring in Northern European populations in about 1/10,000 to 1/15,000 live births. It is characterized, if untreated, by fair hair and pale skin, microcephaly (small head), and profound mental retardation. It is caused by a deficiency of hepatic phenylalanine hydroxylase, which converts phenylalanine to tyrosine, and is characterized biochemically by low plasma tyrosine and high phenylalanine concentrations and by excretion of phenylalanine metabolites such as phenylketones in the urine, giving it a characteristic "mousy" odor. Strict restriction of dietary phenylalanine, if begun early in infancy, can lower plasma phenylalanine levels and prevent mental retardation.

The Guthrie test is based on the observation that β-2-thienylalanine can inhibit the growth of the bacterium *Bacillus subtilis* and this inhibition can be overcome by phenylalanine (Fig. 11.15). A drop of blood collected from a newborn infant (usually at 3 days) is allowed to dry on a piece of filter paper. Disks containing the dried blood are placed on agar containing thienylalanine and *B. subtilis.* In the absence of phenylalanine, bacterial growth is inhibited by the thienylalanine; bacterial growth around a test disk indicates the presence of sufficient phenylalanine in the blood sample to overcome the growth inhibition. The test is standardized by using disks with known amounts of phenylalanine; a positive result is usually set at a phenylalanine concentration over 4 mg/dl. Each positive result must be followed up by a quantitative assay of plasma phenylalanine and tyrosine to establish the diagnosis of PKU.

For every 20 positive Guthrie tests, only one infant will be found to have classical PKU with a phenylalanine level greater than 20 mg/dl

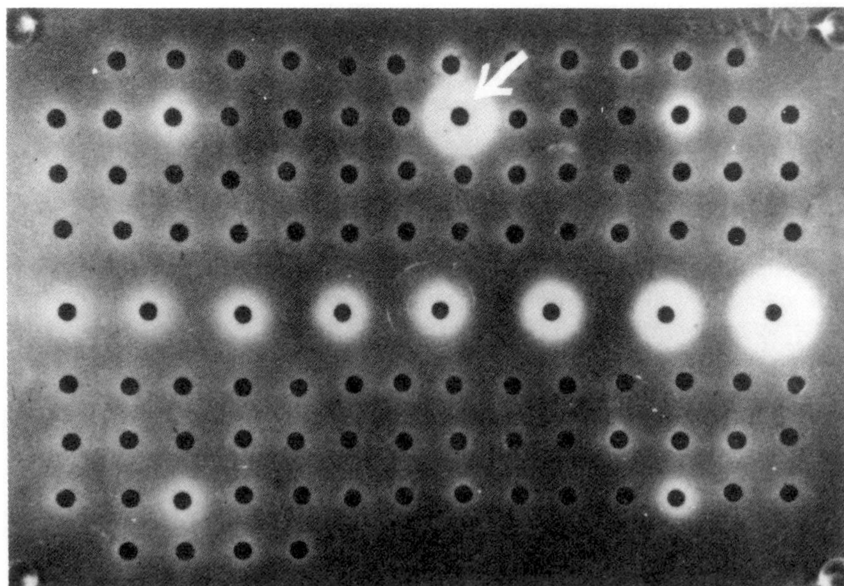

Figure 11.15. Bacterial inhibition assay or Guthrie test. *Row five* shows control discs containing concentrations of phenylalanine from 2 to 50 mg/dl. The *arrow* indicates a positive test in *row two.* (From Levy HL: Genetic screening. Adv Hum Genet 4:1–104, 1973.)

(normal less than 2) and a low plasma tyrosine. These children must be placed on strict phenylalanine restriction in order to prevent mental retardation. A somewhat smaller number of infants have been described who have persistent modest elevations of plasma phenylalanine (usually less than 10 mg/dl) and are characterized as having hyperphenylalaninemia, now known to be secondary to an allelic mutation of phenylalanine hydroxylase, causing a milder deficiency of this enzyme. These children do not require severe dietary restriction and do not become mentally retarded. By far, the most common cause for a false-positive Guthrie test is transient tyrosinemia due to hepatic immaturity. These babies have high levels of plasma tyrosine as well as phenylalanine and both levels will fall with time; they do not require any specific therapy. Finally, newborn screening for PKU has detected a rare condition associated with high levels of blood phenylalanine and severe mental retardation that is not prevented by restricting dietary phenylalanine. These babies have disorders of pteridine biosynthesis, resulting in deficient levels of an essential cofactor of phenylalanine hydroxylase.

Prior to the initiation of widespread neonatal screening for PKU in the 1960s, it was estimated that PKU accounted for approximately 1% of severe mental retardation. The nationwide use of the Guthrie test has virtually eliminated PKU as a major cause of mental retardation. Because there is a very low but finite false-negative rate, some affected babies are missed, particularly if they are tested very early in the neonatal period (before 3 days) before blood phenylalanine levels have had a chance to increase (the fetus is protected from high blood phenylalanine by the maternal metabolism).

The dramatic success of this genetic screening program has produced an unexpected new problem. Women with PKU, successfully treated with dietary therapy in childhood but off phenylalanine restriction as adults, were found to have babies who were microcephalic and severely retarded. Although all of these babies are at least obligate heterozygotes for PKU, only 1% would be expected to have PKU. The retardation was presumably the result of in utero exposure to high phenylalanine levels from the maternal circulation. It may be possible to prevent this form of mental retardation by starting dietary restriction in women prior to the time of conception and maintaining blood phenylalanine levels below 10 mg/dl throughout pregnancy.

Molecular analysis of the phenylalanine hydroxylase locus on 12q24.1 has indicated several allelic mutations causing classical PKU and hyperphenylalaninemia. Population studies have shown that two specific mutations, each associated with a specific RFLP haplotype, may cause 50% of all cases of classical PKU in Northern European populations. These studies open the possibility of widespread carrier detection and allow prenatal diagnosis for selected families at risk of having a child with PKU.

Once programs are in place for screening for PKU, it becomes cost effective to add other newborn screening tests that can be run on spots of dried blood obtained at the same time. The state of Michigan, for example, screens all newborns (approximately 135,000/year) for PKU, congenital hypothyroidism, galactosemia (an inborn error of metabolism also associated with mental retardation as well as severe liver failure), sickle cell anemia, biotinidase deficiency, and maple syrup urine disease (Table 11.9). The latter two conditions are inborn errors of metabolism causing physical and mental retardation that can be treated by pharmacologic doses of biotin or a diet restricting branched-chain

Table 11.9. Michigan Newborn Screening Program

Disease	Inheritance	Incidence	Screening Test	Treatment
Phenylketonuria (PKU)	Autosomal recessive	1/15,000	Bacterial inhibition assay	Dietary restriction of phenylalanine
Congenital hypothyroidism	Usually sporadic	1/5,000	Radioimmunoassay of T4	Thyroid hormone replacement
Sickle cell anemia	Autosomal recessive	1/2,600 (1/400 blacks)	Isoelectric focusing (detects hemoglobins S, C, D, E, and G)	Close medical care, penicillin prophylaxis
Galactosemia	Autosomal recessive	1/50,000 to 1/100,000	Enzymatic assay	Dietary limitation of galactose
Biotinidase deficiency	Autosomal recessive	1/50,000 to 1/100,000	Enzymatic assay	Pharmacologic doses of biotin
Maple syrup urine disease (MSUD)	Autosomal recessive	1/200,000 to 1/250,000	Bacterial inhibition assay (detects leucine)	Dietary restriction of branched-chain amino acids

amino acids, respectively. These six diseases being screened range in frequency from a high of 1 in 2600 (1 in 400 blacks) for sickle cell anemia to 1 in 250,000 for maple syrup urine disease. The cost of the screening program is $18 per infant.

Screening for Carriers of Genetic Diseases

In order to establish a cost effective program for screening carriers of a genetic disease several criteria should be met: (*a*) the disease is clinically significant and severe enough to warrant such a screening program; (*b*) a high risk population can be identified in which to focus screening efforts; (*c*) an inexpensive test is available with adequate sensitivity and specificity; (*d*) definitive tests are available for specific diagnosis in individuals identified as being at high risk by carrier detection tests; and (*e*) reproductive options are available to couples found to be at risk. The best example of the successful application of such a carrier detection test is screening for carriers of Tay-Sachs disease in the Ashkenazi Jewish population. Tay-Sachs disease is an autosomal recessive disorder characterized by a deficiency of the α subunit of *N*-acetyl-β-D-glucosaminidase (hexosaminidase A). Deficiency of this enzyme results in accumulation of G_{M2} gangliosides in neurons, causing a severe neurologic degenerative disease resulting in blindness, loss of neurologic function, and death between the ages of 2 and 4 years. There is no known therapy. Although less than 0.3% of the general population are carriers of this disease, 3% of Ashkenazi Jews are carriers of Tay-Sachs disease; thus, screening programs can be focused on this well-defined population. An inexpensive test is available for measuring heat-labile hexosaminidase A (hex A) activity in blood that is positive in 6–8% of Ashkenazi Jewish individuals. Carrier status can be confirmed by a definitive measurement of hexosaminidase A activity in white blood cells. Because hex A activity can also be measured in cells obtained by amniocentesis or chorionic villus sampling, prenatal diagnosis is available for Tay-Sachs disease, thereby offering couples at risk the option of terminating a pregnancy with an affected fetus. Widespread application of this testing in the Ashkenazi Jewish population has virtually eliminated Tay-Sachs disease in this group over the last 20 years.

Other examples of diseases amenable to such testing are the β-thalassemias in Mediterranean populations, α-thalassemias in Oriental populations, and sickle cell anemia and other hemoglobinopathies in the black population. Advances in the molecular genetics of cystic fibrosis may soon make carrier detection tests available for this, the most common severe autosomal recessive disorder in the white population. The carrier frequency for cystic fibrosis in the United States white population is estimated to be 1 in 22. By the use of RFLPs closely linked to, and in linkage disequilibrium with, the putative cystic fibrosis locus, one could calculate the probability of being a carrier as 1 in 5 for individuals with one specific RFLP genotype and as low as 1 in 500 for those with a different RFLP genotype. The recent cloning of the CF gene and identification of the mutation found in 70% of affected individuals now allows direct accurate detection of carriers of this common mutation.

Screening to Determine the Frequency and Natural History of Genetic Disease

Population screening, including newborn screening, programs may be carried out to obtain epidemiologic information about genetic diseases rather than to identify populations in whom medical intervention is indicated. As discussed in Chapter 8, aneuploidy of the Y chromosome (47,XYY and 48,XXYY) has been associated with a high frequency of social pathology. In order to ascertain whether this was in fact associated with the abnormal karyotype, newborn screening studies were carried out to determine the frequency of sex chromosome aneuploidy in an unselected population. These studies were successful in showing that 47,XYY individuals occur with a frequency of 1 in 1000 in the liveborn population. However, these studies are fraught with hazards including the ethical issues about whether one tells parents the nature of abnormal findings, especially when they are as emotionally charged as the XYY issue. There is also a concern about "self-fulfilling prophecies" if parents, teachers, or others expect antisocial behavior to develop in karyotypically abnormal children.

PRENATAL DIAGNOSIS OF GENETIC DISEASE

The objective of prenatal diagnosis is to offer prospective parents the assurance of having unaffected children when the risk of having an affected child is unacceptably high. This is NOT equivalent to the assurance of having normal children. Prenatal diagnosis allows one to convert a probability statement about the risk of a specific disease to a certainty. It does not address all possible birth defects or genetic diseases.

Prenatal diagnosis represents a paradigm of the application of basic scientific techniques to clinical problems. The development of these diagnostic procedures in the 1960s resulted from advances in obstetrical techniques, in the ability to culture human cells, and in cytogenetics and molecular genetics. Two major techniques are used to obtain fetal cells: amniocentesis and chorionic villus sampling.

Amniocentesis

Amniocentesis involves removal of a small amount (usually 20 ml) of amniotic fluid (Fig. 11.16). The amniotic fluid, which bathes the developing fetus during the early part of pregnancy, is thought to represent a transudate; its composition reflects that of fetal extracellular fluid. Found within this fluid are cells sloughed from the fetal skin and from epithelial linings of the gastrointestinal, respiratory, and genitourinary tract. Later in the pregnancy, as the volume of amniotic fluid increases, the major contributor to the fluid is fetal urine. Amniocentesis must be done early enough to be useful, i.e., to allow a specific diagnostic test to be carried out such that the results may be used to decide whether to continue or terminate a pregnancy within safe and legal limits, and yet late enough to be safe, i.e., so that the removal of a small amount of amniotic fluid does not alter subsequent fetal development.

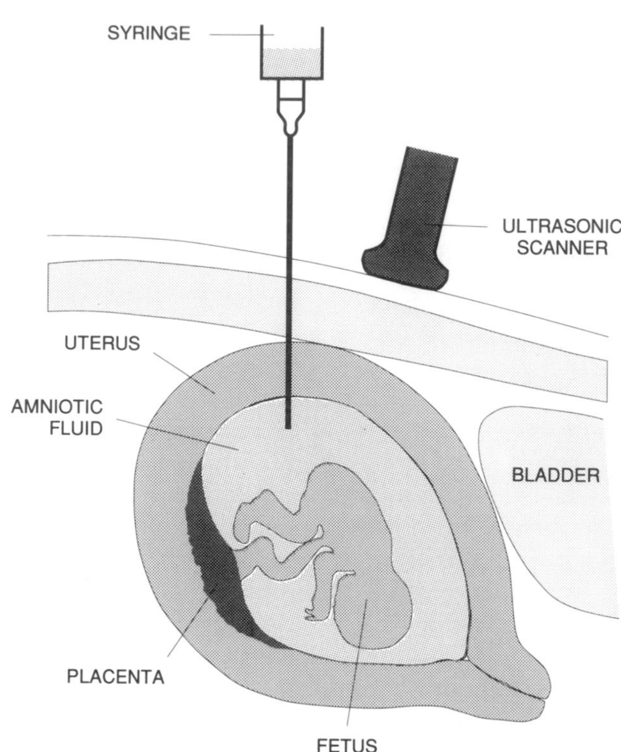

Figure 11.16. Diagram of amniocentesis.

Normally, this is done between 14 and 17 weeks after the last menstrual period.

The amniocentesis procedure itself must begin with supportive and accurate genetic counseling about the indications for the procedure and a consideration of the benefits and risks as well as limitations of amniocentesis. Normally, ultrasound imaging is carried out to determine the location of the fetus and the placenta within the uterus (Fig. 11.17), to establish gestational age accurately, and to determine if there is a multiple pregnancy (twins). The amniocentesis itself is done as an

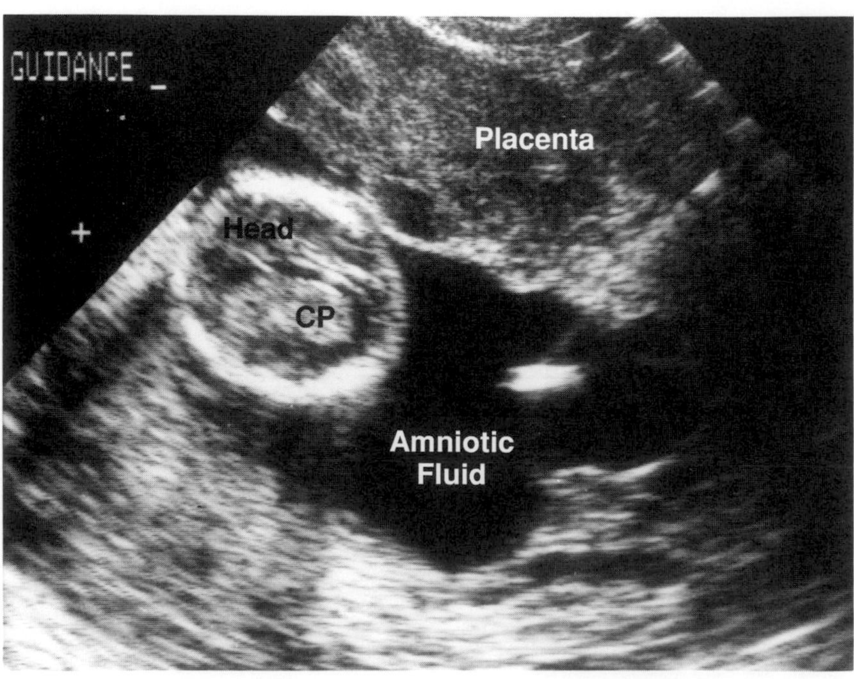

Figure 11.17. Ultrasonogram of an amniocentesis of a normal 16-week gestation. The amniocentesis needle can be seen entering the amniotic cavity from the *upper right;* the *bright area* is a sonic reflection from the tip of the needle. The placenta is *anterior.* The fetal head is seen on the *left. CP,* choroid plexus. (Courtesy of Dr. Richard Bowerman, Department of Radiology, University of Michigan).

Table 11.10. Indications for Amniocentesis

1. Advanced maternal age
2. Chromosomal abnormality
3. Neural tube defect/abnormal maternal serum α-fetoprotein
4. Inborn error of metabolism
5. Disease detectable by DNA analysis

outpatient procedure, using local anesthetic. The fluid removed can be analyzed directly for specific proteins such as α-fetoprotein or can be cultured or analyzed for infectious agents such as rubella virus. More importantly, the cells within the fluid can be collected by centrifugation and either analyzed directly or grown in tissue culture. Most of the cells in the fluid are not viable, but those that are can be used to establish cultures of amniocytes. These cultures can then be examined cytologically, biochemically, or by DNA analysis.

The *indications for amniocentesis* are shown in Table 11.10. More than 80% of amniocenteses are done for chromosomal indications, and, in fact, at the University of Michigan Hospital, more than 80% are done because of "advanced maternal age." This is usually defined as pregnancy in a woman at or over the age of 35 years, at which age the risk of Down syndrome (Fig. 8.16) and other chromosomal trisomies increases sharply. In many centers, the age at which amniocentesis is offered has been declining, and there are studies to indicate that this is a cost-effective procedure by the age of 31. Amniocentesis is also performed for women who have had a previous child with a chromosomal trisomy, have a family history of a chromosome abnormality, or are known to be carrying a balanced translocation. The second most common indication for amniocentesis is the history of a previous child with a neural tube defect (Fig. 11.18) and/or an abnormal maternal serum α-fetoprotein, suggesting an increased risk of carrying a fetus with a neural tube defect. All amniocenteses routinely have chromosome studies done on the cells and α-fetoprotein measured on the fluid because of the frequency of these problems. A third indication is the risk of biochemical defects or inborn errors of metabolism. More than 100 such conditions can now be diagnosed by biochemical assessment of amniocytes; however, most of these diseases are individually rare. Furthermore, a number of the biochemical diagnostic techniques have now been replaced by DNA analysis, which is more reliable and more efficient. Finally, amniocentesis was often performed in the past to determine the sex of the fetus carried by a woman at risk of having a child with an X-linked recessive disease. This is rarely done today, because a number of these diseases can be diagnosed directly by prenatal techniques and because sex can be determined with a reasonably high degree of accuracy by ultrasound examination.

The risks of amniocentesis are often quoted to be approximately 0.5% or less. These include infection or injury to the fetus and/or the mother. In fact, the risks are probably considerably lower. It is important to note that several large controlled studies have shown that there is no statistically significant increase in the risk of miscarriage in women who have undergone amniocentesis compared with a control group of women who have not had this procedure.

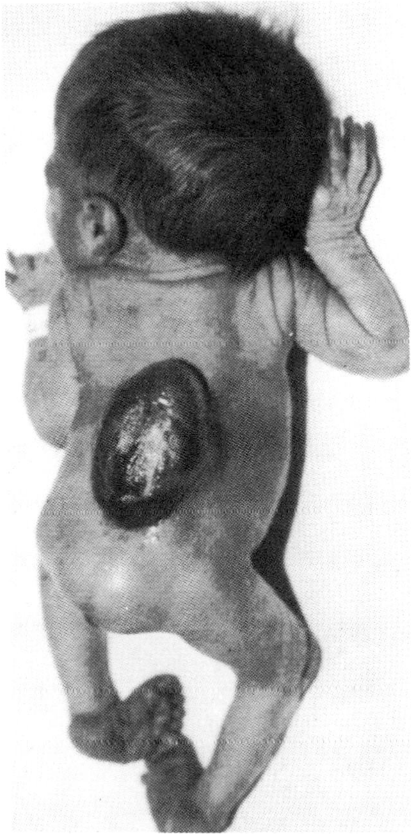

Figure 11.18. Infant with a neural tube defect, a meningomyelocele involving the lower thoracic and upper sacral region. (From Jones KL: *Smith's Recognizable Patterns of Malformation.* 4th Ed. Philadelphia, WB Saunders, 1988, p. 459.)

The probability, in an experienced center, of failure to obtain fluid or to grow cells from the fluid is less than 0.1%. Problems that can arise after amniocentesis include delay in being able to grow the cells from the fluid, failure of growth and/or contamination of the cells, contamination of amniocytes by maternal cells that would confuse the results, chromosomal mosaicism, or other laboratory errors. Fortunately, amniocentesis has proven to be a highly accurate and reliable diagnostic technique, and the error rate is well under 1%. It is important to remember, howcvcr, that critical decisions (possible termination of a pregnancy) are being based on a laboratory diagnosis without physical examination of the patient. This is a situation physicians try to avoid in clinical medicine, but is generally unavoidable in the setting of prenatal diagnosis.

Chorionic Villus Sampling

An alternative approach to prenatal diagnosis is chorionic villus sampling (CVS). This technique involves passing a fine, flexible, polyethylene catheter through the cervix and into the uterus under ultrasound guidance and removing, by suction, small amounts of the chorion frondosum, a tissue that will subsequently become the placenta (Fig. 11.19). Alternatively, a transabdominal approach is being used in some centers. The fetal chorionic villi can be dissected away from maternal tissue and examined by a variety of techniques. The fetal cytotrophoblasts are rapidly dividing (1 of 400 cells is undergoing mitotic division) so that these cells can be examined karyotypically without the need for growing them in tissue culture. Although the quality of karyotype is not as good as in cells cultured from amniotic fluid, a result can be obtained within hours, versus days to weeks as in the case of amniocentesis. Furthermore, the cytotrophoblasts can be grown in tissue culture and studies repeated on larger numbers of cells. Biochemical analysis may also be carried out on the cultured cells. Most importantly, DNA analysis can be carried out readily on chorionic villi. The yield of DNA is greater than that obtained from the cells in 20 ml of amniotic fluid, often allowing direct DNA analysis without a requirement for first culturing the cells.

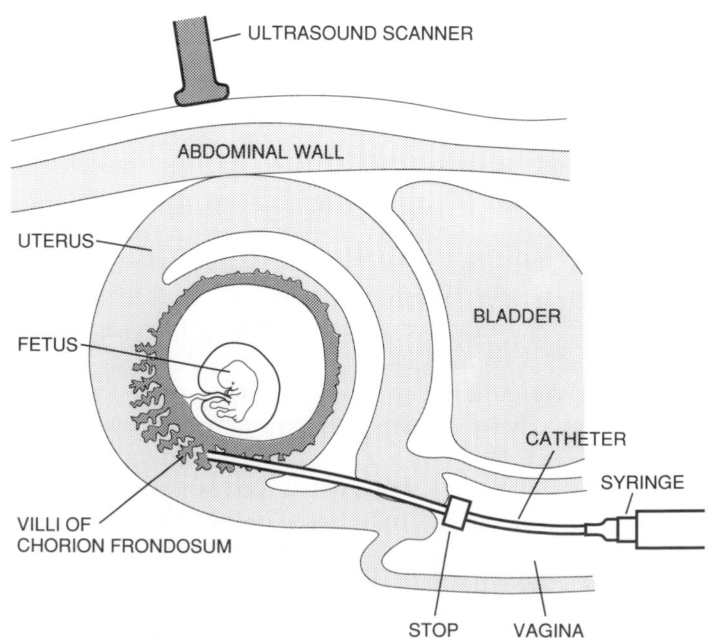

Figure 11.19. Technique of transcervical chorionic villus sampling.

Chorionic villus sampling is normally carried out at 8–10 weeks of gestation. This allows results of the tests to be available at a time when termination of pregnancy, should it be chosen, is medically safer and emotionally easier than the midtrimester termination that might follow amniocentesis. The rapidity with which results can be obtained from chorionic villus sampling and the fact that culturing cells is unnecessary can markedly reduce the cost of this test. A disadvantage of the procedure is that it is not possible to diagnose neural tube defects, as it is from amniocentesis. Although there may be a slightly increased risk of procedure failure and of fetal loss in women who undergo chorionic villus sampling compared to those who have amniocentesis, a recent prospective study of 2278 CVS procedures concluded that it is a safe and effective technique for early prenatal diagnosis. As of October 1989, nearly 66,000 CVS procedures at 182 centers worldwide had been performed. The rate of failure to obtain adequate samples was approximately 1.8%, and the rate of fetal loss was just under 3.2%.

An exciting prospect for the future is the possible isolation of fetal trophoblastic cells from the maternal circulation. Amplification of the DNA by polymerase chain reaction (PCR) from a small number of cells might allow DNA-based fetal diagnosis without even the small risks associated with amniocentesis or CVS.

Interestingly, the frequency of chromosomal abnormalities in CVS samples is 2–5 times higher than it is in amniotic fluid samples, in which, in turn, it is about twice as high as among liveborn infants. This is consistent with selection acting upon karyotypically abnormal fetuses throughout the course of pregnancy. While most severe chromosomally abnormal fetuses will be spontaneously aborted before the time of chorionic villus sampling, these data suggest that continuing fetal loss occurs throughout the course of pregnancy.

Other techniques available for prenatal diagnosis include fetal visualization. The most important of these is ultrasonography (Fig. 11.20). Ultrasound imaging can often be used to determine fetal sex (by detecting the phallus in male fetuses) by 18–20 weeks of gestation. Anatomical defects including major congenital abnormalities can be detected by high-resolution ultrasonography. Open neural tube defects

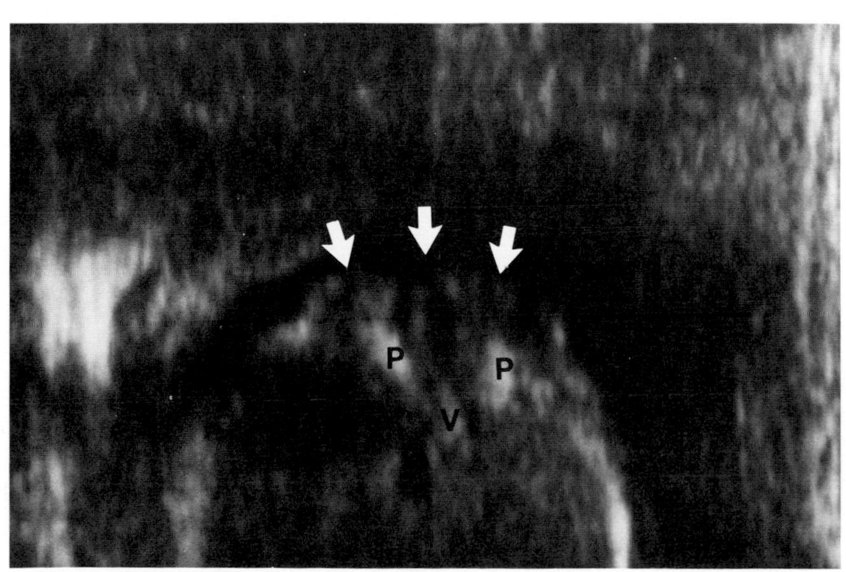

Figure 11.20. Ultrasonogram of a 22-week-old fetus with a neural tube defect. This is a transverse section through the upper abdomen of the fetus; the posterior surface of the fetus is toward the *top* of the figure. *V*, vertebral body; *P*, vertebral pedicles. The *dark areas* represent fluid. Note that the vertebral pedicles are splayed out and the overlying skin *(arrows)* is bulging outward, findings indicative of a neural tube defect. (Courtesy of Dr. Richard Bowerman, Department of Radiology, University of Michigan.)

can be detected with a sensitivity approaching 90%. Preliminary data suggest that even Down syndrome may be detected or suspected on the basis of ultrasound examination.

Applications of DNA Analysis to Prenatal Diagnosis

Most genes are expressed in a tissue-specific manner. This limits biochemical diagnostic techniques to those diseases for which the gene products are expressed in amniocytes. Deficiency of gene products expressed only in specialized tissues such as liver (e.g., ornithine transcarbamylase) could not be diagnosed by such biochemical techniques. Because the DNA in all somatic cells is essentially the same, the ability to detect mutations at the DNA level overcomes this limitation. Several techniques can be used for DNA analysis (Table 11.11).

If a single base change causes an altered restriction site, then one can readily diagnose the condition prenatally by restriction enzyme analysis. The best example of this is sickle cell anemia in which the causative mutation causes the loss of an *Mst*II site (see Chapter 6).

A more useful technique at present is to detect known single base changes by the use of allele-specific oligonucleotides (see Chapter 5). This technique is particularly useful when most cases of a disease are caused by one or a limited number of mutations, as is the case for α_1-antitrypsin deficiency, PKU, and cystic fibrosis. In the case of β-thalassemia, where there are multiple mutations, the technique can still be applied in situations in which a small number of particular mutations is especially common in a defined population (e.g., the splice mutation at position 110 of IVS-I in certain Mediterranean populations or the β^{39} nonsense mutation in Sardinia).

Major deletions or rearrangements can be detected by Southern blot analysis. Currently, this technique may be most useful in the prenatal diagnosis of Duchenne muscular dystrophy, in which more than 60% of cases are the result of deletions in this very large gene.

Allele-linked RFLPs may be very useful in defined populations in which there is linkage disequilibrium between specific RFLP haplotypes and mutant alleles (known or unknown), and in which there is limited allelic heterogeneity. This technique was first applied to sickle cell anemia in which a specific *Hpa*I polymorphism was shown to be associated with the β^S mutation. This technique has also been used in the case of phenylketonuria, α_1-antitrypsin deficiency and cystic fibrosis in Northern European populations.

Locus-linked RFLPs require family study to be useful, but this is the most generally applicable technique for prenatal diagnosis for single-gene defects. This technique can be used when the specific mutation is unknown, as long as the gene has been mapped and there are closely linked RFLPs. Numerous examples in which this technique has been

Table 11.11. Prenatal Diagnosis by DNA Analysis

1. Restriction endonuclease analysis to detect point mutations that alter restriction sites
2. Allele-specific oligonucleotides to detect known point mutations
3. Southern blot analysis to detect deletions or other major structural rearrangements
4. Allele-linked RFLPs to detect unknown mutations known to be in linkage disequilibrium with specific RFLP haplotypes
5. Locus-linked RFLPs to detect unknown mutations whose map position is known

Table 11.12. Selected Single-gene Diseases Amenable to Prenatal or Presymptomatic Diagnosis by DNA Analysis

Autosomal dominant
Adult polycystic kidney disease
Huntington disease
Neurofibromatosis-1
Autosomal recessive
Sickle cell anemia
β-Thalassemia, α-thalassemia
Cystic fibrosis
Phenylketonuria
α_1-Antitrypsin deficiency
Tay-Sachs disease
X-linked recessive
Hemophilia A and B
Duchenne and Becker muscular dystrophy
Ornithine transcarbamylase deficiency

used include hemophilia, Duchenne muscular dystrophy, α_1-antitrypsin deficiency, and adult polycystic kidney disease.

The list of diseases diagnosable by DNA analysis (Table 11.12) is growing rapidly and includes the hemoglobinopathies, hemophilia A and B, OTC deficiency, α_1-antitrypsin deficiency, PKU, Duchenne muscular dystrophy, and cystic fibrosis, as well as such late-onset diseases as adult polycystic kidney disease and Huntington disease. In many cases a combination of the above techniques can be, and are, used to make the diagnosis.

Newer developments should further expand these diagnostic possibilities. Most important is the ability to amplify specific DNA segments enzymatically more than 1 million-fold by the technique of polymerase chain reaction (PCR) described in Chapter 5. This technique and its refinements allow the use of small DNA samples (the amount obtained in chorionic villus samples or amniotic fluid samples) without purification of the DNA. Because the amplified DNA can be visualized by chemical staining techniques, radioactive probes may not be needed. This means the technique can be more rapid, inexpensive, and applicable in situations in which handling radioactivity can be a problem. DNA amplification may also allow direct genomic sequencing of the PCR product to discover the specific mutation causing the disease, without the need to clone the entire gene. Newer techniques are also expanding the ability to detect novel mutations causing disease. These include DNA denaturing gradient gel electrophoreses and RNase cleavage techniques, both of which take advantage of mismatches between specific DNA or RNA probes and mutant sequences. These two techniques, especially when coupled with DNA amplification, should allow the definition of virtually all mutations found in genes that have been cloned.

Ethical Questions

A major ethical issue raised by prenatal diagnosis is that related to abortion. Should a couple undergoing prenatal diagnosis have made a commitment to terminate a pregnancy carrying an affected fetus? At a time when the safety of amniocentesis (and of chorionic villus sampling) was unknown, this was not an unreasonable expectation because physicians do not wish to expose patients to hazardous procedures unless the results of the procedure will affect therapeutic decisions. Now that it is known that amniocentesis is a very safe procedure (and CVS appears to be as well) this commitment seems inappropriate. Furthermore, it should be noted that less than 5% of fetuses examined by prenatal diagnostic techniques are, in fact, affected with the disease being sought. Therefore, the outcome for the vast majority of women undergoing prenatal diagnosis is reassurance that they are carrying a fetus that is not affected with the disease in question.

A second issue is how to handle unrequested or unexpected information. Because a karyotype and α-fetoprotein analysis are done on all amniocenteses whatever their primary indication, unexpected information may be obtained. However, the same consideration holds for any medical diagnostic test, and most genetic counselors feel that full disclosure with appropriate supportive counseling should be provided. How does one handle the situation of twin pregnancies and specifically, twins discordant for a serious genetic disease? For example, what if one twin has Down syndrome and the other does not? A number of such cases have been reported in which it has been possible to selectively abort the affected fetus, allowing the birth of the unaffected twin. The situation emphasizes again the limitation of prenatal diagnosis; it is possible to terminate the life of a fetus affected with a genetic disease, but not yet possible to treat the affected fetus. For the couple faced with the anguish of carrying a fetus with a severe or lethal genetic disease, this option nevertheless may be a more humane and satisfactory one than any of the alternatives.

Effect of Prenatal Diagnosis on Gene Frequency and Disease Frequency

Prenatal diagnosis coupled with therapeutic abortion of affected fetuses has no effect per se on the gene frequency of an otherwise lethal genetic disease. Without prenatal diagnosis, an affected child would die without reproducing. The effect on gene frequency of an autosomal recessive trait would depend on whether carriers would have more children if they could avoid having affected children, and thus, might actually pass more mutant alleles on to the next generation. Although this might be seen as a danger of increasing the mutant allele frequency, as long as prenatal diagnostic techniques are available to detect the affected fetus this problem can be dealt with.

The effect on disease frequency depends on whether one is able to carry out primary or only secondary prevention. For example, the frequency of neural tube defects in the general population is about 1 in 1000; for a woman who has had a child with a neural tube defect, the recurrence risk is approximately 2–5%. Prenatal detection and therapeutic abortion of affected fetuses, if limited to couples who have already had one affected child, will have a very small impact on the overall frequency of neural tube defects in the population. (This is not to say that it will not have a major emotional and medical impact on specific families.) If, however, prenatal diagnosis is coupled with genetic screening programs (e.g., maternal α-fetoprotein screening to detect women at higher risk of carrying a fetus with a neural tube defect), then one can carry out primary prevention and make a significant impact on the population frequency of this very severe birth defect.

Finally, prenatal diagnosis can be seen as the paradigm of contemporary medical genetics. Successful prenatal diagnostic procedures require a knowledge of Mendelian genetics, of population genetic considerations, and of the application of molecular genetic techniques. Knowledge gained from human gene mapping and linkage studies is critical in many prenatal diagnoses. The technology must be coupled with appropriate genetic counseling programs and, in order to provide primary prevention, requires appropriate genetic screening programs. The application of prenatal diagnosis allows couples at risk for having a child with a genetic disease to choose among reproductive options and to avoid the birth of an affected child.

TREATMENT OF GENETIC DISEASE

Principles

Treatment of genetic diseases, parodoxically, usually involves *environmental* manipulation rather than genetic manipulation (the beginnings of gene therapy are discussed in the next chapter). Prevention of genetic disease by genetic screening, counseling, prenatal diagnosis, and early intervention is closely intertwined with treatment. Medical genetics offers a notable example of the emphasis on preventive medicine rather than treatment of established disease. Finally, treatment of genetic diseases at the environmental level generally involves a combination of the application of the three R's: restriction, replacement, and removal. It should be kept in mind that genetic diseases are no less treatable than most nongenetic diseases faced by the physician.

Restriction of Potentially Toxic Environmental Agents

Dietary therapy is an important part of the treatment of several genetic metabolic diseases. The restriction of dietary phenylalanine in PKU can prevent the development of profound mental retardation. Protein restriction in children with urea cycle defects is an important adjunct to more specific therapy. Similarly, in familial hypercholesterolemia, restriction of dietary cholesterol and saturated fats is helpful in lowering serum cholesterol. Restriction of drugs and toxins is critically important in certain other diseases. For example, individuals with G6PD deficiency must avoid oxidant stresses such as antimalarial drugs and certain antibiotics. In α_1-antitrypsin deficiency, cigarette smoking (a serious hazard for any individual) is a particular hazard and can be shown to accelerate the destruction of lung tissue and the development of severe emphysema.

Replacement

Replacement of deficient products or even organs can be therapeutic or even curative. In hemophilia A, replacement of factor VIII has been a successful therapy in the great majority of patients. In the case of α_1-antitrypsin deficiency, clinical trials are under way to replace purified α_1-antitrypsin. There is evidence that intravenous administration of human α_1-antitrypsin can result in levels of this inhibitor in alveolar fluid sufficient to neutralize elastase (Fig. 11.21). By using recombinant DNA techniques, genetically engineered α_1-antitrypsin derivatives less susceptible to oxidative damage are being developed (see Chapter 7) and will be tested as therapeutic agents. In addition, alternative, low molecular weight inhibitors of elastase are also being considered as therapy for this condition. It is noteworthy that replacement of deficient or abnormal α_1-antitrypsin will not be expected to prevent the liver damage that occurs in some patients with this disease secondary to the accumulation of the abnormal protein in that organ.

Organ replacement by transplantation has also been used as a ther-

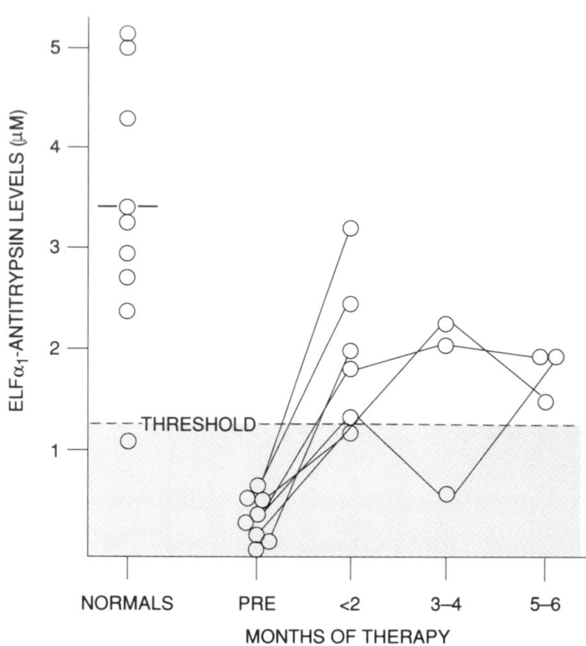

Figure 11.21. Effect of intravenous administration of purified human α_1-antitrypsin on levels of this inhibitor in alveolar fluid. Patients with α_1-antitrypsin deficiency received weekly infusions of purified inhibitor for the times indicated. The *red dashed line* represents the theoretical protective level of α_1-antitrypsin in lung epithelial lining fluid (ELF). (From Wewers MD, Cosolaro MA, Sellers SE, Swayze SC, McPhaul EM, Witts JT, Crystal RG: Replacement therapy for α_1-antitrypsin deficiency associated with emphysema. N Engl J Med 316:1055–1062, 1987. Reprinted by permission from *The New England Journal of Medicine.*)

apeutic measure. Kidney transplantation in cystinosis (in which the kidney is damaged by accumulation of intracellular cystine) can correct the most severe problem associated with this disease. Liver transplantation has been carried out in patients with homozygous familial hypercholesterolemia with successful reversal of the metabolic defect. Bone marrow transplantation with HLA-matched marrow is curative in some patients with severe combined immunodeficiency disease secondary to adenosine deaminase deficiency. Experimentally, fibroblast transplantation has been attempted in experimental models of such diseases as α_1-antitrypsin deficiency. Fibroblasts can be transfected with DNA or retroviruses containing and expressing genes for specific human products. This is a potentially promising approach to gene therapy and is discussed in Chapter 12.

Removal

Removal of toxic substances or organs at risk of damage has also been used successfully. Wilson disease is an autosomal recessive disease characterized by hepatic and neurologic damage secondary to copper accumulation. Chelation of copper by penicillamine is a highly effective treatment to prevent the damage associated with this disease and has even been shown to reverse liver cirrhosis in a limited number of patients. Neurologic symptoms are often reversed if treatment is begun early enough (Fig. 11.22). Similarly, phlebotomy to remove iron in hemochromatosis can successfully prevent the progressive damage to liver, heart, pancreas, and other organs (see Chapter 9). In familial polyposis of the colon there is a virtually 100% risk of malignant degeneration of the multiple polyps leading to cancer of the colon. Although not trivial therapy, removal of the colon can completely prevent cancer of the colon from developing and can be a lifesaving procedure.

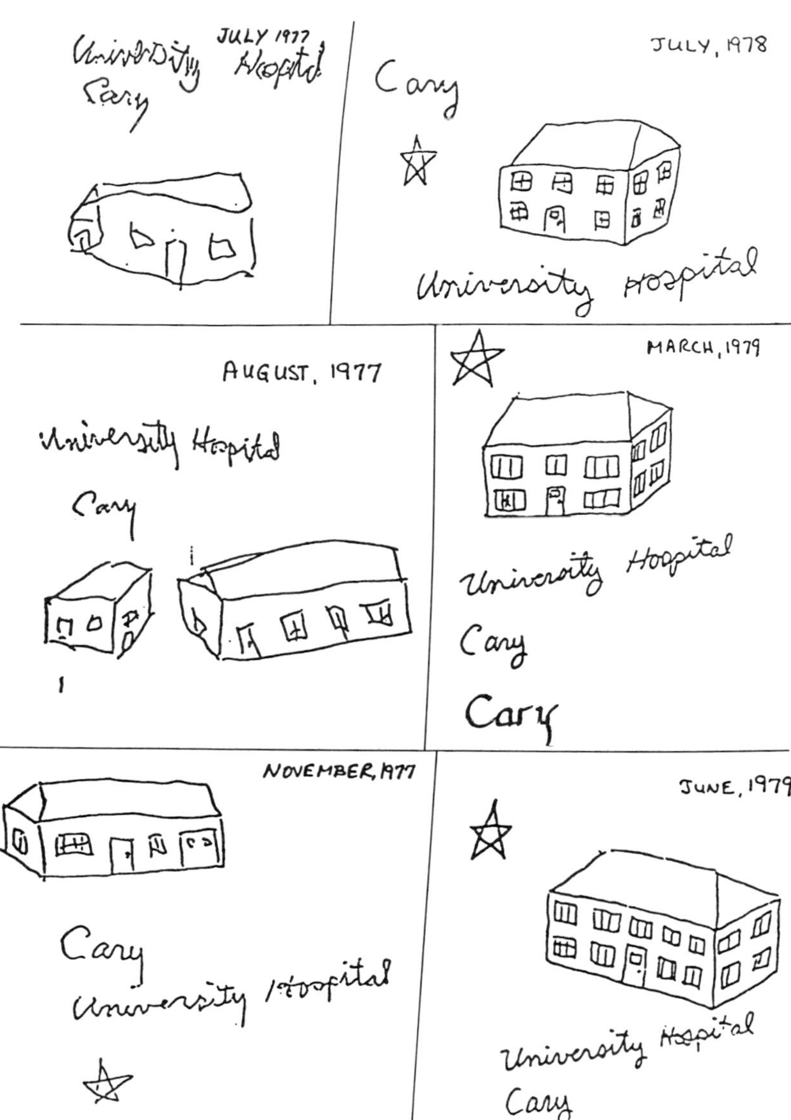

Figure 11.22. Samples of handwriting and drawing by a 21-year-old man with Wilson disease treated with penicillamine to chelate and remove copper. The first sample of writing was obtained before initiation of therapy (July, 1977); the subsequent samples, over the first 2 years of his treatment. This is a convenient method for assessing the degree of tremor and dystonia (abnormal muscle tone).

In addition to the three R's, a number of metabolic tricks can be used to treat genetic metabolic diseases. These have often involved the application of rational biochemical and molecular approaches. For example, in OTC deficiency, alternative metabolic pathways for elimination of nitrogen have been used with considerable success in reversing the metabolic abnormalities and hyperammonemia of this condition. The administration of sodium benzoate and phenylacetate to conjugate glycine and glutamine, respectively, and cause their urinary excretion has been a major advance in the treatment of this severe disease (see Fig. 7.19). In familial hypercholesterolemia secondary to LDL-receptor deficiency, endogenous cholesterol biosynthesis can be blocked by lovastatin, a competitive inhibitor of HMG-CoA reductase, which in turn causes an increase in cellular LDL receptors and normalization of serum cholesterol (see Fig. 7.13).

In summary, rapid and dramatic advances in medical genetics, particularly in the area of molecular genetics, have indeed propelled the geneticist from the role of "bookie" to that of "fixer." Nowhere is this more striking than in the area of prenatal diagnosis. Clinical genetics has benefited from impressive progress in gene mapping and in recombinant DNA technology and from parallel advances in nongenetic medical diagnosis and therapy. The diagnosis, treatment, and prevention of genetic diseases has moved to the mainstream, and indeed forefront, of medical practice.

SUGGESTED READINGS

Genetic Counseling

Edwards JH: The importance of genetic disease and the need for prevention. Phil Trans R Soc Lond B 319:211–227, 1988.

Emery AEH, Pullen IM (eds): *Psychological Aspects of Genetic Counselling.* New York, Academic Press, 1984.

Gelehrter TD: The family history and genetic counseling: Tools for preventing and managing inherited disorders. Postgrad Med 73:119–126, 1983.

McKusick VA: *Mendelian Inheritance in Man.* 8th Ed. Baltimore, Johns Hopkins University Press, 1988.

Murphy EA, Chase GA: *Principles of Genetic Counseling.* Chicago, Year Book Medical Publishers, 1975.

Genetic Screening

Holtzman NA: The future of genetic testing. Prog Med Genet 7:220–245, 1988.

Holtzman NA: *Proceed with Caution. Predicting Genetic Risks in the Recombinant DNA Era.* Baltimore, Johns Hopkins University Press, 1989.

Kerem B-S, Rommens JM, Buchanan JA, et al.: Identification of the cystic fibrosis gene: Genetic analysis. Science 245:1073–1080, 1989.

Kidd KK: Phenylketonuria. Population genetics of a disease. Nature 327:282–283, 1987.

Levy HR: Molecular genetics of phenylketonuria and its implications. Am J Hum Genet 45:667–670, 1989.

Screening and Counseling for Genetic Conditions. President's commission for the study of ethical problems in medicine and biomedical and behavioral research. (Abram MB, Chairman), Washington, D.C., United States Government Printing Office, 1983.

Scriver CR: Population screening: Report of a workshop. Prog Clin Biochem Res 163B:89–152, 1985.

Prenatal Diagnosis

Antonarakis S: Diagnosis of genetic disorders at the DNA level. N Engl J Med. 320:153–163, 1989.

Boehm CS: Prenatal diagnosis and carrier detection by DNA analysis. Prog Med Genet 7:143–179, 1988.

Kazazian HH: Diagnosis by gene amplification. J Lab Clin Med 114:95–96, 1989.

Landegren U, Kaiser R, Caskey CT, Hood L: DNA diagnostics—Molecular techniques and automation. Science 242:229–237, 1988.

Milunsky A, Alpert E: Results and benefits of a maternal serum α-fetoprotein screening program. J Am Med Assoc 252:1438–1442, 1984.

Ramiro R, Pilu G, Jenaty P, Ghidini A, Hobbins JC: *Prenatal Diagnosis of Congenital Anomalies.* Norwalk, CT, Appleton & Lange, 1988.

Rhoads GG, Jackson LG, Schlesselman SE, et al.: The safety and efficacy of chorionic villus sampling for early prenatal diagnosis of cytogenetic abnormalities. N Engl J Med 320:609–617, 1989.

Weatherall DJ: *The New Genetics and Clinic Practice.* 2nd Ed. Oxford, England, Oxford University Press, 1985.

Therapy of Genetic Diseases

Valle D: Genetic disease: An overview of current therapy. Hosp Pract 22:167–182, 1987.

11/ Study Questions

1/ Interview with Thomas Smith, Jr.:

Doctor, my wife Alice and I are planning on starting a family and we would like to know whether there is any risk to our children for having the nerve problem that seems to be in my family.

My oldest brother, Don, started having muscle weakness and loss of sensation in his legs and feet when he was a teenager. These got progressively worse until he had to go on disability 10 years ago when he was 55-years-old. When his problems first began, my mother told us that these problems seemed very similar to ones that her husband's brother Fred Smith (age 68) and sister Sally (age 63) have, although our father, Tom, and his half brother and sister, the twins Eddie and Jane (age 73), never were bothered with these problems.

My cousins Frank and Bill seem healthy. They are in their 20's. Their father, my uncle Fred Smith, is one of my relatives with the leg muscle weakness and numbness. Cousin Frank, the older one, is married but doesn't have any children although I think his wife had a miscarriage last year. My aunt Sally has one daughter, Linda, who also seems to have the leg weakness problem and is worried about her two children, Dick and Bob.

My father, Thomas Smith, Sr., died in an auto accident when he was 40-years-old. He was the youngest in the family. His parents are dead. His father, William, was a healthy man who died of some heart problem in his 80's. His first wife died in childbirth with Eddie and Jane. His second wife, Mary, was my grandmother. I never knew her but everyone said she always complained of 'pins and needles' in her feet and she got so weak at the end that she was in a wheelchair.

Alice's family is very healthy. Her father and mother are still alive, as are her three sisters and two brothers.

Draw the pedigree of the family portrayed above. What kind of inheritance pattern do you think the described trait is following? What else do you learn about the disease from taking this family history?

2/ Why take a family history?

*** 3/** Analyze each of the following clinical vignettes by identifying for parents and offspring the risks and burdens of different reproductive decisions. These cases are presented to stimulate discussion and do not necessarily have clear-cut "correct" answers.

a. A pregnant woman, known to be a heterozygote for a severe X-linked form of hydrocephalus, seeks counseling prior to prenatal sex determination.
b. A young woman, an aspiring show-business performer, wishes to start a family and is concerned about the medications she takes for acne.
c. A young man, about to be married, is concerned about the impact on his family plans of his radiation therapy and chemotherapy for testicular cancer.
d. A 30-year-old pregnant woman with no history of having children with birth defects wants amniocentesis to detect chromosomal aneuploidies.
e. A 32-year-old female machine operator is concerned about having a family while taking medication for seizures.

4/ A woman has a brother with a rare autosomal recessive disorder that affects 1 in 160,000 individuals. She is unaffected. She marries an unrelated person and comes to you for genetic counseling. What is her chance of having an affected child?

You learn of a test that is abnormal in 90% of carriers of this disorder, although a small percentage (3%) of the general population may also give an abnormal result. You test the woman and her husband and find they both give a positive result. What is now her chance of being a carrier? What is her husband's chance? What is the risk of having an affected child?

12

Looking Toward the Future

"The recombinant DNA line of research is already upsetting, not because of the dangers now being argued about but because it is disturbing, in a fundamental way, to face the fact that the genetic machinery in control of the planet's life can be fooled around with so easily."

—Lewis Thomas, 1977

The preceding 11 chapters of this text have reviewed what might be considered the mainstream of modern medical genetics. In this chapter, we will take the luxury of speculating a bit about where the field is going and what issues will face physician-geneticists of the 21st century. Making such predictions is fraught with pitfalls, as the rapid pace of progress in the field has made most such previous predictions only vaguely accurate. But certain issues are almost certain to represent major topics in medical genetics in the coming 1 or 2 decades and therefore deserve inclusion here. In future editions of this text, it is likely that these topics may emerge to occupy entire chapters of their own.

THE HUMAN GENOME PROJECT

The concepts of linkage analysis and reverse genetics of human disease, outlined in Chapter 9, have led to a major emphasis in developing a complete genetic and physical map of the human genome. Certain small segments of particular chromosomes in the area of important disease genes such as cystic fibrosis and Duchenne muscular dystrophy are being intensively studied already. There is an emerging consensus in the medical and biological communities, however, that it is now appropriate to plan to map and sequence the entire 3 billion bp of the human genome once and for all, in order to provide the ultimate DNA data base for an assault on a genetic understanding of our species. Such a proposal has not been without controversy. However, after much discussion, many leaders in the field have concluded that the value of the project outweighs its possible drawbacks, including the considerable expense (estimated at 3 billion dollars) that will be involved. The National Institutes of Health and the Department of Energy are both initiating major efforts to get the project underway, and plans are being made to encourage international cooperation.

The four phases of the Human Genome Project are diagrammed in Figure 12.1, although they may not necessarily be carried out consecutively. The first phase is to develop a more powerful genetic map, with the goal being an increase in the density of RFLP markers to an average spacing of 1 cM. Although enormous progress has been made already in developing such a panel, as outlined in Chapter 9, prior to the onset of the Human Genome Project the average spacing between markers was about 8–10 cM. This is insufficiently dense to carry out fine mapping of disease genes, and hence this component of the project is an essential one. Whereas the labor involved is considerable, the technology to develop such markers is now well established.

A second component of the effort is to develop a complementary physical map of the human chromosomes, so that the genetic markers can be placed on actual restriction maps in order to assess their real physical distances from each other. Recalling that on the average 1 cM is about 1 million bp, it should be clear that such physical maps will not be trivial. In fact, maps of regions as large as 20 million bp have already been constructed in specific areas of interest where numerous probes were available. The method of carrying this out depends on a technique known as pulsed field gel electrophoresis, which is capable of reliably and reproducibly separating DNA fragments as large as 10 million bp. Combined with restriction enzymes that cut very rarely in the human genome, and therefore generate fragments of the order of 1 million bp in size, this approach is capable of generating the kind of map shown schematically in Figure 12.1.

If one is interested in cloning a disease gene, however, it is necessary to have the entire candidate region available in overlapping clones.

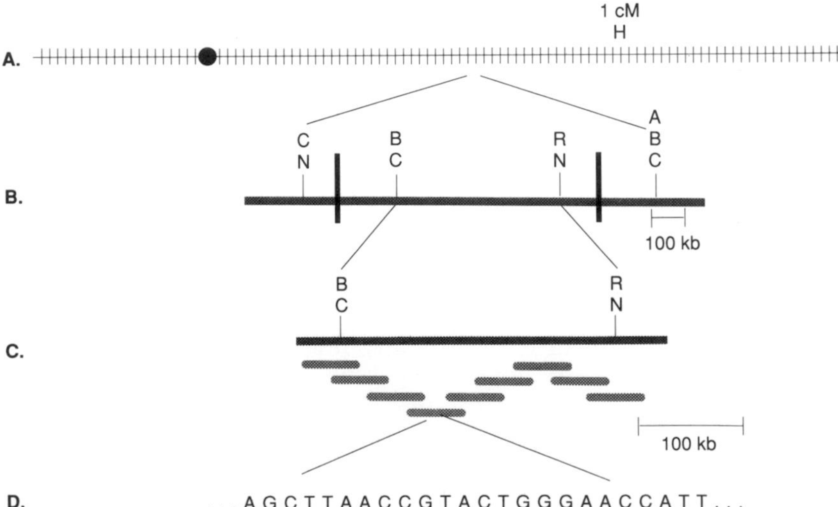

Figure 12.1. **Schematic of the proposed steps in the Human Genome Project.** This includes: **A**, Construction of a 1-cM genetic map. The diagram shows a typical chromosome, with the *hatch marks* representing genetic markers. About 150 evenly spaced markers are needed to give a 1-cM resolution for an average chromosome. **B**, Construction of a physical map. The *large hatch marks* indicate the location of a pair of genetic markers from **A**, and the *capital letters* represent the location of restriction sites, as determined by pulsed field gel electrophoresis. **C**, Development of an ordered overlapping array of clones *(horizontal lines)*. **D**, Determination of the complete nucleotide sequence.

This represents the next phase of the Human Genome Project. To obtain a set of clones covering the entire genome is not difficult; in fact, generating such a library is a routine exercise in everyday molecular genetics. The major challenge is to develop a technology capable of identifying overlaps between clones so that a completely arrayed and ordered set can be generated. If one were able to identify flanking genetic markers for a disease gene, one could simply use the physical map and the set of overlapping clones to completely define the area within which the gene of interest must reside. Developing a technique that is capable of ordering a set of 100,000 or so clones is, so far, a difficult challenge. The proposals to carry out such an effort depend on generating fingerprints of DNA clones, which can be investigated for similarities in an automated analysis. The identification of a significant similarity would then lead to the conclusion that two clones share DNA sequence. Obviously, repetitive sequences can create some difficulties with this sort of analysis. The exact nature of the overlapping clone set also remains to be defined. These clones might be cosmids, which include 30–45 kb of continuous human DNA. Alternatively, a new technology involving cloning longer stretches of DNA as artificial chromosomes in yeast may be applied. Obviously, the larger the stretch of DNA in each clone, the fewer that will need to be used to develop a complete overlapping set.

The final and most laborious stage of the Human Genome Project will be to actually determine the sequence of this overlapping set of clones. To be practical, this major undertaking will require considerable advances in technology, as currently it is difficult for one person to generate more than 100,000 bp of sequence per year. At that rate, approximately 30,000 person-years of effort would be required. Advances in automated sequencing technology are likely to greatly reduce this rate over the next decade.

The consequences of knowing the normal sequence of the human genome, which can be thought of as the ultimate genetic map, are profound. Focusing again on the effort to identify important disease genes, if one has narrowed down a region where the gene must reside, using linkage analysis, to 1 or 2 million bp, and if the sequence of that region has been determined already, it is possible by computer methods (though these need to be refined) to scan that region for the presence of coding regions. This utilizes the fact that exons of expressed genes do not contain stop codons and also are likely to use certain codons more frequently than others. This latter effect, referred to as a "codon usage bias," can be used to identify a stretch of DNA that encodes a protein and distinguish it from noncoding regions. Of course, once a coding region has been located by this method, the protein sequence is immediately predictable, which may give clues to the function of the gene. Such clues will often be useful in deciding whether a coding region could represent a candidate for a particular disease gene. Furthermore, if one then wishes to investigate individuals with a particular disease for mutations in a candidate gene, the availability of the normal sequence makes sequencing the DNA from an affected individual vastly easier, using the polymerase chain reaction discussed in Chapter 5.

The value of carrying out the Human Genome Project is not limited to human disease genes that occur in families and are inherited in Mendelian fashion. Somatic genetic events are felt to play a major role in the development of cancer (see Chapter 10), and these could be much more efficiently approached if the complete map and sequence of the human genome were obtained. For example, there are a large number of chromosomal translocations that are characteristic of particular tumors. Examples mentioned in Chapter 10 include the t(8;14) translocation in Burkitt lymphoma and the t(9;22) translocation (the Philadelphia chromosome) in chronic granulocytic leukemia. Unlike these two examples, however, in the vast majority of such translocations no information exists as to the mechanism by which the translocation produces malignancy. Having a complete map and sequence of the genome would make the cloning of breakpoints and the identification of the biology of such translocations a much more straightforward task and would undoubtedly shed important light on the mechanism of malignancy.

For these various reasons, the Human Genome Project appears certain to proceed. With the help of international collaboration, the anticipated improvements in technology, and an anticipated budget of 200 million dollars a year, the project is targeted for completion by the year 2005. The consequences for medicine and biology are likely to be enormous. The information achieved will be greater because of the intention to sequence the genomes of several other important organisms such as the mouse, the fruit fly, and yeast. Comparative analysis of such genomes will reveal a great deal about the evolution of chromosome structure and genome complexity. It is important, however, not to overstate the information that will derive from this massive effort. Understanding the regulation of gene expression will still be a major task; it is worth noting, for example, that the 90 kb of DNA sequence surrounding the human β-globin cluster (Chapter 6) have not led to an immediate understanding of the control of expression of these genes.

MAPPING COMMON DISEASE GENES

Another major frontier in human genetics is the identification of loci making a major contribution to such common diseases as hypertension, coronary artery disease, adult onset diabetes, and various types of cancer. Analysis of families has indicated that there is a strong genetic component to such disorders, but, as outlined in Chapter 4, more than one locus is involved, as well as a potential environmental component in many of these disorders. The identification of the loci responsible for the genetic component is a difficult but potentially attainable goal. Three things are required: (*a*) a large number of families with a high incidence of the trait; (*b*) a large number of polymorphic DNA markers covering essentially the entire genome; and (*c*) powerful mathematical methods to allow the detection of multiple simultaneously contributing loci.

These three components are currently being actively pursued. Efforts are already under way to collect families. The 1 cM genetic map identified as a major goal of the Human Genome Project (see above) will provide a sufficiently dense map of markers. Very recently, considerable progress has been made in the mathematics of multilocus analysis, although successful application to a major human disease problem has not yet been achieved. Shown in Figure 12.2 is an interesting example of such an analysis to detect the location of important genes controlling tomato phenotype. Several loci that play a role in tomato mass, soluble solids, and pH have been identified in this analysis. The obvious advantage that was used in those experiments was the ability to carry out selective breeding, which of course is not practical in human disease mapping.

An attractive alternative to mapping genes for quantitative traits

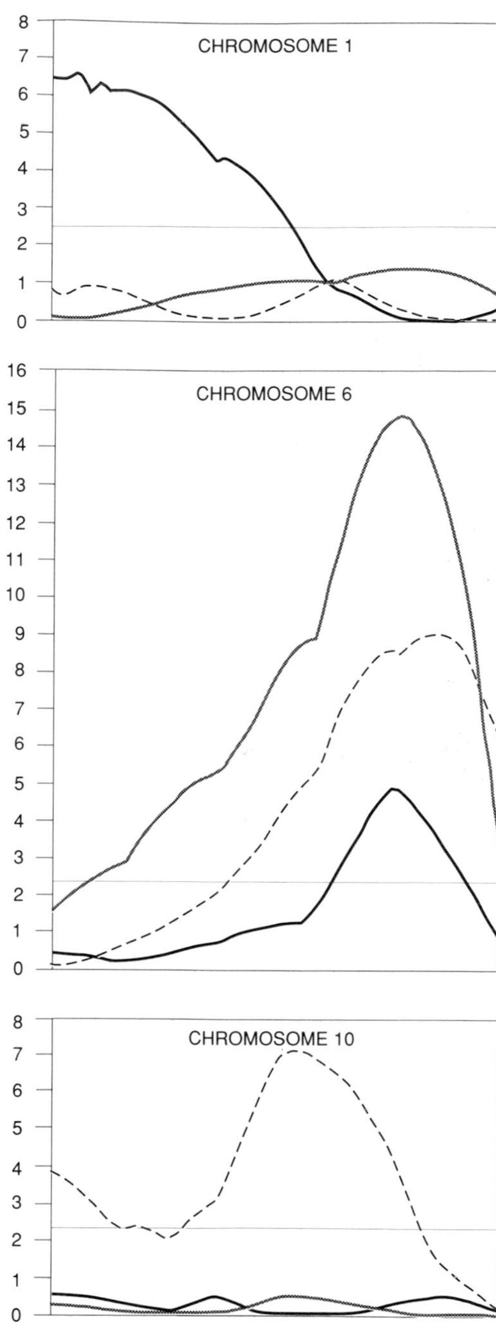

Figure 12.2. An example of the simultaneous mapping of multiple loci contributing to quantitative traits. Using controlled breeding experiments in the tomato and RFLP analysis of the progeny, it was possible to define several loci contributing to fruit mass *(solid gray lines),* soluble solids *(solid red lines),* and pH *(dashed red lines).* Only the results for chromosomes 1, 6, and 10 are shown here, but additional loci were identified on other tomato chromosomes as well. In *each panel* the *horizontal axis* represents map units along the chromosome; the *vertical axis* indicates the significance of a genetic contribution, with the *horizontal line* at 2.4 indicating statistical significance. A gene for fruit mass is located on chromosome 1, a gene (or genes) controlling all three parameters is present on chromosome 6, and at least one gene for pH is on chromosome 10. (From Peterson AH, Lander ES, Hewitt JD, et al.: Resolution of quantitative traits into Mendelian factors by using a complete linkage map of restriction fragment length polymorphisms. Nature 335:721, 1988.)

such as hypertension is to initially carry out these studies in an animal model such as mouse or rat. Genes identified in such a search are likely to have homologs in humans.

The goal of common disease gene mapping is 2-fold. In the first place, the identification of such loci, even though an arduous task, may be the only direct route to a complete biological understanding of the mechanism of disease and may, therefore, lead to more effective treatment. In the shorter run, however, identification of such loci should allow identification of individuals at risk for a particular disorder. Because many of the common diseases likely to be studied in this fashion can be modified by appropriate environmental or life-style alterations, the availability of such a "genetic physical" to identify specific predispositions will become an extremely important component of preventive medicine of the future. Thus, an individual known by such an analysis to be at risk for colon cancer could be advised to alter diet and undergo yearly colonoscopy in order to detect and treat early lesions. Similarly, a person genetically at risk for coronary artery disease could be advised with great certainty that smoking would be a very dangerous activity. Obviously, great care will have to be taken that such information is not abused and confidentiality is not breached. To some extent, however, such screening already takes place as part of well-patient care: the serum cholesterol measurement, which nearly every young and middle-aged adult now undergoes, is a good example, because serum cholesterol is a strong indicator of coronary artery disease.

SOMATIC CELL GENE THERAPY

With the ability to clone and study genes that are responsible for human disease, a dream of many physicians and geneticists is to insert a normal gene into the appropriate tissues of an individual affected with a recessive genetic disease, in order to precisely and permanently correct the disorder. As described in the opening quotation of this chapter, however, such shuffling about of genetic material has created concern. It is extremely important in these discussions to draw a distinction between *somatic cell gene therapy,* which is likely to be carried out in the near future and which involves no novel ethical concerns, and *germline gene therapy,* which most investigators feel should not be applied to human beings. Somatic cell gene therapy refers to the insertion of new DNA material into a particular tissue of an affected individual (for example, the bone marrow), but in such a way that the inserted DNA does not enter the germline and is, therefore, not transmitted to future generations. While this sort of therapy, as any new form of medical therapeutics, must be studied carefully in terms of risks and benefits, it can be considered actually less disruptive genetically than accepted forms of organ transplantation, which of course involve replacement of the entire genetic makeup of a particular organ with the genes from another individual. The goal of somatic cell gene therapy is to correct *only* the defective gene, with the anticipated benefit of avoiding the serious complications of organ rejection.

Germline gene therapy, on the other hand, is an approach that carries such risks of unknown damage to future generations that virtually all geneticists and lay organizations have concluded that it would not be appropriate to attempt it in humans.

Several scientific hurdles must be crossed before a realistic attempt at somatic cell gene therapy can be initiated. A major challenge is the development of efficient methods of transferring the normal gene into the tissue where its expression is required. Most methods of DNA transfer, as discussed in Chapter 5, are not efficient enough for this purpose, and much current effort is devoted to the engineering of retroviruses to get around this difficulty. Figure 10.6 depicts the normal life cycle of an RNA retrovirus, which is very efficiently designed to infect cells and integrate its genome into the host chromosome. The normal life cycle of a retrovirus involves a productive infection, however; obviously such ongoing virus production would be an unacceptable outcome of a therapeutic effort. Accordingly, a number of clever schemes have been designed that allow engineering of the desired gene into a defective retrovirus. The recombinant retrovirus is incapable of self-replication but can be packed into retroviral particles using a "packaging cell line."

A likely target for the first gene therapy experiments is the rare disease adenosine deaminase (ADA) deficiency, which causes severe combined immunodeficiency in children. The absence of ADA leads to an accumulation of adenosine monophosphate in the immune cells of such an individual, which is toxic and leads to the premature destruction of cells. The disease is autosomal recessive, and it is known that as little as 5% of normal levels of ADA would probably be curative. The feature of this disorder that makes it particularly attractive for the gene therapy approach is that natural selection would exist for immune cells that have been successfully transfected with a normal ADA gene. That is, immune cells that have received the normal ADA gene and express acceptable amounts of it will be protected against premature destruction and will have a survival advantage over their nontransfected neighbors.

A major challenge of this approach is the need to transfer the gene to stem cells in the lymphoid lineage in order for the beneficial effects to be realized. Such stem cells, which by definition are capable of giving rise to lymphoid cells over months and even years, have not yet been purified and represent only a tiny fraction of the cells in the bone marrow. Furthermore, retroviral DNA transfer can be carried out successfully only in dividing cells, and at any given moment only a small proportion of stem cells are involved in cell division. This represents a major stumbling block for the application of this dramatic form of therapy to human disease, and current efforts are focused on methods of identifying stem cells and promoting their movement into the cell cycle at the time of DNA transfer. Some of these problems are beginning to yield to a concerted effort. At the time of this writing, it has been possible to transfer the ADA gene to mice by retroviral transfection of bone marrow, followed by reinfusion of the treated marrow. Long-term, high level expression of ADA has occurred in at least some of these animals, raising hopes that this protocol can be applied to human disease in the relatively near future.

The bone marrow is not the only possible target organ, and efforts are being made also to carry out gene transfer into other sites. For example, skin fibroblasts can be transfected with a gene of interest and then reimplanted under the skin to generate small localized factories for a particular gene product, as long as its presence in circulating blood would be sufficient to correct a disease. Efforts are under way, for example, to use this approach to treat α_1-antitrypsin deficiency and hemophilia B, which is due to factor IX deficiency. Another attractive cellular target is the endothelial cell lining of blood vessels, because putting a gene into this site will allow ready access to the blood circulation. Targeting a gene to the airway epithelium has been proposed as the potential mode of gene therapy now that the cystic fibrosis gene has been cloned, and even the liver may be approachable, which would be necessary to treat disorders such as familial hypercholesterolemia. It is not clear that retroviruses will provide the best vehicles for all of these settings, and harnessing other viruses with particular tropisms, such as hepatitis virus for the liver, may provide significant advantages if reliable methods of inactivating their pathogenicity can be developed. The difficulties of these various hurdles should not be underestimated, however, and it seems likely that the full range of gene therapy approaches will require some time to develop.

With any new therapy, there are concerns about risks versus benefits. As noted above, as long as the germline is not involved, the ethics of somatic cell gene therapy do not propose particularly new or troubling issues. Any proposed new treatment, however, will have to be assessed in view of the possible availability of more conventional therapies. It is likely that initial trials of somatic cell gene therapy will involve disorders that currently are untreatable and lethal.

Advances in molecular biology also may have more direct implications for therapy, as in the production of purified human proteins (for example, clotting factors). In some instances, this development may make somatic cell gene therapy unnecessary.

For those who may be concerned about the potential risks of this new approach, it is worth pointing out that a careful review system already exists. The Recombinant DNA Advisory Committee of the National Institutes of Health is charged with reviewing any human experimentation involving gene transfer. This provides ample opportunity for scientific review and public discussion before new experiments are carried out.

CONCLUSION

The pace of research in human medical genetics is accelerating. This is a field where one must not only learn the current principles, but learn how to keep on learning as new techniques and applications are discovered in rapid succession. The present era will be viewed a few generations hence as a golden age in medical molecular biology, a time when the genetic basis of human disease evolved from a descriptive to a pathophysiologic and even therapeutic science. While making possible the tremendous advances of the present and future, the increasing technology that surrounds this field carries with it an ever present risk of creating a distance between physician and patient. This must be resisted if the healing profession is to maintain its true effectiveness and significance. The challenge to tomorrow's physician will be, more than ever, to balance this technology with a warm and empathetic approach to patients struggling with difficult issues of illness or the threat of illness. Physicians of the coming years would be well advised to heed the Russian proverb, "Let your brain be loving, and your heart be wise." We owe to ourselves and our patients, both present and future, nothing less.

SUGGESTED READINGS

Lander ES, Botstein D: Strategies for studying heterogeneous genetic traits in humans by using a linkage map of restriction fragment length polymorphisms. Proc Natl Acad Sci USA 83:7353–7357, 1986.

Friedmann T: Progress toward human gene therapy. Science 244:1275–1281, 1989.

National Research Council: *Mapping and sequencing the human genome.* Washington D.C., National Academy Press, 1988.

Glossary

Acrocentric chromosome—a chromosome in which the centromere lies near the end of the chromosome.

Additivity principle—if two events are mutually exclusive, the probability of obtaining one or the other is the sum of their separate probabilities.

Allele—alternative forms of a gene at a given locus.

Allelic heterogeneity—similar or identical phenotypes caused by different mutant alleles at the same genetic locus.

α_1-Antitrypsin—a serine protease inhibitor that inhibits the activity of elastase. Absence of this inhibitor as in α_1-antitrypsin deficiency results in chronic severe pulmonary disease and liver disease.

Alu repetitive sequence—moderately repetitive sequence located within intergenic or intronic DNA, containing a recognition site for the restriction enzyme *Alu*I. These sequences are about 300 bp long, and occur about 500,000 times in the human genome.

Amniocentesis—a prenatal diagnostic procedure, generally performed during the second trimester of pregnancy, whereby amniotic fluid is withdrawn from the amniotic sac surrounding the fetus.

Amplification—the production of multiple copies of a DNA sequence.

Aneuploid—any chromosome number that is not an exact multiple of the haploid number. Usually aneuploid refers to an extra copy of a single chromosome (trisomy) or the absence of a single chromosome (monosomy), resulting from nondisjunction during meiosis or mitosis.

Antisense strand (of DNA)—the noncoding strand of double-stranded DNA. It is complementary to the mRNA and serves as the template for mRNA synthesis.

Ascertainment—the selection of individuals for inclusion in a genetic study.

Association—in a population the occurrence together of two or more different phenotypes more often than expected by chance (not the same as linkage).

Assortative mating—nonrandom mating in which a member of a particular subpopulation is more likely to mate with other members of that subpopulation (positive) or less likely (negative).

Autoimmune disorder—a disorder characterized by the presence of antibodies directed against the individual's own antigens.

Autosomal disease—a disease encoded by a gene on one of the 22 pairs of autosomes.

Autosome—any chromosome other than the sex chromosomes or the mitochondrial chromosome.

Auxotrophic mutants—mutant cells dependent on an exogenous nutrient because they lack the ability to catalyze a specific metabolic step.

B cells—small lymphocytes that respond to antigenic stimulation by producing humoral antibodies.

Bacteriophage—bacterial virus. In molecular biology, these are used as vectors in cloning.

Barr bodies—sex chromatin as seen in female somatic cells (derived from the inactivated X chromosome).

Base pair (bp)—in double-stranded DNA there is complementary purine-pyrimidine hydrogen bonding (adenine must always pair with thymine, and guanine with cytosine). The hydrogen-bonded residue pair designates 1 bp. This unit is used for measuring the length of pieces of DNA.

Bayes' theorem—a theorem using conditional probability to incorporate all pertinent information relevant to estimating the likelihood that an individual at risk is affected with, or a carrier of, a genetic disorder. See text for explanation.

Cap—a modified nucleotide, 7-methylguanosine, added at the 5′ end of the growing mRNA chain which appears to be necessary for normal processing, stability, and translation of mRNA.

Cap site—site of initiation of transcription.

Carrier—an individual heterozygous for a mutant allele that generally causes disease only in the homozygous state.

CCAAT box—a region found 75–80 bp upstream from the transcription initiation site of many, but not all, genes that seems to be important for quantitatively efficent transcription.

CentiMorgan (cM)—a unit of genetic distance. Two loci are 1 cM apart if there is a 1% chance of recombination between them in a given meiotic event.

Centromere—central constriction of the chromosome, a heterochromatic region by which the chromatids are held together and to which the kinetochore is attached.

Chain terminator mutations—nonsense or frameshift mutations that result in premature cessation of translation of the mRNA.

Chorionic villus sampling—a procedure used for prenatal diagnosis at 8–10 weeks gestation. Fetal tissue for analysis is aspirated under ultrasonic guidance from the villous area of the chorion (chorion frondosum).

Chromatids—the two parallel identical strands, connected at the centromere, of the doubled chromosome after chromosomal replication but before anaphase.

Chromatin—the nucleic acids and proteins of which chromosomes are made.

Chromosomal disorder—disorders that are the results of addition or deletion of entire chromosomes or parts of chromosomes (e.g., Down syndrome, trisomy 21).

Chromosome aberration—an abnormality of chromosome number or structure.

Clone—a group of genetically identical cells derived by mitosis from a single ancestral cell.

Codon—a triplet of three bases in a DNA or RNA molecule, specifying a single amino acid.

Coefficient of relationship (r)—the probability that two persons have inherited a particular allele from a common ancestor. Also, the proportion of all genes that are identical by descent from a common ancestor.

Complementary—the interaction of purine-pyrimidine base pairs of a nucleic acid by hydrogen bonding (thus adenine with thymine, guanine with cytosine) to provide the geometry for nucleic acid secondary structure.

Complementary DNA (cDNA)—DNA synthesized from a mRNA template, using reverse transciptase.

Complementation analysis—a genetic test for whether two mutations producing a similar phenotype are allelic or not.

Compound heterozygote—an individual with two different mutant alleles at a given locus.

Concordant—a twin pair in which both members exhibit the same phenotype or trait.

Conditional probability—the probability of the joint occurrence of two nonindependent events is the product of the probability of one event times the probability of the second event given that the first event has occurred.

Consanguinity (consanguineous)—genetically related by descent from a common ancestor (literally of the same blood.)

Consensus sequence—a nucleotide sequence, such as CCAAT, TATA, or the splice donor, which plays an important functional role in gene expression. Such sequences may not be identical from gene to gene, but tend to share certain features, which are denoted as consensus sequences.

Consultand—the individual seeking, or referred for, genetic counseling.

Contact inhibition—the condition whereby normal cells will stop growth when they touch each other.

Crossing over—reciprocal breaking and rejoining of homologous chromosomes in meiotic prophase I that results in exchange of chromosomal segments.

Cytotrophoblast—rapidly dividing cells obtaincd from fetal chorionic villi by chorionic villus sampling; used for karyotyping and DNA analysis.

Degeneracy of the code—several codons code for the same amino acid.

Diploid—the number of chromosomes in most somatic cells, which is double the number found in the gametes (the haploid number). In humans the diploid chromosome number is 46.

Discordant—a twin pair in which one member exhibits a certain trait and the other does not.

Dizygotic—the product of fertilization of two separate eggs by two separate sperm; nonidentical twin pair.

DNA, deoxyribonucleic acid—the ultimate molecule of life. The polymer of which eukaryotic genes are composed.

DNA ligase—enzyme that catalyzes religation of two fragments of DNA.

DNA methylation—covalent attachment of methyl groups to DNA. Most commonly in eukaryotes this involves methylation of cytosine residues and is associated with reduced levels of transcription of a gene.

DNA polymerase—enzyme responsible for replication of DNA, which is accomplished by using each complementary strand of the DNA double helix as a template for the synthesis of a new strand.

DNA rearrangements—somatic recombination of DNA segments. In cells of the immune system, the variable (V), diversity (D), and joining (J) regions rearrange to generate functional antibody genes.

Domain—a region of the amino acid sequence of a protein that can be equated with a particular function, or a corresponding segment of a gene.

Dominant (trait)—those conditions that are expressed in heterozygotes (i.e., individuals with one copy of the mutant gene and one copy of the normal allele).

Dosage compensation—mechanism to account for the observation that the amount of a product encoded by a gene on the X chromosome is the same in males and females.

Double heterozygote—an individual with one mutant allele at each of two different loci.

Duffy blood group locus—the first autosomal gene placed on a chromosome (chromosome 1) by Donahue in 1968.

Dystrophin—the protein encoded by the X-linked gene, which, when mutated, causes Duchenne or Becker muscular dystrophy. Dystrophin is presumed to be involved in anchoring the contractile apparatus of striated and cardiac muscle to the cell membrane.

Ecogenetic disorder—a disorder resulting from the interaction of a common environmental factor with a specific genetic predisposition to disease (e.g., cigarette smoking causing emphysema in α_1-antitrypsin deficiency).

Electroporation—application of a short high-voltage electric pulse to cells in the presence of DNA to permit DNA to enter the cells.

Empirical recurrence risks—recurrence risks for siblings or offspring, calculated using actual observed frequency of the trait in families rather than on knowledge of the exact inheritance pattern of the trait.

Endonuclease—an enzyme that cuts DNA at an internal site. Restriction endonucleases cut DNA at specific nucleotide sequences.

Enhancers—DNA sequences that act in *cis* to increase transcription of a nearby gene. Enhancers can act in either orientation, may be either 5′ or 3′ to the gene, and may act at considerable distance from the gene.

Env gene—encodes capsule or envelope protein of a retrovirus.

Euchromatin—the chromatin that is light staining with trypsin G banding and is thought to contain genes that are, or have the potential to be, actively transcribed.

Euploid—any exact multiple of the number of chromosomes in a normal haploid gamete. In a normal somatic cell, the number of chromosomes is 2N, or diploid.

Exon—the transcribed regions of the gene that are present in mature mRNA and usually contain coding information.

Expressivity—the nature and severity of the phenotype of a mutant allele are a reflection of its expressivity. Variable expressivity is a frequent characteristic of autosomal dominant traits.

False-positive rate—proportion of all positive tests occurring in individuals who are not affected.

False-negative rate—proportion of all negative results in individuals with the trait or disease.

Familial—any trait that is more common in relatives of an affected individual than in the general population; could be due to genetic and/or environmental causes.

Familial hypercholesterolemia—an autosomal dominant disease in which there is a deficiency of low density lipoprotein (LDL) receptors, resulting in elevated serum cholesterol and LDL-cholesterol.

Favism—acute hemolytic anemia in certain G6PD-deficient individuals, resulting from ingestion of fava beans.

α-Fetoprotein—a protein produced by the fetus and found in amniotic fluid. The amounts increase during normal pregnancy up to the 34th week, but abnormally high levels are found under certain normal (i.e., multiple births) or pathologic (i.e., neural tube defects, fetal death) conditions.

Fitness (f)—a measure of fertility and therefore of the contribution to the gene pool of the succeeding generation. For a given genotype, the number of offspring surviving to reproductive age relative to the number for the wild-type genotype.

Founder effect—the high frequency of a mutant gene in a rapidly expanding population founded by a small ancestral group when one or more of the founders was, by chance, a carrier of the mutant gene.

Frameshift mutation—a mutation involving a deletion or insertion that is not an exact multiple of 3 bp, which changes the reading frame of the gene. All coding regions 3′ to the frameshift mutation will thus be read as gibberish, usually soon encountering a stop codon.

gag gene—encodes the core protein of a retrovirus.

Gene flow—gradual diffusion of genes from one population to another, as a result of migration and intermarriage.

Gene map—placement of genes in correct linear arrangement on specific chromosome regions.

Genetic code—the base triplets that specify the 20 different amino acids.

Genetic counseling—a communication process, the intent of which is to provide individuals and families having a genetic disease or at risk of such a disease with information about their condition and to provide information that would allow couples at risk to make informed reproductive decisions. (For details, see text.)

Genetic drift—random fluctuations in gene frequencies, most evident in small populations.

Genetic heterogeneity—different mutations can cause a similar phenotype; *allelic heterogeneity* refers to different mutations at the same locus, whereas *locus heterogeneity* refers to mutations at a different loci.

Genetic lethal—a genetic disease that prevents fertility. It need not cause illness or death, but must prevent reproduction.

Genetic locus—a specific position or location on a chromosome.

Genetic marker—a locus whose alleles are readily detectable. It may or may not be part of an expressed gene.

Genetic screening—testing on a population basis to identify a subset of individuals at high risk of having a specific disorder, or of transmitting a specific genetic disorder.

Genome—the complete DNA sequence of an organism containing its complete genetic information.

Genotype—the genetic constitution of an individual or, more specifically, the alleles at specific genetic loci.

Giemsa banding—characteristic light and dark bands, unique for each human chromosome, obtained by staining with Giemsa stain after gentle trypsin treatment.

Glucose-6-phosphate dehydrogenase (G6PD)—enzyme catalyzing the first step in the hexose monophosphate shunt pathway.

Guthrie test—bacterial inhibition test used to screen for the presence of phenylketonuria.

Haploid—the chromosome number of a normal gamete, with only one member of each chromosome pair. In humans, the haploid number is 23.

Haplotype—genotype of a group of alleles from two or more closely linked loci on one chromosome, usually inherited as a unit, e.g., the HLA complex.

Hardy-Weinberg equilibrium—the law that relates gene frequency to genotype frequency in a population at equilibrium and permits determination of allele frequency and heterozygote carrier frequency in a population for which the frequency of a trait is known.

Hemoglobinopathies—disorders of hemoglobin in which the mutation has caused a qualitative abnormality, e.g., a missense mutation in the β-globin gene, which results in valine replacing glutamic acid at position 6, resulting in sickle cell anemia.

Heterochromatin—chromatin that stains darkly with trypsin and Giemsa and is composed of repetitive DNA.

Heteromorphism—a normal variant of a chromosome.

Heteropyknotic—dense and dark staining, suggestive of inactive chromatin.

Heterozygote (heterozygous)—an individual who has two different alleles at a given locus on a pair of homologous chromosomes.

Histones—proteins associated with DNA in the chromosomes, rich in basic amino acids (lysine or arginine) and virtually unchanged throughout eukaryote evolution.

Homozygote (homozygous)—an individual possessing a pair of identical alleles at a given locus on a pair of homologous chromosomes.

Housekeeping genes—genes that encode enzymes required for basic functions that are present in virtually all cells.

Human Genome Project—the plan to map and sequence the entire 3 billion bp of the human genome.

Hybridization (or reannealing)—in molecular genetics, complementary pairing of an RNA and a DNA strand or of two different DNA strands. In somatic cell genetics, fusion of two somatic cells to form a hybrid cell containing genetic information from both parental cells.

In situ hybridization—one of the most direct means for mapping a gene; the molecular hybridization of a cloned DNA sequence to metaphase chromosomes spread on a microscope slide.

Inborn error of metabolism—a genetically determined biochemical disorder in which a specific enzyme defect produces a metabolic block that may have pathological consequences. The concept put forward by Archibald Garrod in 1908 that, in effect, established the field of biochemical genetics.

Independence principle—the probability of a joint occurrence of two or more independent events is the product of their separate probabilities.

Index case—proband.

Insertion—a structural chromosomal abnormality in which part of the material from one chromosome is inserted into a nonhomologous chromosome.

Intergenic DNA—relatively long stretches of DNA in between the transcribed genes, without known function.

Intervening sequence (IVS)—an intron.

Intron—a segment of a gene that is initially transcribed into RNA but is then removed from the primary transcript by splicing together the exon sequences on either side of it. Intronic sequences are not found in mature mRNA.

Inversion—a structural abnormality of a chromosome in which a segment of a chromosome is reversed end to end; may be pericentric when inverted segment includes the centromere, or paracentric when it does not.

Isochromosome—an abnormal chromosome in which one arm is duplicated (so that two arms of equal length are formed with the same loci in reverse sequence) and the other arm is deleted.

Karyotype—the chromosome constitution of an individual (number of chromosomes, sex chromosome constitution, and any abnormalities in number or morphology). Also commonly used term for a photomicrograph of the chromosomes of an individual arranged in the standard classification and for the process of preparing such a photomicrograph (karyotyping).

Kilobase (kb)—one thousand base pairs in a DNA sequence.

Kinetochore—a structure at the centromere to which the spindle fibers are attached.

Library—a large collection of recombinant DNA clones, in which genomic or cDNA fragments have been inserted into a particular vector.

Linkage—co-inheritance of two or more nonallelic genes because their loci are in close proximity on the same chromosome, such that after meiosis they remain associated more often than the 50% expected for unlinked genes.

Linkage disequilibrium—the preferential association of a particular allele, for example, a mutant allele for a disease with a specific allele at a nearby locus more frequently than expected by chance.

Linkage map—a chromosome map showing the relative positions of genetic markers of a given species, as determined by linkage analysis; not the same as a physical map or a gene map that uses linkage analysis, cytogenetic examination, and physical techniques to generate the map.

Locus heterogeneity—similar phenotypes caused by mutations at different genetic loci.

Lod score—a statistical method that tests whether a set of linkage data indicates two loci are linked or unlinked. The lod score is the base 10 logarithm of the odds favoring linkage. By convention, a lod score of +3 (1000:1 odds) is taken as proof of linkage; a score of −2 (100:1 odds against) indicates no linkage.

Lyonization—one of the two X chromosomes in female somatic cells is randomly inactivated early in embryonic development. As a result, the female is a mosaic of cells each functionally hemizygous for one or other X chromosome.

Major histocompatibility complex (MHC)—the complex of human leukocyte antigen (HLA) genes on the short arm of chromosome 6. Because it is so polymorphic, this complex is an ideal marker for linkage studies.

Maxam-Gilbert method—method for determining the exact nucleotide sequence via a chemical degradation process.

Meiosis—special type of cell division occurring in the germ cells of sexually reproducing organisms during which gametes containing the haploid chromosome number are produced from diploid cells. Two meiotic divisions occur, meiosis I and meiosis II; reduction in number takes place during meiosis I.

Messenger RNA (mRNA)—the template upon which polypeptides are synthesized; the crucial connecting link between information contained in a gene and its end result as the specific amino acid sequence of a protein.

Metacentric chromosome—chromosome in which the centromere is in the middle of the chromosome.

Missense mutation—a single DNA base substitution resulting in a codon specifying a different amino acid.

Mitochondrial DNA—The DNA in the circular chomosome of the mitochondria, cytoplasmic organelles that possess their own unique DNA. Mitochondrial DNA is present in many copies per cell, is maternally inherited, and evolves five to ten times as rapidly as genomic DNA.

Mitosis—process of nuclear division, occurring in five stages (prophase, prometaphase, metaphase, anaphase, and telophase) whereby one cell divides to give rise to two that are genetically identical to the parent.

Molecular hybridization—the ability of a single-stranded DNA or RNA to anneal to its complementary single strand by Watson-Crick base pairing.

Monosomy—a condition in which one chromosome of a pair is missing, as in 45,X Turner syndrome.

Monozygotic—arising from a single zygote or fertilized egg; genetically identical twin pair.

Mosaicism—condition in which an individual has two or more genetically distinct cell lines derived from a single zygote, but differing because of mutation or nondisjunction.

Multifactorial inheritance—those traits resulting from interplay of multiple environmental factors with multiple genes.

Mutagen—a chemical or physical agent that increases the mutation rate by causing changes in DNA.

Mutation—any permanent heritable change in the sequence of genomic DNA.

Mutation rate (u)—the frequency of mutation expressed as the number of mutations/locus/gamete/generation.

Nondisjunction—the failure of two homologous chromosomes to disjoin during meiosis I, or two chromatids of a chromosome to separate in meiosis II or mitosis, so that both pass to the same daughter cell and the other daughter cell receives neither.

Nonpenetrance—lack of clinical expression of the mutant phenotype in an individual with the appropriate genotype.

Nonsense mutation—a single DNA base substitution resulting in a stop (termination) codon.

Northern blot—blotting technique, analogous to Southern blotting, for detecting RNA fragments by hybridization. The blot reveals the size and abundance of the RNA complementary to the probe used.

Nucleosome—the basic structural units of chromatin. They consist of 146 bp of DNA wrapped around a core of eight histone molecules.

Nude mice—immunologically deficient mice used to permit growth of tumor cells from mouse and other species, such as human.

Obligate heterozygote—an individual who is clinically unaffected but, on the basis of pedigree analysis, must carry the mutant allele. (See text for discussion.)

Oligogenic diseases—diseases or traits that result from the effects of relatively few genes, some of which have rather large effects.

Oncogenes—normal genes of vertebrates that are involved in control of cell growth and have been preserved throughout evolution. When mutated, overexpressed or amplified in somatic cells, oncogenes may cause neoplastic transformation.

p—designation for the short arm of a chromosome, from the French *petit*.

Palindrome—a DNA sequence that contains the same 5′ to 3′ sequence on both strands, e.g., 5′ GAATTC 3′ / 3′ CTTAAG 5′.

Pedigree—from "pied de grue" or crane's foot; a diagram of a family history indicating the family members, their relationship to the proband, and their status with respect to a particular hereditary condition.

Penetrance—an all-or-none phenomenon that refers to the observable expression, or lack of it, of the mutant gene; for a dominant disease, defined quantitatively by determining the proportion of obligate gene carriers (heterozygotes), for a mutant gene, who express the phenotype.

Peptide fingerprint—chromatographic pattern of peptides obtained after partial hydrolysis of a protein or polypeptide. The technique may also be applied to DNA and RNA.

Pharmacogenetics—study of the genetic basis for differences in response to drugs.

Phenocopy—a phenotype produced by environmental factors that mimics a genetically determined trait.

Phenotype—the observed result of the interaction of the genotype with environmental factors, the observable expression of a particular gene or genes.

Philadelphia chromosome (Ph^1)—structurally abnormal chromosome 22, a reciprocal translocation between the distal portion of this chromosome and of chromosome 9, occurring in a proportion of bone marrow cells in patients with chronic myelogenous leukemia.

Phytohemagglutinin—lectin from the red bean used to agglutinate red blood cells and stimulate lymphocytes to divide; used in preparation of peripheral blood karyotypes.

Plasmid—independently replicating, extrachromosomal circular DNA molecules often bearing antibiotic resistance genes and propagated in bacteria; used in recombinant DNA technology as vectors to carry cloned DNA segments.

Platelet-derived growth factor (PDGF)—a protein, produced by platelets and other cells, that strongly stimulates cell growth and division and is involved in normal wound healing. The gene for PDGF is identical to the proto-oncogene *sis*.

Pleiotropy—the diverse effects of a single gene or gene pair on several organ systems and functions.

Point mutation—substitution of one nucleotide for another.

pol gene—encodes reverse transcriptase on a retrovirus.

Polyadenylation—the addition of about 200 adenosine residues at the 3′ end of messenger RNAs, apparently involved in their transport out of the nucleus and stability.

Polygenic diseases—diseases (or traits) that result from the interaction of multiple genes, each of which has a relatively minor effect.

Polymerase chain reaction (PCR)—a technique for amplifying a short stretch of DNA. The method depends on the use of two flanking oligonucleotide DNA primers and repeated cycles of primer extension using DNA polymerase.

Polymorphism—in a population the occurrence of two or more genetically determined alternative phenotypes at such a frequency that the rarest could not be maintained by recurrent mutation alone. In practice, a genetic locus is considered polymorphic if the rare allele (alleles) has (have) a frequency of at least 0.01, such that heterozygotes carrying this allele occur at a frequency greater than 2%.

Polysome (polyribosome)—structures composed of multiple ribosomes attached to mRNA in the process of translation.

Population genetics—the study of distribution of genes in populations and of the factors that maintain or change the frequency of genes and genotypes from generation to generation.

Primary transcript—the direct RNA transcript of a gene, containing introns as well as exons.

Proband (propositus; proposita)—index case; the affected person through which a pedigree is discovered and explored.

Probe—in molecular genetics, a labeled DNA or RNA sequence used to detect the presence of a complementary sequence by molecular hybridization; a reagent capable of recognizing the desired clone in a complex mixture of many DNA or RNA sequences.

Promoter—the sequence elements located 5′ to the gene. These elements fix the site of initiation of transcription and control mRNA quantity and sometimes tissue specificity.

Protein suicide mechanism—in dominant disorders, one mutant subunit leads to the loss of function of an entire multimeric protein, e.g., collagen.

Proto-oncogenes—normal genes that are found in normal eukaryotic cells concerned with various aspects of cell division. If amplified, mutated, rearranged, or picked up by a retrovirus, they may give rise to oncogenes that can cause cancer.

Pseudogenes—DNA sequences that have the structures of expressed genes, and were presumably once functional, but have acquired one or more mutations during evolution that render them incapable of producing a protein product.

q—designation for the long arm of a chromosome.

Quasidominance—the pattern of inheritance produced by the mating of a homozygous affected individual with an individual heterozygous for the same recessive trait, so that homozygous affected members appear in two or more successive generations.

Reading frame—one of the possible ways of reading a nucleotide sequence as a series of triplets. An open reading frame contains no termination codons and thus is potentially translatable into protein.

Recessive (trait)—those conditions that are clinically manifest only in individuals homozygous for the mutant gene (i.e., carrying a double dose of the abnormal gene).

Reciprocal translocation—exchange of material between two nonhomologous chromosomes.

Recombinant chromosome—chromosome in an offspring that has a genotype not found in either parent, due to crossing over in meiosis.

Recombinant DNA technology—techniques of genetic analysis whereby the DNA from one gene or part of a gene from one organism is inserted into the genome of another organism.

Recombination—the formation of new combinations of linked genes by crossing over (breakage and rejoining) between their loci.

Recombination fraction (θ)—in linkage analysis, the fraction of meiotic events that show a recombination between two loci.

Recurrence risk—the probability that a genetic disorder that has occurred in a family will recur in another member in the same or in future generations.

Restriction enzymes—endonucleases purified from bacteria that can cut double-stranded DNA at a specific nucleotide sequence. Each enzyme is designated by the organism from which it was obtained, e.g., *Eco*RI from *Escherichia coli* RY13, which cleaves at the sequence GAATTC.

Restriction fragment length polymorphism (RFLP)—a variation in DNA sequence that alters the length of a restriction fragment. These may be simple point mutations, which create or destroy a restriction site, or variable length regions (so-called VNTRs, for variable number of tandem repeats). RFLPs provide convenient markers for linkage analysis.

Restriction map—a map of a DNA sequence, usually in base pairs, indicating the location of restriction sites.

Reticulocyte—precursor of mature erythrocyte.

Retrovirus—RNA viruses that encode a reverse transcriptase so that they are transcribed into DNA on entering a host cell.

Reverse genetics—the application of human gene mapping to clone the gene responsible for a disease, when no information about the biochemical basis of the disease is available.

Reverse transcriptase—an enzyme that catalyzes the synthesis of DNA on an RNA template.

Ribosome—cytoplasmic organelle composed of ribosomal RNA and protein, on which polypeptide synthesis from messenger RNA occurs.

Ring chromosome—a structurally abnormal chromosome in which the end of each arm has been deleted and the broken arms have rejoined in ring formation.

RNA polymerases—DNA-template-dependent transcription enzymes that synthesize RNA from ribonucleoside triphosphate precursors.

RNA, ribonucleic acid—the ribonucleotide polymer, containing ribose instead of deoxyribose, into which DNA is transcribed.

Robertsonian translocation—a translocation between two acrocentric chromosomes by fusion at the centromere with loss of the short arm and satellites.

Sanger method—enzymatic method for determining the exact nucleotide sequence of a cloned fragment of DNA.

Segregation—in genetics, the separation of allelic genes at meiosis. Because allelic genes occupy the same locus on homologous chromosomes, they pass to different gametes; that is, they segregate.

Selection—the action of environmental factors on a particular phenotype, and hence its genotype, based on differences in biological fitness.

Semiconservative replication—as applied to DNA, each daughter DNA strand contains one parental strand and one newly synthesized strand.

Sensitivity—as applied to a diagnostic test, the frequency with which the test yields a positive result when the disease is present.

Sex chromosomes—X and Y chromosomes.

Sibship—group comprising all the siblings (brothers and sisters) in a family.

Silent gene—a mutant gene that has no detectable phenotypic effect.

Single-gene disorders—disorders due to single mutant genes with a large effect on the patient's phenotype (e.g., sickle cell anemia).

Sister chromatids—two identical strands of DNA generated during the S phase (DNA synthesis) of the cell cycle and held together at the centromere until mitosis or meiosis II anaphase.

Somatic cell—any cell of an organism not involved in the germline.

Somatic cell gene therapy—insertion of new DNA material into a particular tissue of an affected individual in such a way that the inserted DNA does not enter the germline.

Somatic cell hybrid—a hybrid cell made by fusing different cells (usually from different species) together. For human gene mapping, human and rodent cell hybrids are commonly used.

Southern blot—a technique, devised by Edward Southern, for transferring DNA fragments separated by agarose gel electrophoresis to a nitrocellulose filter, on which specific DNA fragments can then be detected by their hybridization to radioactive probes.

Specificity—as applied to a diagnostic test, the frequency with which the test is negative when the disease is absent.

Splicing—removal of introns in the generation of mature mRNA.

Submetacentric chromosome—a chromosome in which the centromere is somewhat distant from the center of the chromosome.

Synapsis—in meiosis, the pairing of homologous chromosomes in meiotic prophase I.

Syntenic genes—genes with loci on the same chromosome.

TATA box—a conserved sequence 25–30 bp upstream from the start site of transcription, in many but not all genes, apparently involved in the initiation of transcription.

T cells—small lymphocytes committed by the influence of the thymus gland to be responsible for cell-mediated response to antigens.

Telomere—the tips of chromosomes.

Teratogen—a chemical or physical agent that produces or raises the incidence of congenital malformations.

Termination (or stop) codon—one of the three codons, UAG, UAA, or UGA, that cause termination of protein synthesis (also called a nonsense codon).

Thalassemias—disorders of hemoglobin in which the mutation has caused a quantitative abnormality, e.g., deficiency of α-globin, α-thalassemia; deficiency of β-globin, β-thalassemia.

Transcription—the synthesis of a single-stranded RNA molecule from a double-stranded DNA template in the cell nucleus, catalyzed by RNA polymerase.

Transfection—transfer of a specifically altered gene or segment of a gene into prokaryotic or eukaryotic cells.

Transfer RNA (tRNA)—in cooperation with the ribosomes, transfer RNAs bring amino acids into position along the messenger RNA template and are used to carry out the translation from mRNA sequence to protein sequence.

Transforming retrovirus—a retrovirus carrying an additional DNA sequence (often an oncogene) that confers the ability to transform infected cells to a malignant phenotype.

Transgenic—containing foreign DNA in the germline.

Translation—the process of synthesizing a polypeptide directed by the sequence of a specific mRNA.

Translocation—exchange of chromosomal material between two or more nonhomologous chromosomes; may be balanced or unbalanced.

Trisomy—the state of having an additional copy of a chromosome or three copies instead of the normal two.

Unequal crossing over—crossing over between similar DNA sequences on chromosomes that are misaligned, resulting in a deletion or duplication of nucleotides. Such unequal crossing over accounts for several variants of hemoglobin, e.g., α-thalassemia and Lepore hemoglobins. (See text for explanation.)

Variable expressivity—refers to the variable severity of a genetic trait. Individuals with the same mutant gene with pleiotropic effects frequently show variable expressivity due to either environmental effects or effects of other genes modifying the expression of the mutant gene.

Vector—a DNA segment capable of autonomous replication. In cloning, the plasmid or phage used to carry the cloned DNA segment.

Virion—the complete extracellular virus particle.

Western blot—blotting technique, analoguous to Southern blotting, for detecting proteins, usually by immunological methods.

X-autosome translocation—reciprocal translocation between the X chromosome and one of the autosomes.

X-chromosome inactivation—*see* lyonization.

X-linked disease—a disease encoded by a mutant gene on the X chromosome.

Zinc finger proteins—transcription-activator proteins containing finger-like structures containing a zinc atom.

zygote—the diploid cell resulting from the union of the haploid male and female gametes.

Index

Page numbers in *italics* denote figures; those followed by "t" denote tables.